1998
YEAR BOOK OF
NEUROLOGY AND NEUROSURGERY®

Statement of Purpose

The YEAR BOOK Service

The YEAR BOOK series was devised in 1901 by practicing health professionals who observed that the literature of medicine and related disciplines had become so voluminous that no one individual could read and place in perspective every potential advance in a major specialty. In the final decade of the 20th century, this recognition is more acutely true than it was in 1901.

More than merely a series of books, YEAR BOOK volumes are the tangible results of a unique service designed to accomplish the following:

- to *survey* a wide range of journals of proven value
- to *select* from those journals papers representing significant advances and statements of important clinical principles
- to provide *abstracts* of those articles that are readable, convenient summaries of their key points
- to provide *commentary* about those articles to place them in perspective.

These publications grow out of a unique process that calls on the talents of outstanding authorities in clinical and fundamental disciplines, trained literature specialists, and professional writers, all supported by the resources of Mosby, the world's preeminent publisher for the health professions.

The Literature Base

Mosby and its editors survey more than 1,000 journals published worldwide, covering the full range of the health professions. On an annual basis, the publisher examines usage patterns and polls its expert authorities to add new journals to the literature base and to delete journals that are no longer useful as potential YEAR BOOK sources.

The Literature Survey

The publisher's team of literature specialists, all of whom are trained and experienced health professionals, examines every original, peer-reviewed article in each journal issue. More than 250,000 articles per year are scanned systematically, including title, text, illustrations, tables, and references. Each scan is compared, article by article, to the search strategies that the publisher has developed in consultation with the 270 outside experts who form the pool of YEAR BOOK editors. A given article may be reviewed by any number of editors, from one to a dozen or more, regardless of the discipline for which the paper was originally published. In turn, each editor who receives the article reviews it to determine whether or not the article should be included in the YEAR BOOK. This decision is based on the article's inherent quality, its probable usefulness to readers of that YEAR BOOK, and the editor's goal to represent a balanced picture of a given field in each volume of the YEAR BOOK. In addition, the editor indicates when to include figures and tables from the article to help the YEAR BOOK reader better understand the information.

Of the quarter million articles scanned each year, only 5% are selected for detailed analysis within the YEAR BOOK series, thereby assuring readers of the high value of every selection.

The Abstract

The publisher's abstracting staff is headed by a seasoned health care professional and includes individuals with training in the life sciences, medicine, and other areas, plus extensive experience in writing for the health professions and related industries. Each selected article is assigned to a specific writer on this abstracting staff. The abstracter, guided in many cases by notations supplied by the expert editor, writes a structured, condensed summary designed so that the reader can rapidly acquire the essential information contained in the article.

The Commentary

The YEAR BOOK editorial boards, sometimes assisted by guest commentators, write comments that place each article in perspective for the reader. This provides the reader with the equivalent of a personal consultation with a leading international authority—an opportunity to better understand the value of the article and to benefit from the authority's thought processes in assessing the article.

Additional Editorial Features

The editorial boards of each YEAR BOOK organize the abstracts and comments to provide a logical and satisfying sequence of information. To enhance the organization, editors also provide introductions to sections or individual chapters, comments linking a number of abstracts, citations to additional literature, and other features.

The published YEAR BOOK contains enhanced bibliographic citations for each selected article, including extended listings of multiple authors and identification of author affiliations. Each YEAR BOOK contains a Table of Contents specific to that year's volume. From year to year, the Table of Contents for a given YEAR BOOK will vary, depending on developments within the field.

Every YEAR BOOK contains a list of the journals from which papers have been selected. This list represents a subset of the more than 1,000 journals surveyed by the publisher and occasionally reflects a particularly pertinent article from a journal that is not surveyed on a routine basis.

Finally, each volume contains a comprehensive subject index and an index to authors of each selected paper.

The 1998 Year Book Series

Year Book of Allergy, Asthma, and Clinical Immunology: Drs. Rosenwasser, Borish, Gelfand, Leung, Nelson, and Szefler

Year Book of Anesthesiology and Pain Management®: Drs. Tinker, Abram, Chestnut, Roizen, Rothenberg, and Wood

Year Book of Cardiology®: Drs. Schlant, Collins, Gersh, Graham, Kaplan, and Waldo

Year Book of Chiropractic®: Dr. Lawrence

Year Book of Critical Care Medicine®: Drs. Parrillo, Balk, Calvin, Franklin, and Shapiro

Year Book of Dentistry®: Drs. Meskin, Berry, Jeffcoat, Leinfelder, Roser, Summitt, and Zakariasen

Year Book of Dermatologic Surgery®: Drs. Greenway, Papadopoulos, Whitaker, and Barrett

Year Book of Dermatology®: Dr. Thiers

Year Book of Diagnostic Radiology®: Drs. Osborn, Groskin, Dalinka, Maynard, Pentecost, Rebner, Ros, Smirniotopoulos, and Young

Year Book of Drug Therapy®: Drs. Lasagna and Weintraub

Year Book of Emergency Medicine®: Drs. Wagner, Dronen, Davidson, King, Niemann, and Roberts

Year Book of Endocrinology®: Drs. Bagdade, Braverman, Horton, Kannan, Landsberg, Molitch, Morley, Nathan, Odell, Poehlman, Rogol, and Ryan

Year Book of Family Practice®: Drs. Berg, Bowman, Davidson, Dexter, and Scherger

Year Book of Gastroenterology®: Drs. Aliperti and Fleshman

Year Book of Geriatrics and Gerontology®: Drs. Beck, Burton, Ostwald, Rabins, Reuben, Roth, Shapiro, and Whitehouse

Year Book of Hand Surgery®: Drs. Amadio and Hentz

Year Book of Hematology®: Drs. Spivak, Bell, Ness, Quesenberry, Wiernik, and Horowitz

Year Book of Infectious Diseases: Drs. Keusch, Barza, Bennish, Poutsiaka, Skolnik, and Snydman

Year Book of Medicine®: Drs. Klahr, Cline, McCallum, Frishman, Utiger, Malawista, Mandell, and Jett

Year Book of Neonatal and Perinatal Medicine®: Drs. Fanaroff, Maisels, and Stevenson

Year Book of Nephrology, Hypertension, and Mineral Metabolism: Drs. Schwab, Bennett, Emmett, Hostetter, Kumar, and Toto

Year Book of Neurology and Neurosurgery®: Drs. Bradley and Gibbs

Year Book of Nuclear Medicine®: Drs. Gottschalk, Blaufox, Neumann, Strauss, and Zubal

Year Book of Obstetrics, Gynecology, and Women's Health: Drs. Mishell, Herbst, and Kirschbaum

Year Book of Occupational and Environmental Medicine®: Drs. Emmett, Frank, Gochfeld, and Hessl

Year Book of Oncology®: Drs. Ozols, Eisenberg, Glatstein, Loehrer, Tallman, and Wiersma

Year Book of Ophthalmology®: Drs. Wilson, Augsburger, Cohen, Eagle, Grossman, Laibson, Maguire, Nelson, Penne, Rapuano, Sergott, Spaeth, Tipperman, Ms. Gosfield, and Ms. Salmon

Year Book of Orthopedics®: Drs. Morrey, Beauchamp, Currier, Tolo, Trigg, and Swiontkowski

Year Book of Otolaryngology–Head and Neck Surgery®: Drs. Paparella and Holt

Year Book of Pathology and Laboratory Medicine®: Drs. Raab, Cohen, Olson, Sirgi, and Stanley

Year Book of Pediatrics®: Dr. Stockman

Year Book of Plastic, Reconstructive, and Aesthetic Surgery®: Drs. Miller, Bartlett, Garner, McKinney, Ruberg, Salisbury, and Smith

Year Book of Psychiatry and Applied Mental Health®: Drs. Talbott, Ballanger, Frances, Lydiard, Meltzer, Schowalter, and Tasman

Year Book of Pulmonary Disease®: Drs. Jett, Maurer, Ryu, Strollo, and Wenzel

Year Book of Rheumatology®: Drs. Panush, Hadler, LeRoy, Liang, Reichlin, Simon, and Weinblatt

Year Book of Sports Medicine®: Drs. Shephard, Drinkwater, Eichner, Torg, Alexander, and Mr. George

Year Book of Surgery®: Drs. Copeland, Bland, Deitch, Eberlein, Howard, Luce, Seeger, Souba, and Sugarbaker

Year Book of Thoracic and Cardiovascular Surgery®: Drs. Ginsberg, Wechsler, and Williams

Year Book of Urology®: Drs. Andriole and Coplen

Year Book of Vascular Surgery®: Dr. Porter

1998

The Year Book of NEUROLOGY AND NEUROSURGERY®

"Published without interruption since 1902"

Neurology

Editor

Walter G. Bradley, D.M., F.R.C.P.

Professor and Chairman, Department of Neurology, University of Miami School of Medicine, Florida

Neurosurgery

Editor

Scott R. Gibbs, M.A., M.D.

Director of Brain and NeuroSpine Center Division of Neurosurgery, Southeast Missouri Hospital, Cape Girardeau, Missouri

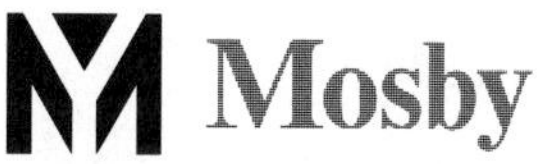

St. Louis Baltimore Boston Carlsbad Naples New York Philadelphia Portland London
Madrid Mexico City Singapore Sydney Tokyo Toronto Wiesbaden

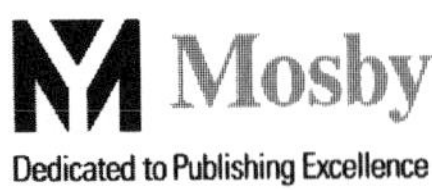

Mosby

Dedicated to Publishing Excellence

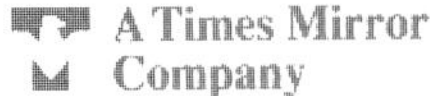

A Times Mirror
Company

Associate Publisher: Gretchen C. Murphy
Developmental Editor: Jaime Chatman
Manager, Periodicals Editing: Kirk Swearingen
Manuscript Editor: Amanda Maguire
Project Supervisor, Production: Joy Moore
Production Assistant: Laura Bayless
Manager, Literature Services: Idelle L. Winer
Illustrations and Permissions Specialist: Steve Ramay
Illustrations and Permissions Coordinator: Chidi C. Ukabam

1998 EDITION
Copyright © June 1998 by Mosby, Inc.

Printed in the United States of America
Composition by Reed Technology and Information Services, Inc.
Printing/binding by Maple–Vail

Mosby, Inc.
11830 Westline Industrial Drive
St. Louis, MO 63146
Customer Service: customer.support@mosby.com
www.mosby.com/Mosby/CustomerSupport/index.html

International Standard Serial Number: 0513–5117
International Standard Book Number: 0–8151–9648–2

Associate Editors

Joseph R. Berger, M.D.
Professor of Neurology and Internal Medicine, University of Kentucky College of Medicine; Chairman, Department of Neurology, University of Kentucky Medical Center, Kentucky Clinic, Lexington, Kentucky

John P. Blass, M.D., Ph.D.
Burke Professor of Neurology, Medicine and Neuroscience, Cornell University Medical College, New York; Director, Dementia Service, Burke, Burke Rehabilitation Hospital; White Plains, New York Hospital, New York, New York

Charles Bondurant, M.D.
Clinical Assistant Professor, Division of Neurosurgery, University of Missouri-Columbia, School of Medicine, Columbia, Missouri

H. Alan Crockard, F.R.C.S.
Consultant Neurosurgeon, Department of Surgical Neurology, The National Hospital for Neurology and Neuorosurgery, London, England

Robert A. Davidoff, M.D.
Professor of Neurology, University of Miami School of Medicine; Chief, Neurology Service UAMC Miami, Jackson Memorial Hospital, Miami, Florida

Myron D. Ginsberg, M.D.
Peritz Schinberg Professor of Neurology, University of Miami School of Medicine; Attending Neurologist, Jackson Memorial Hospital, Miami, Florida

David Jimenez, M.D.
Assistant Professor, Department of Surgery, Division of Neurosurgery, University of Missouri-Columbia, School of Medicine, Columbia, Missouri

Professor Igor Kachkov
MONIKI, Department of Neurosurgery, Moscow, Russia

Eduardo A. Karol, M.D.
Assistant Professor of Neurosurgery, University of Buenos Aires; Neurosurgeon, Buenos Aires University Hospital "José de San Martin", Buenos Aires, Argentina

Andrew H. Kaye, M.D.
The Royal Melbourne Hospital, Department of Surgery, Division of Neurosurgery, University of Melbourne, Parkville, Victoria, Australia

Dr. Boris Klun, M.D., Ph.D.
Professor of Neurosurgery, University of Ljubljana Medical School, Medical Center, Department of Neurosurgery, Ljubljana, Slovenia

Rodrigo Kuljis, M.D.
Associate Professor of Neurology, Division of Behavioral Neurology, University of Miami School of Medicine, Miami, Florida

Richard Leblanc, M.D., M.S.C., F.Q.C.F.C.
Assistant Professor, Department of Neurosurgery, Montreal Neurological Institute, McGill University, Montreal, Quebec

Philippe Maeder, M.D.
Maitre D'Enseignement et de Recherche (Mer), Medecin Adjoint, Lausanne, Switzerland

Raul Marino, Jr., M.D.
Professor and Chairman, Neurosurgery, University of São Paulo Medical School; Chief of Neurosurgery, Hospital das Clínicas University of São Paulo Medical School, São Paulo-SP-Brazil

Marc R. Mayberg, M.D.
Professor of Neurological Surgery, Department of Neurological Surgery, University of Washington, Seattle, Washington

Bruce Nolan, M.D.
Associate Professor of Neurology, University of Miami; Director, Sleep Disorders Center, University of Miami/Jackson Memorial Hospital, Miami, Florida

John H. Noseworthy, M.D., F.R.C.P.C.
Professor and Chairman; Chair, Department of Neurology, Mayo Clinic/Mayo Foundation, Rochester, Minnesota

Stan Pelofsky, M.D.
Assistant Professor, Division of Neurosurgery, Oklahoma Memorial Hospital, Veteran's Administration Hospital, Oklahoma Children's Hospital; Chief of Neurosurgery, Saint Anthony Hospital; President of the Neuroscience Specialists, Oklahoma City ,Oklahoma, Secretary of the American Association of Neurological Surgeons

Miguel-A. Perez-Espejo, M.D., Ph.D.
University Hospital "V. Arrixaca", Servicio Regional de Neurocirugia, Murcia, Spain

George Pjura, M.D.
Neuroradiologist, Department of Radiology, Southeast Missouri Hospital and St. Francis Medical Center, Cape Girardeau, Missouri

Ryszard M. Pluta, M.D., Ph.D.
Visiting Scientist, Surgical Neurology Branch, NINDS, NIH, Bethesda, Maryland

Jerome D. Posner, M.D.
Evelyn Frew American Cancer Society Clinical Research Professor, George C. Cotzias Chair in Neuro-oncology; President of the American Neurological Association, Memorial Sloan-Kettering Cancer Center, New York, New York

Robert M. Quencer, M.D.
Chairman and Professor, University of Miami School of Medicine; Chief of Radiology Service, University of Miami/Jackson Memorial Medical Center, Miami, Florida

Eugene R. Ramsay, M.D.
Professor of Neurology, Department of Neurology, University of Miami School of Medicine; Director International Center for Epilepsy, Miami, Florida

Dr. Jean Regis
Service de Neurochirurgie Fonctionnelle et Stereotaxique, C.M.U. LaTimone, Marseille, France

Damianos E. Sakas, M.D.
Clinical Senior Lecturer, Section of Surgery, Postgraduate Medical School, University of Warwick; Consultant Neurosurgeon and Chairman, Department of Clinical Neurosciences, Walsgrave General Hospital, Coventry, England

Juan A. Sanchez-Ramos, M.D., Ph.D.
Ellis Professor of Neurology, University of South Florida, Tampa General and James Haley Veterans Administration Medical Center, Tampa, Florida

Keiji Sano, M.D., D.M.Sc., F.A.C.S.
Emeritus Professor of Neurosurgery, University of Tokyo; Director of the Fuji Brain Institute, Fuji Brain Institute, Fujinomiya, Japan

Norman J. Schatz, M.D.
Voluntary Professor of Clinical Neurology and Ophthalmology, University of Miami School of Medicine, University of Pennsylvania, Mercy Neuroscience Institute; Clinical Professor of Ophthalmology/Neurology, Miami, Florida

Nina Felice Schor, M.D., Ph.D.
Professor of Pediatrics, Neurology, and Pharmacology, University of Pittsburgh; Attending Physician, Children's Hospital of Pittsburgh, Pennsylvania

Julio Sotelo, M.D.
Director, National Institute of Neurology and Neurosurgery, Mexico City, Mexico

David Stumpf, M.D., Ph.D.
Chairman and Professor of Neurology; Professor of Pediatric Neurology, Northwestern University Medical School; Chairman and Professor of Neurology, Northwestern Memorial Hospital, Chicago, Illinois

Vincent C. Traynelis, M.D.
Associate Professor, Department of Surgery, Division of Neurosurgery, University of Iowa, Iowa City, Iowa

Nicolas de Tribolet, M.D.
Professor and Chairman, Centre Hospitalier Universitaire Vaudois, Service de Neurochirurgie de CHUV, Lausanne, Switzerland

Ronald J. Tusa, M.D., Ph.D.
Professor of Neurology and Otolaryngology; Bascom Palmer Eye Institute, University of Miami, Anne Bates Leech Hospital, Miami, Florida

Olivier Vernet, M.D.
Maitre D'Enseignement et de Recherches (Mer), University of Lausanne; Medecin Associe, Centre Hospitalier Universitaire Vaudois (CHUV), Lausanne, Switzerland

Clark Watts, M.D., J.D.
Clinical Professor, Surgery, University of Texas Health Sciences Center, San Antonio, Texas

Table of Contents

Journals Represented

Mosby and its Editors survey more than 1,000 journals for its abstract and commentary publications. From these journals, the Editors select the articles to be abstracted. Journals represented in this YEAR BOOK are listed below.

Acta Neurochirurgica
Acta Neurologica Scandinavica
Acta Radiologica
Age and Ageing
American Journal of Human Genetics
American Journal of Medicine
American Journal of Neuroradiology
American Journal of Ophthalmology
American Journal of Otology
American Journal of Roentgenology
American Surgeon
Anaesthesia
Anesthesia and Analgesia
Annals of Neurology
Annals of Oncology
Annals of Otology, Rhinology and Laryngology
Annals of Surgical Oncology
Anuals of Vascular Surgery
Archives of Neurology
Archives of Physical Medicine and Rehabilitation
Archives of Surgery
Biological Psychiatry
Blood
Brain
British Medical Journal
Canadian Journal of Neurological Sciences
Canadian Medical Association Journal
Cancer
Cancer Research
Cephalalgia
Chest
Childs Nervous System
Circulation
Clinical Orthopaedics and Related Research
Clinical Radiology
Critical Care Medicine
Developmental Medicine and Child Neurology
Epilepsia
International Journal of Radiation, Oncology, Biology, and Physics
Journal of Clinical Immunology
Journal of Clinical Oncology
Journal of Computer Assisted Tomography
Journal of Infectious Diseases
Journal of Laryngology and Otology
Journal of Neurology
Journal of Neurology, Neurosurgery and Psychiatry
Journal of Neuropathology and Experimental Neurology

Journal of Neuropsychiatry and Clinical Neurosciences
Journal of Neurosurgery
Journal of Nuclear Medicine
Journal of Otolaryngology
Journal of Pain and Symptom Management
Journal of Pediatrics
Journal of Rheumatology
Journal of Spinal Disorders
Journal of Urology
Journal of Vascular Surgery
Journal of the American Geriatrics Society
Journal of the American Medical Association
Journal of the Neurological Sciences
Journal of the Royal College of Surgeons of Edinburgh
Lancet
Medical Care
Neurology
Neuropediatrics
Neuroradiology
Neurosurgery
New England Journal of Medicine
Ophthalmology
Otolaryngology - Head and Neck Surgery
Pediatric Neurology
Pediatrics
Science
Spinal Cord
Spine
Sports Medicine
Stroke
Surgical Neurology
Western Journal of Medicine

STANDARD ABBREVIATIONS

The following terms are abbreviated in this edition: acquired immunodeficiency syndrome (AIDS), cardiopulmonary resuscitation (CPR), central nervous system (CNS), cerebrospinal fluid (CSF), computed tomography (CT), deoxyribonucleic acid (DNA), electrocardiography (ECG), health maintenance organization (HMO), human immunodeficiency virus (HIV), intensive care unit (ICU), intramuscular (IM), intravenous (IV), magnetic resonance (MR) imaging (MRI), and ribonucleic acid (RNA).

NOTE

The YEAR BOOK OF NEUROLOGY AND NEUROSURGERY is a literature survey service providing abstracts of articles published in the professional literature. Every effort is made to assure the accuracy of the information presented in these pages. Neither the editors nor the publisher of the YEAR BOOK OF NEUROLOGY AND NEUROSURGERY can be responsible for errors in the original materials. The editors' comments are their own opinions. Mention of specific products within this publication does not constitute endorsement.

To facilitate the use of the YEAR BOOK OF NEUROLOGY AND NEUROSURGERY as a reference tool, all illustrations and tables included in this publication are now identified as they appear in the original article. This change is meant to help the reader recognize that any illustration or table appearing in the YEAR BOOK OF NEUROLOGY AND NEUROSURGERY may be only one of many in the original article. For this reason, figure and table numbers will often appear to be out of sequence within the YEAR BOOK OF NEUROLOGY AND NEUROSURGERY.

Introduction: "The Winds and Waves Are Always on the Side of the Ablest Navigators"*

Our YEAR BOOK is a "snapshot" capturing the sum and substance of new developments in the neurology and neurosurgery literature, and it continues to serve as a compass to navigate position and chart our course. The YEAR BOOK series was born in 1902 out of a need to distill the morass of medical literature because, even at the beginning of this century, it was more than any one individual could read and place in perspective in a major specialty. In 1946, this YEAR BOOK began, and without question, the breadth, depth, and pace of neurosurgical research has since burgeoned.

In his introduction for this Year Book at the midpoint of this century, Percival Bailey wrote that he expected further discoveries that would relieve even more human suffering. He noted, "But two clouds appear on the horizon: one is the alarming increase in the number of neurosurgeons which may bring doubtful practices in its wake, and the other is the incredible stupidity of the human race which seems to be unable to devise any way to save itself from suicide." Some may agree with Bailey's concerns; however, at this juncture on the precipice of the 21st century, the view is far and wide, and we have reason to be more optimistic, despite the fact that we have our own challenges and concerns.

We are living in a time of profound change and interconnection. The Internet's World Wide Web is a brilliant example that is rapidly affecting the practice of medicine. If the current trend persists, we will most surely witness its evolution into something monumental with arresting combinations of text, sound, and video. On the new horizon, the Internet is clearly rising and now looms as the dominant forum for rapid global communication and dissemination of information. This presents a unique opportunity for an interconnected world-wide neurospecialist community, positioned to assimilate information from a variety of sources appearing in a rapidly moving window of opportunity. Perhaps the most useful neurosurgical technology globally available in 2000 A.D. will be the Internet. This communication system is already being used in close partnership by researchers, academicians and private practitioners alike, to improve the quality of, and accessibility to, neurosurgical care throughout the world. Contemporaneous reporting of results combined with collective, cumulative, and collaborative scholarship over the Internet will speed the advancement of neuroscience and the result will ultimately be accessed and transmitted by fiber optics at the speed of light to you, your peers, and even your patients. Accomplishing this ideal requires that enough individuals embrace the change with an imaginative and innovative spirit.

To prepare the YEAR BOOK for an international perspective on each year's selections, I established its first International Board of Neurosurgeons. As you know, the developments in neurosurgery have been traditionally printed and chronicled in the Year Book, but soon the Year Book will be available on-line to announce faster the arrival of new technologies

---

*Edward Gibbon, *The Rise and Fall of the Roman Empire*, Strahan and Cadel, London, 1776, p. 68.

and developments and communicate them more widely to the world's neurosurgeons. This will facilitate further synergistic, interdisciplinary exchange, and advancement.

Despite enormous advances in neuroscience, our understanding of the basic brain functions and their importance to the individual and humanity were known well and revealed by Hippocrates' eloquent description more than 2,000 years ago.

Men ought to know that from the brain, and from the brain only, arise our pleasures. joys, laughter and jest, as well as our sorrows, pains, griefs and tears. Through it, in particular, we think, see, hear, and distinguish the ugly from the beautiful, the bad from the good, the pleasant from the unpleasant ... It is the same thing which makes us mad or delirious, inspires us with dread and fear, whether by night or day, brings sleeplessness, inopportune mistakes, aimless anxieties, absent-mindedness, and acts that are contrary to habit. These things that we suffer all come from the brain, when it is not healthy, but becomes abnormally hot, cold, moist, or dry, or suffers any other unnatural affection to which it was not accustomed. Madness comes from moistness. When the brain is abnormally moist, of necessity it moves, and when it moves neither sight nor hearing are still, but we see or hear now one thing and now another, and the tongue speaks in accordance with the things seen and heard on occasion. But all the time the brain is still, a man can think properly.[1]

Clearly, the brain is more than an amorphous mass of insubstantial electricity—it is the bower of human communication and guidance. Its care is the neurosurgeon's venue, as, by virtue of our knowledge, training and experience we have been entrusted as guardians of the highest level of intelligence known to man. Cerebral aneurysms, brain and spinal tumors, arteriovenous malformations and other complex neurological maladies require the unique application of our art and science for each individual. Neurosurgeons have this professional duty to their individual patients and, likewise, they have a duty to the public to protect the integrity of the health care system. There has been a proliferation of third party involvement in patient care decisions that is, at the very least, unsettling. Much of this third party activity is pecuniarily motivated, but ostensibly it is done in the name of "quality." We must beware that health care sold on the margin may lead to marginal health care.

The value of years of postgraduate education, research and development, and new technology is simply too great to be repackaged and sold wholesale like bulk commodities. Neurosurgery does not lend itself to assembly line techniques as some governments, insurance companies, and managed care organizations appear to believe. In the final analysis, it is the physician's duty to the patient that must prevail, whatever the delivery system. Neurosurgeons, not third parties, know first-hand the complexity, trials, triumphs and tragedies that we experience in our practices. It is incumbent upon us to educate the various constituencies involved in the design, development and maintenance of the health care system so that finite resources may be properly allocated. When public and private leaders have a better understanding of our work, they will be more likely to enact health care legislation and design insurance products that more accurately reflect our value and the resources needed to assure continued access to quality neurosurgery programs.

If government and business leaders could spend one day experiencing a neurosurgeon's life, it could radically affect the way they think about health care. This is one vicarious experience where "virtual reality" meets the real world. With your patient's permission, invite those who should know, to learn first hand about our work. Suit them in a white coat and have them accompany you on rounds to the intensive care units and the emergency center. Introduce them to your patients, let them don scrubs and observe an operation. In other words, give them an opportunity that many only imagine by allowing them to witness our work first-hand as an "Ambassador of Neurosurgery."

Although it has become nearly unfashionable, and almost priggish, to talk about virtues, the virtues of self-discipline, compassion, responsibility, courage, perseverance, honesty, loyalty, and faith are integral to our practice. These immutable basics are the heart and soul of our profession, and we must not allow technology, delivery systems, governments, or businesses to diminish their importance. When our ambassadors, and potential advocates, witness these virtues applied, we will effectively prevent further erosion of confidence and appreciation, and restore our position. We have an opportunity to chart a course of understanding and advocacy for our profession; but we can not develop advocates among those who do not know our work or our issues.

The "winds and waves" of change in science, medicine, communications, and politics are lashing furiously. And, we must use these vectors to ably navigate through these tumultuous times. Clearly, the Internet holds the potential for unprecedented unity among the world's neurosurgeons, and this sum of intellectual capital, combined with a steadfast effort to demystify and reveal neurosurgery, will allow us to create more than a ripple of influence that may be felt at the change of the next millennium.

Scott R. Gibbs, M.A., M.D.

Reference

1. Attributed to Hippocrates, 5th Century B.C., *Principles of Neural Science*, 2nd Edition, Elsevier Science Publisher, Inc., New York, 1985.

NEUROLOGY

WALTER G. BRADLEY, D.M., F.R.C.P.

The Neurological Revolution in the Third Millennium

I am sitting watching the billowing spinnakers of a regatta of sailboats on the Rio de la Plata in Buenos Aires on my way to be a guest of the annual meeting of the Asociacion Argentina de Neurosiencias. The Asociacion, founded in 1921, combines the Argentinian societies for neurology, psychiatry, neurosurgery, and neurobiology. This visit, and the recent annual meeting of the American Academy of Neurology, prompts me to consider how neurology has advanced in the last 20 years throughout the world, and to look forward to the continuing neurological revolution in the third millennium.

The World Federation of Neurology, founded in 1957, is now a federation of 75 national societies comprising more than 20,000 neurologists. It has 30 research groups that promote the advance of knowledge across the whole range of neurological diseases. The World Federation of Neurology is responsible for organizing the quadrennial World Congress of Neurology.

The American Neurological Association, the senior neurological organization in the United States was founded in 1875. Its membership is by election based on academic criteria, and there are 156 overseas members currently among its 1,232 members. The leadership of the American Neurological Association has brought about considerable rejuvenation of the annual meetings in the last 5 years by introducing an increasing number of scientific symposia and attracting attendees from neurologists around the world.

The American Academy of Neurology (ANN), founded in 1948, will have its golden anniversary meeting in Minneapolis on April 23, 1998. The AAN with almost 15,000 members, about 10% overseas, is the largest single association of neurologists in the world. The annual meeting of the AAN has become *the* major international clinical neuroscience meeting, combining the latest in neuroscience research, extensive educational courses, and a great deal of work related to the practice of neurology, its administration, and its advancement in the political and legislative arenas. At the annual meeting in Boston in April 1997, there were nearly 6,500 attendees.

As chair of the Scientific Issues Committee of the AAN, I am responsible for putting together the entire scientific program, and I have the unique opportunity to overview the latest clinical neuroscience developments presented at the meeting. The scientific program includes two symposia. The Presidential Symposium includes several AAN awards, the most notable of which was the Wartenberg Lecture. Dr. John Mazziotta, this year's recipient, presented a superb demonstration of the latest techniques for imaging and investigating the functional anatomy of the brain. The Decade of the Brain Symposium highlights advances in neuroscience of relevance to clinical neurologists. This year, Dr. Mark Hallett reviewed the latest information on dystonia, including writer's cramp; Dr. William Mobley reviewed recent discoveries on neurotrophic factors and their use in neurological therapy; Dr. Bruce Ransom reviewed recent information on the interrelationship of glia and neurons, and Dr. Karen Hsiao reviewed the use of transgenic mice to study neurogenetic diseases, in particular, Alzheimer's disease.

In addition, at the AAN annual meeting a number of important prizes are presented, including the Potamkin Prize for Research into Pick's Disease, Alzheimer's Disease and Related Disorders. The Prize for 1997 was jointly awarded to Dr. Sangram S. Sisodia, for his molecular genetic research into the genes responsible for familial Alzheimer's disease, and Drs. Pierluigi Gambetti and Elio Lugaresi, for their discovery and elucidation of the molecular basis of the prion disease, fatal familial insomnia. The Sheila Essey Award for Amyotrophic Lateral Sclerosis went to Dr. Jeffrey Rothstein, for his discoveries of the role of abnormalities of glutamate transport.

The powerhouse of the annual scientific meeting of the AAN is the scientific presentations by members and guests. About 2,000 scientific abstracts are submitted for consideration, of which only about 1,200 can be accepted because of space constraints. About one third of these are given as platform presentations and two thirds as posters.

The 1997 meeting included reports of many significant advances in neurological therapy. There were several presentations on new acetylcholinesterase inhibitors that produce a limited reduction in mental deterioration. Vitamin E and selegiline were reported to reduce the rate of regression in Alzheimer's disease. Of greater magnitude were reductions of over 60% in the risk of developing Alzheimer's disease with postmenopausal estrogen replacement according to one report, and with moderate intakes of alcohol (three glasses of wine per day) in another report.

Several presentations in the AAN scientific sessions in Boston described advances in the surgical treatment of Parkinson's disease. Pallidotomy is clearly confirmed to produce benefit, but bilateral pallidotomy is accompanied by unacceptable morbidity. Of greater efficacy, probably is bilateral deep brain stimulation of the globus pallidus internus.

Therapy of multiple sclerosis continues to advance. Cladribine, an antineoplastic agent that causes a prolonged decrease of peripheral blood lymphocytes, was reported to decrease the burden of gadolinium-enhanced plaques in chronic progressive multiple sclerosis, though the study did not show a significant clinical benefit. A new non-amphetamine agent, Modafinil, was reported to be of benefit in narcolepsy.

Unfortunately, not all therapeutic trials reported at the annual meeting were positive. Enlimomab (anti-ICAM1 monoclonal antibodies) actually worsened the prognosis of acute ischemic stroke when given within 6 hours of onset. Brain-derived neurotrophic factor given subcutaneously was not effective in amyotrophic lateral sclerosis, though post hoc analyses suggested benefit to patients who had diarrhea with the drug or who had low plasma chloride on entry. Further trials of the administration of neurotrophins into the cerebrospinal fluid and of low-molecular-weight neurotrophin agonists taken by mouth are underway and may in the end prove to be beneficial.

There was a challenging report on 29 patients with familial amyloid polyneuropathy treated with liver transplantation. Twenty-six percent of patients died within the first year, and of the 10 patients followed up for more than 3 years, only 50% saw their condition stabilized. Progression of the other 50% was presumably caused by ongoing damage from the amyloid load that is not affected by removing the mutant transthyretin from the blood by replacing the source of its synthesis in the liver.

Molecular genetics continues to produce a host of new advances in our understanding of neurological diseases. Several reports characterized the molecular basis of Friedreich's ataxia. It is clear that more than 95% of patients with classic Friedreich's ataxia have increased triplet repeats in the Frataxin gene on chromosome 9q, and probably many of the remaining patients have point mutations in that gene. However, the reports also showed that similar mutations in the Frataxin gene with a relatively low number of triplet repeat expansions were responsible for a proportion of patients with later onset spinocerebellar ataxias, and for familial ataxia with preservation of tendon reflexes.

Several presentations clarified the complex molecular genetics of the dominantly inherited spinocerebellar ataxias. Machado-Joseph disease is responsible for about 40% of these families in different parts of the world, but SCA1, 2 and 6, and dentatorubro-pallido-Luysian atrophy make up different proportions of cases in different parts of the world. All of these are triplet repeat diseases, with evidence of anticipation relating to meiotic instability, similar to that which has now been established for myotonic dystrophy and Huntington disease.

A series of reports on genotype-phenotype correlations were of particular interest to those involved in the classification of neurological disease. We are now clearly beyond the debate between "lumpers" and "splinters." We are now in the "era of the overlap." This is illustrated by the fact that the same gene mutation, such as in Machado-Joseph disease, can give rise to very different phenotypes, while the same clinical syndrome of spinocerebellar ataxia can be caused by mutations of several different SCA genes. Gene therapy remains the holy grail of molecular genetic research. It was reported that targeted liposomes can introduce DNA and genes into cells. This can now be added to the use of incomplete viral vectors as potential therapeutic modalities for gene therapy.

Neuroscience research continues to increase our understanding of neurological disease. Several reports confirmed previous observations of decreased N-acetyl-aspartate (NAA) to creatine (Cr) ratio in the motor cortex and corticospinal tracts of amyotrophic lateral sclerosis patients, particularly those with upper motor neuron disease. It is generally thought that this reduction of NAA/Cr is due to loss of motor neurons, but the report of a rise in NAA/Cr in the temporal lobe of patients whose seizures were controlled by antero-temporal lobectomy raised the possibility that a decreased ratio can be related to neurons being "sick" but still alive, rather than dead and disappeared.

The neurological complications of HIV infection are becoming increasingly important in the treatment of AIDS as opportunistic infections are brought under control. There were several papers at the 1997 AAN meeting dealing with neurological disease of the central and peripheral nervous system in HIV infection. Though there is some debate, it is possible that CSF RNA load may be related to the development of the AIDS-dementia complex.

The highlights that I have outlined from the 1997 Annual Scientific Meeting of the AAN are a very personal selection. The addition of these highlights to the papers selected from the literature for inclusion in this volume of the YEAR BOOK OF NEUROLOGY AND NEUROSURGERY makes clear that neurology continues to advance ever more rapidly as we move toward the third millennium. These advances give to all of us in clinical neurology greater understanding and greater therapeutic tools that we can bring to our patients. Despite all the pressures, financial and organizational, that neurologists the world over are exposed to, the neurological revolution in the third millennium appears assured.

Walter G. Bradley, D.M., F.R.C.P.

1 Neuromuscular Disorders

Autosomal Recessive Hereditary Motor and Sensory Neuropathy With Focally Folded Myelin Sheaths: Clinical, Electrophysiologic, and Genetic Aspects of a Large Family
Quattrone A, Gambardella A, Bono F, et al (School of Medicine, Catanzaro, Italy; Istituto G Gaslini, Genova, Italy; Unità Operativa, Italy; et al)
Neurology 46:1318–1324, 1996   1–1

Introduction.—There is ongoing discussion regarding how to classify the demyelinating hereditary motor and sensory neuropathies (HMSN). The autosomal recessive varieties of HMSN account for a number of different disorders of varying clinical severity. Cases of HMSN with focally folded myelin sheaths have been reported but have not been clearly de-

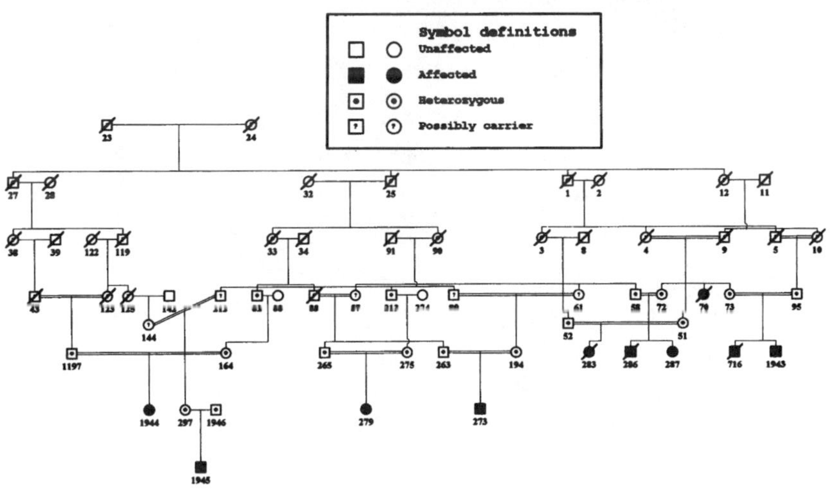

FIGURE 1.—Simplified pedigree of the family. (Courtesy of Quattrone A, Gambardellla A, Bono F, et al: Autosomal recessive hereditary motor and sensory neuropathy with focally folded myelin sheaths: Clinical, electrophysiologic, and genetic aspects of a large family. *Neurology* 46:1318–1324, 1996, by permission of Little, Brown and Company, Inc.)

fined. The clinical, electrophysiologic, pathologic, and natural history findings in a large family with this form of HMSN was reported.

Methods.—Ten patients from 1 Italian family with early onset motor and sensory neuropathy were studied (Fig 1). Six patients were still living; another 4 similarly affected patients were dead. Clinical information was available in all patients, and some living patients underwent nerve conduction studies, auditory brainstem response testing, MRI, and sural nerve and muscle biopsy. Geneologic and molecular investigations were performed as well.

Findings.—All patients reached early motor milestones before the development of symptoms at a mean age of 34 months. The initial symptoms included progressive distal and proximal weakness of the muscles of the lower limbs, with weakness of the upper limbs and severe limb deformities developing later on. Three of the living patients were adults, and all were wheelchair bound. All patients were intellectually normal; 4 had slight facial weakness, 1 with bilateral facial dyskinesia, but none had evidence of peripheral nerve thickening. The patients died in their thirties or forties.

On ancillary testing, the youngest patients had upper limb motor nerve conduction velocities of 15 to 17 m/sec; by adulthood, no detectable conduction velocities were recorded. Few patients had detectable sensitive action potentials, and all had abnormally delayed interpeak I–III latencies on auditory evoked potentials testing. The myelin deformity in these

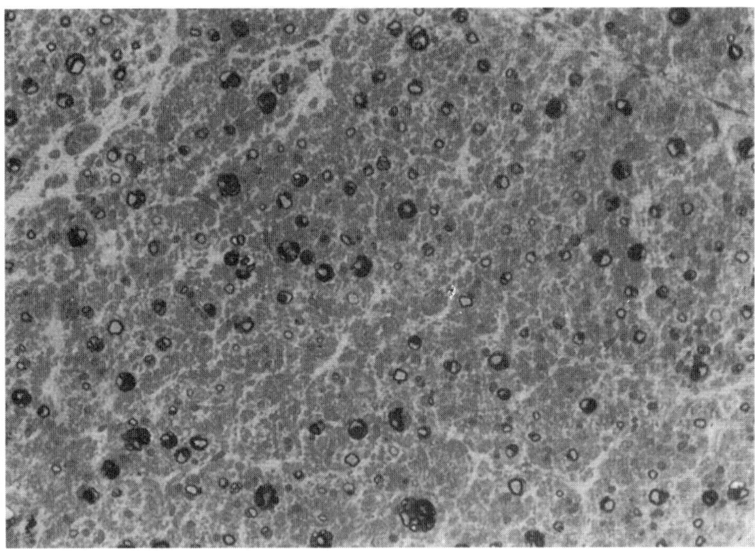

FIGURE 2.—Transverse section of sural nerve biopsy specimen in 1 patient. There is severe fiber loss; most fibers show irregular myelin proliferation; few fibers reveal a thin myelinated sheath; toluidine blue; original magnification, ×540. (Courtesy of Quattrone A, Gambardellla A, Bono F, et al: Autosomal recessive hereditary motor and sensory neuropathy with focally folded myelin sheaths: clinical, electrophysiologic, and genetic aspects of a large family. *Neurology* 46:1318–1324, 1996, by permission of Little, Brown and Company, Inc.)

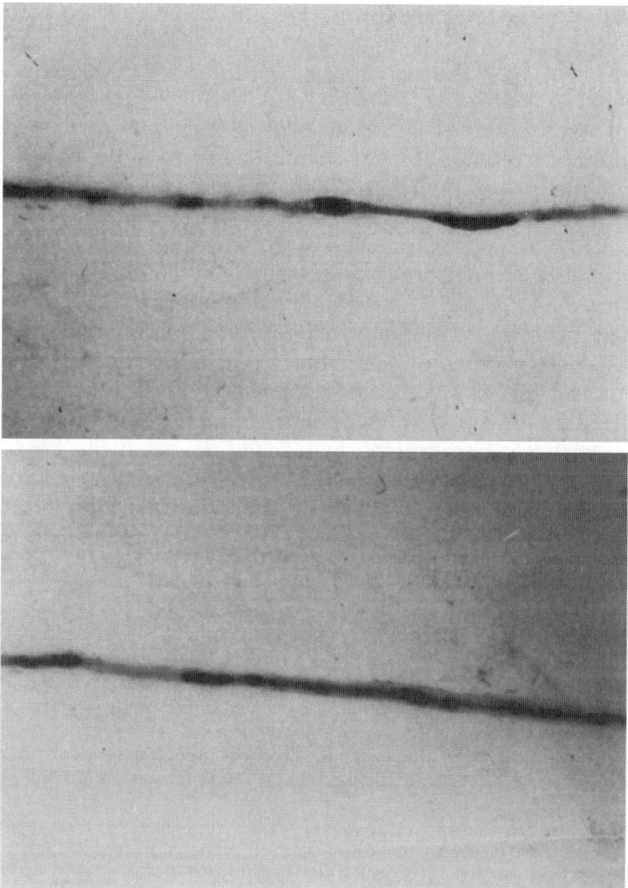

FIGURE 3.—Consecutive portions of a teased fiber from the same patient. Note segmental demyelination and focal areas of irregular myelin folding; original magnification, ×300. (Courtesy of Quattrone A, Gambardellla A, Bono F, et al: Autosomal recessive hereditary motor and sensory neuropathy with focally folded myelin sheaths: Clinical, electrophysiologic, and genetic aspects of a large family. *Neurology* 46:1318–1324, 1996, by permission of Little, Brown and Company, Inc.)

patients consisted of irregular redundant loops with folding of the myelin sheath (Figs 2 and 3). The genealogical study suggested an autosomal recessive inheritance pattern. Molecular analysis produced no evidence of the mutations noted in other forms of HMSN.

Conclusion.—These findings will serve as a starting point for finding the causative gene for an autosomal recessive form of HMSN associated with focally folded myelin sheaths, thus permitting unambiguous diagnosis and providing useful insight into the process of myelinogenesis. The mechanism of the very unusual myelin findings in these patients could involve abnormal expression of structural proteins responsible for compacting myelin.

▶ Autosomal recessive demyelinating HMSN, or Dejerine-Sottas disease, is a heterogeneous group of disorders seen in childhood with a slowly progressive demyelinating neuropathy. Some cases have been reported to be caused by mutations of the *PMP-22* gene,[1, 2] and of the *connexin-32* gene,[3] whereas others have been caused by mutations of the P_O gene.[4, 5] Some have been found to have a gene mapped to chromosome 8q 13–21.1[6] although the gene product is unknown.

Morphologic studies of the peripheral nerve are also heterogeneous. Some cases have classical onion bulbs with circumferential Schwann cell lamellae. Some have onion bulbs with circumferential double basal lamina membranes lacking Schwann cell cytoplasm; and some, like the large pedigree described in this paper, have focally folded myelin sheaths. The morphology is relatively striking (see Figs 2 and 3), but might be easily overlooked (see Fig 1). Quattrone et al. appear to have excluded linkage to all the above genes, and hence, the molecular basis remains to be discovered.

W.G. Bradley, D.M., F.R.C.P.

References

1. Valentijn LJ, Ouvrier RA, van den Bosch NH, et al: Dejerine-Sottas neuropathy is associated with a de novo PMP22 mutation. *Hum Mutat* 5:76–80, 1995.
2. Suter U, Snipes GJ: Peripheral myelin protein 22: Facts and hypotheses. *J Neurosci Res* 40:145–151, 1995.
3. Ionasescu V, Searby C, Ionasescu R, et al: New point mutations and deletions of the connexin 32 gene in X-linked Charcot-Marie-Tooth neuropathy. *Neuromuscul Disord* 5:297–299, 1995.
4. Rautenstrauss B, Nelis E, Grehl H, et al: Identification of a de novo insertional mutation in P_O in a patient with a Dejerine-Sottas syndrome (DSS) phenotype. *Hum Mol Genet* 3:1701–1702, 1994.
5. Ikegami T, Nicholson G, Ikeda H, et al: A novel homozygous mutation of the myelin P_O gene producing Dejerine-Sottas disease (hereditary motor and sensory neuropathy type III). *Biochem Biophys Res Commun* 222:107–110, 1996.
6. Othmane KB, Hentati F, Lennon F, et al: Linkage of a locus (CMT4A) for autosomal recessive Charcot-Marie-Tooth disease to chromosome 8q. *Hum Mol Genet* 2:1625–1628, 1993.

Pathologic Alterations in the Diabetic Neuropathies of Humans: A Review

Dyck PJ, Giannini C (Mayo Clinic and Mayo Found, Rochester, Minn)
J Neuropathol Exp Neurol 55:1181–1193, 1996   1–2

Background.—The study of pathologic changes in diabetic neuropathies is important to characterize the interstitial nerve changes that cannot be inferred from clinical or electrophysiologic assessment; to gain insight into mechanisms and causes; to correlate morphometric abnormalities with changes in clinical impairment and nerve conduction, quantitative sensory testing, and quantitative autonomic testing abnormality; and to correlate neuropathologic findings with metabolic derangements. Pathologic changes in diabetic neuropathies were reviewed.

Discussion.—The natural history and pathologic changes among diabetic neuropathies vary greatly, suggesting that they are heterogeneous. Two possible mechanisms underlying diabetic polyneuropathy have been described. In the first, hyperglycemia is assumed to induce metabolic derangements directly affecting Schwann cells or myelin, nodes of Ranvier, or axons. In the second, hyperglycemia and metabolic derangement are assumed to affect the structure and function of endoneurial microvessels, which in turn induce alterations in fiber by changing the blood-nerve barrier, inducing hypoxia or ischemia, or by unknown mechanisms. In proximal diabetic neuropathy, increasing evidence suggests that the characteristic lesion is an inflammatory vasculitis inducing ischemic nerve fiber degeneration. Truncal radiculopathy may result from an inflammatory polyganglionopathy. The monophasic course and pathologic changes of ischemia in cranial nerve III neuropathy suggest that localized vasculitis needs to be excluded. Many upper limb mononeuropathies associated with diabetes mellitus are associated with carpal or cubital tunnel syndromes. These mononeuropathies may result from repetitive shear forces, anatomical factors, and excessive stiffness of connective tissues (Figs 1 and 4).

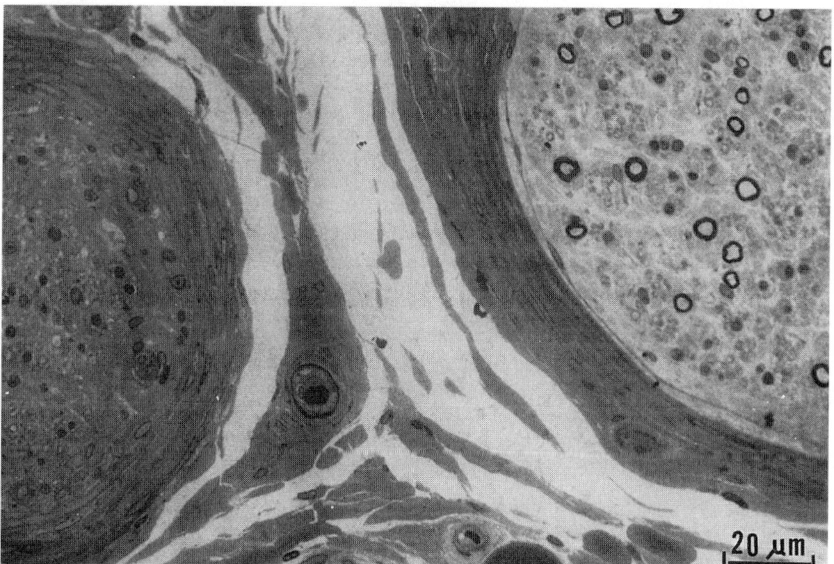

FIGURE 1.—A portion of a transverse section of a sural nerve from a patient with diabetic polyneuropathy illustrates the striking focal absence of myelinated fibers sometimes encountered in this condition. The nerve fascicle (**left**) is without fibers; the fascicle on the **right** has many fibers. Such a striking loss of myelinated fibers is usually attributable to ischemia. (From Dyck PJ, Giannini C: Pathologic alterations in the diabetic neuropathies of humans: A review. Reproduced with permission from the *Journal of Neuropathology and Experimental Neurology* 55:1181–1193, 1996. Courtesy of *Annals of Neurology* 19:425–439, 1986 by permission of Little, Brown and Company Inc.)

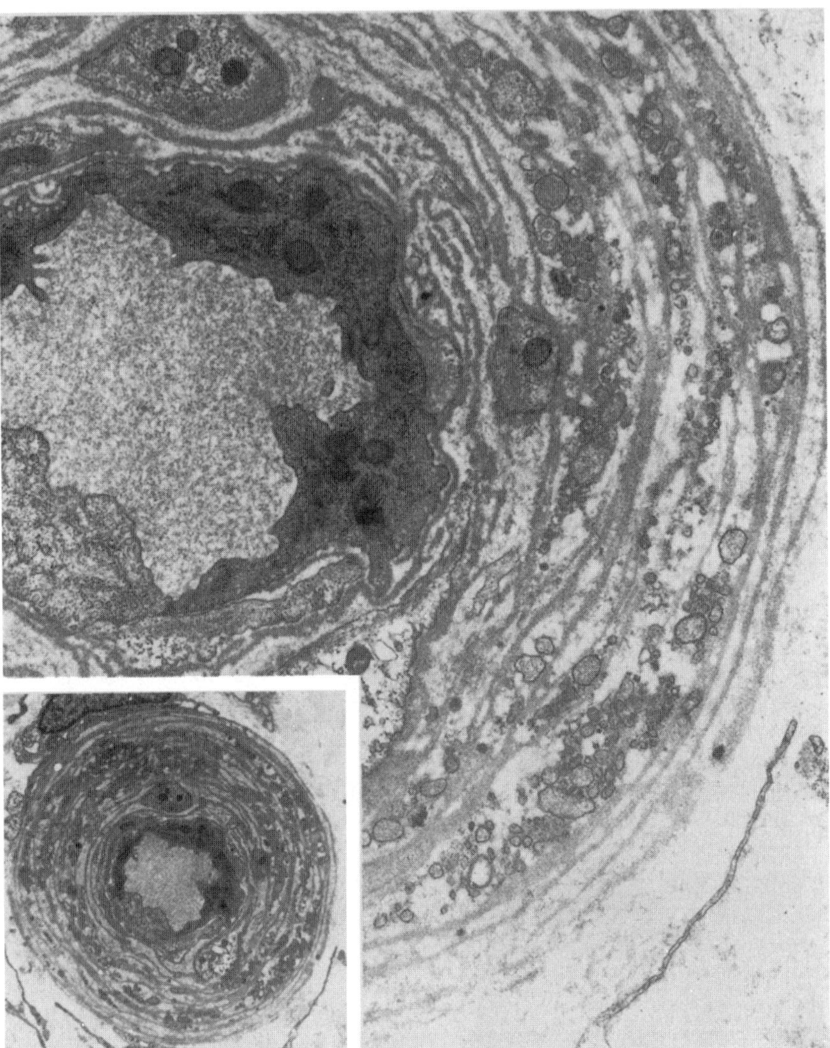

FIGURE 4.—Electron micrographs of a transverse section of an endoneurial microvessel from the sural nerve of a patient with diabetic polyneuropathy illustrates pericyte degeneration (cytoplasmic debris) and reduplicated basement membranes outside of the endothelial cells and lumen. The transverse section of the entire microvessel at low power is shown in the **inset**. It has been shown that these changes precede the development of polyneuropathy and are significantly associated with severity of neuropathy. The functional significance of these changes is not entirely understood, but alterations of the blood-nerve barrier are known to occur in diabetic neuropathy. (From Dyck PJ, Giannini C: Pathologic alterations in the diabetic neuropathies of humans: A review. Reproduced with permission from the *Journal of Neuropathology and Experimental Neurology* 55:1181–1193, 1996. Courtesy of *Annals of Neurology* 36:408–415, 1994 by permission of Little, Brown and Company Inc.)

▶ The range of involvement of the peripheral nervous system in patients with diabetes mellitus is considerable, and the mechanism of nerve damage is still somewhat uncertain. It is always important to exclude treatable conditions that are associated more commonly with diabetes but do not, in themselves, constitute diabetic neuropathy. These include vitamin B12 deficiency, chronic inflammatory demyelinating polyneuropathy, and vasculitic neuropathy. Even in what appears to be classic diabetic polyneuropathy, there is a possibility that autoimmune processes play a role and that treatments such as IV immunoglobulin may be of value. This review gives an excellent outline of the current state of knowledge regarding the types of neuropathy associated with diabetes.

W.G. Bradley, D.M., F.R.C.P.

Vasculitis Confined to Peripheral Nerves

Davies L, Spies JM, Pollard JD, et al (Royal Prince Alfred Hosp, Camperdown, Australia)
Brain 119:1441–1448, 1996   1–3

Introduction.—Commonly seen in association with systemic vasculitis, vasculitic neuropathy most frequently occurs in the polyarteritis nodosa group of disease or rheumatoid vasculitis. This devastating illness has a

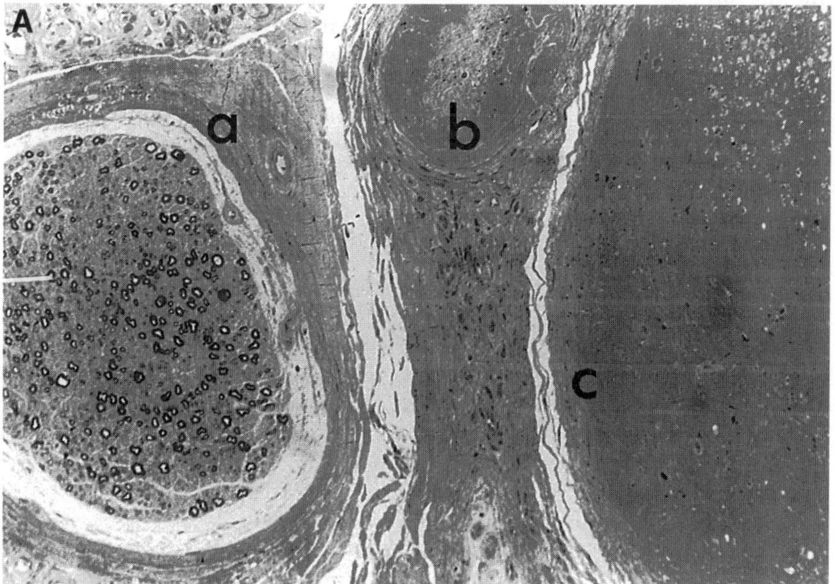

FIGURE 1A.—A, transverse section of sural nerve in isolated peripheral nervous system vasculitis showing evidence of segmental nerve infarction. At this level, 1 fascicle (a) shows a mild reduction of myelinated fibers, whereas in other fascicles no fibers remain and the endoneurium shows homogenous hyaline change consistent with infarction. *Bar* = 50 μm. (Courtesy of Davies L, Spies JM, Pollard JD, et al: Vasculitis confined to peripheral nerves. *Brain* 119:1441–1448, 1996.)

5–year survival in 37% of patients and may occur with lesions confined to 1 organ system. Isolated angiitis has been reported in the brain, in skin, and in the peripheral nervous system. To determine response to therapy and the prognosis, the clinical and pathologic features of 25 patients with isolated peripheral nervous system vasculitis were examined.

Methods.—Case records of 25 patients with evidence of a vasculitic process affecting the peripheral nervous system without any historical, clinical, or serologic evidence of systemic involvement by the same process were reviewed. Clinical data were reviewed, nerve biopsy and histology were performed, nerve pathology was classified, and a statistical analysis was done.

Results.—When seen initially, 6 of 25 patients had a symmetric neuropathy clinically and on neurophysiologic testing. Whereas most patients had a history of mononeuritis multiplex or an asymmetric neuropathy. No patients had signs of accompanying systemic vasculitis. Segmental nerve infarction was seen on a transverse section of sural nerve (Fig 1, A). In 9 of 21 patients there was an elevated erythrocyte sedimentation rate, and 4 of 20 patients had a low titer of antinuclear antibodies. On nerve biopsy, most patients had a necrotizing vasculitis. On immunofluorescence studies, some patients received a diagnosis of inflammatory cell infiltrates with extensive axonal degeneration and immune complex deposition. From symptom onset of diagnosis, the mean time was 46 weeks. Corticosteroids was the predominant form of treatment, and most patients also had immunosuppressive therapy.

Conclusions.—With 24 of 25 survivors at a mean of 176 weeks, the prognosis was good, in contrast to vasculitic neuropathy associated with systemic vasculitis. On a 6-point disability scale, there was a mean improvement of 1.4 units. According to this disability scale, 20 of 23 patients were ambulant and self-caring without walking aids.

▶ Neurologists will inevitably see vasculitis that is preferentially confined to the peripheral nervous system, whereas internists and rheumatologists will see the polysystemic classic variety of polyarteritis nodosa. This monosystemic syndrome undoubtedly has a better prognosis than polysystemic polyarteritis nodosa.

This review of 25 such patients gives a good outline of the problems. The treatment is similar to that for polyarteritis nodosa with mononeuritis multiplex, namely, high-dose corticosteroids plus immunosuppressant drugs. In my experience, cyclophosphamide at a dose sufficient to lower the total lymphocyte count to about 750/mm^3 is the treatment of choice when combined with high-dose corticosteroids. Twenty-five years ago, polyarteritis nodosa had an 80% 2–year mortality rate, whereas now with the combination of cyclophosphamide and high-dose prednisone, the 5–year *cure* rate is about 60% to 70%. However, the treatment of such patients requires considerable experience and care.

W.G. Bradley, D.M., F.R.C.P.

Contribution of Nerve Biopsy Findings to the Diagnosis of Disabling Neuropathy in the Elderly: A Retrospective Review of 100 Consecutive Patients
Chia L, Fernandez A, Lacroix C, et al (Universitaire de Bicêtre, Paris)
Brain 119:1091–1098, 1996

1–4

Background.—The peripheral nervous system is known to change with age. Among the elderly, peripheral neuropathy is an important factor in disability. The value of intensive assessment of elderly patients with subacute or chronic disabling peripheral neuropathy was investigated.

Methods and Findings.—The clinical and nerve biopsy findings of 100 patients older than 65 years were reviewed. All patients had a peripheral neuropathy severe enough to warrant nerve biopsy for diagnosis or prognosis.

In 3 patients, normal nerve biopsy findings led to a diagnosis of lower motor neuron disease. In another 6, findings suggested lesions of the spinal roots. In 23 patients, biopsy specimens demonstrated necrotizing arteritis. Nonnecrotizing vasculitis was documented in 5.

In another 5 patients, vasculitic neuropathy was diagnosed despite noncontributive biopsy findings. Vasculitis also was found in the biopsy specimens of 2 patients with diabetes with a multifocal neuropathy. Altogether, 35% of the patients in the current series had some form of vasculitic neuropathy. Chronic inflammatory demyelinating polyneuropathy was documented in 14 patients. Neuropathy was associated with monoclonal gammopathy in 11 patients. Two of the 6 patients with diabetes initially had a multifocal neuropathy and were found to have vasculitis in the nerve specimen. In the other 4, biopsy was done because of uncommonly severe pains or motor involvement caused by an extremely severe diabetic neuropathy.

Six patients had a long-lasting disability from drug-induced neuropathy. The other 15% had neuropathies of different origins. These included amyloidosis, lepromatous leprosy, carcinomatous neuropathy, and alcoholic neuropathy. Six patients had a mild, nonprogressive, or slowly progressive axonopathy of unknown origin. Peripheral nervous system aging may have played a role in the development of this.

Conclusions.—Vasculitis is an important and treatable cause of disabling neuropathy among the elderly. Only a small proportion of patients have severe neuropathy of unknown origin.

▶ For many years it has been accepted that nerve biopsy is positively diagnostic in a relatively small proportion of patients with peripheral nerve disease. In most series, at least 50% of patients with chronic progressive sensorimotor polyneuropathies remained undiagnosed despite nerve biopsy. Detailed investigations of these patients and their families reveal that about half may have a familial neuropathy. A proportion of the remainder can be shown to have chronic inflammatory demyelinating polyneuropathy by detailed electrophysiologic studies, including the presence of slowed nerve conduction and multifocal block.

This article by Said and colleagues identified a surprisingly high proportion of elderly patients with neuropathies having a vasculitis. Additionally, the subset of patients with a final definitive diagnosis is surprisingly high, compared with general experience. It does appear that the elderly may be a more fertile ground for diagnostic nerve biopsies than was previously thought.

W.G. Bradley, D.M., F.R.C.P.

Randomised Trial of Plasma Exchange, Intravenous Immunoglobulin, and Combined Treatments in Guillain-Barré Syndrome

Hughes RAC, and the Plasma Exchange/Sandoglobulin Guillain-Barré Syndrome Trial Group (Guy's Hosp, London)
Lancet 349:225–230, 1997
1–5

Background.—The relative effectiveness of plasma exchange (PE) and IV immunoglobulin (IVIg) in patients with Guillain-Barré syndrome has not been determined. An international, multicenter, randomized trial compared PE with IVIg and with a combination of PE and IVIg.

Methods.—Three hundred eighty-three adults with Guillain-Barré syndrome were assigned randomly to five 50 mL/kg PEs for 8–13 days, 0.4 g/kg of IVIg daily for 5 days, or the PE regimen followed immediately by the IVIg regimen. All patients had had severe disease and onset of neuropathic symptoms within the previous 14 days. The follow-up was 48 weeks.

Findings.—Four weeks after randomization, the mean improvement on a 7-point disability scale was 0.9 in the PE group, 0.8 in the IVIg group, and 1.1 in the combined treatment group. The differences among groups were nonsignificant. The 3 groups were also comparable in recovery of unaided walking, time to discontinuation of ventilation, and trend describing the recovery from disability for up to 48 weeks. A nonsignificant trend toward more favorable outcomes was observed in some outcome measures with combined treatment.

Conclusion.—The efficacies of PE and IVIg appear to be equivalent in the treatment of severe Guillain-Barré syndrome in the first 2 weeks after onset. Combining PE and IVIg did not seem to have a significant advantage.

▶ The demonstration that PE significantly improved the short-term and long-term prognosis of Guillain-Barré syndrome in the late 1970s was a significant breakthrough. When it was later shown, by a number of studies, that IVIg infusion was also effective, there was a need for a controlled trial comparing these 2 treatments. This paper not only shows that the 2 treatments are of similar efficacy but that PE followed by IVIG offers little or no additional benefit. It has been suggested, by a number of authorities, that there is a greater frequency of progression of the disease or relapses after IVIG compared with PE. Our experience has shown the opposite, namely, that more relapses occur after plasma exchange.

Despite the importance of the therapy considered in this study, the article also highlights the fact that the major features bearing upon prognosis are age, the severity of the disease, and the rapidity of progression; IVIg and PE have a relatively minor effect compared with these other prognostic features.

W.G. Bradley, D.M., F.R.C.P.

Chronic Inflammatory Demyelinating Polyradiculoneuropathy: Unusual Clinical Features and Therapeutic Responses

Midroni G, Dyck PJ (Mayo Clinic and Mayo Found, Rochester, Minn)
Neurology 46:1206–1212, 1996

1–6

Background.—Patients with chronic inflammatory demyelinating polyradiculopathy (CIDP) usually demonstrate a sensorimotor polyradiculopathy, varying in symmetry and progression, with predominant motor deficits and diffuse hyporeflexia or areflexia. The condition commonly responds to corticosteroids and other immune-modulating therapies, and this response is sometimes considered to confirm the diagnosis. The true range of clinical and pathologic features of CIDP is probably wider than suggested in recent reports. Three cases of atypical, treatment-resistant CIDP were reported.

Patients.—The patients were all men aged 29 to 46 years. The first patient had severe demyelinating neuropathy accompanied by severe pseudotumor cerebri syndrome. This patient had pupillary involvement and myelopathy caused by massive nerve root enlargement (Figs 1 and 3). The early course of disease was very aggressive, requiring 2 operations—urgent lumboperitoneal shunting and cervical laminectomy—followed by prolonged treatment with plasma exchange.

The clinical presentation in the second patient was focal brachial plexus neuropathy and hypertrophy; a gadolinium-enhanced MRI scan of the cauda equina showed lower extremity involvement as well. This patient apparently failed to respond to initial corticosteroid treatment. Only after IV immune globulin and plasma exchange were tried, without success, was the patient given a more aggressive trial of corticosteroid treatment. This regimen produced dramatic improvement.

The third patient had an apparently "typical" case of CIDP but showed no apparent response to IV immune globulin, plasma exchange, and corticosteroid therapy. The patient was referred for further evaluation, which found no alternative cause of his condition. Intravenous immune globulin was repeated, this time in a once-weekly, 8-week regimen, which produced a response.

Discussion.—Chronic inflammatory demyelinating polyradiculopathy may appear in atypical and/or treatment-resistant forms, as this experience illustrates. When treating patients with CIDP, it is important to observe the need for intensive and prolonged treatment and for objective assessments

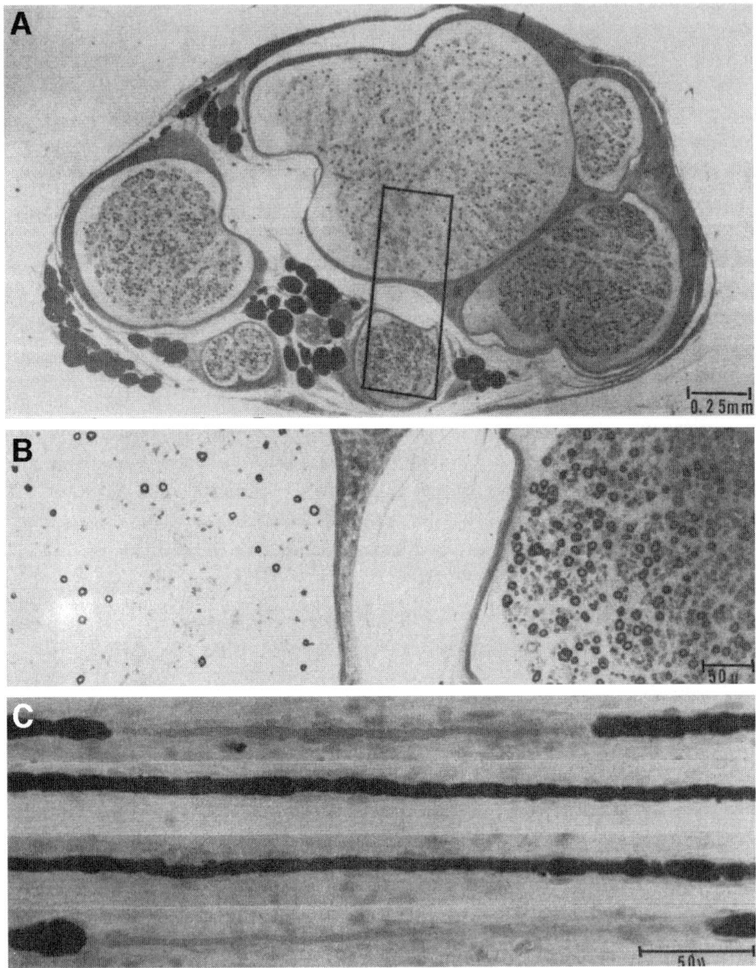

FIGURE 1.—A: Cross section of sural nerve biopsy specimen reveals marked focality of pathology. B: Many denervated onion bulbs are present in the most severely affected fascicle. C: Consecutive lengths of a teased fiber show 2 demyelinated internodes. (Courtesy of Midroni G, Dyck PJ: Chronic inflammatory demyelinating polyradiculopathy: Unusual clinical features and therapeutic responses. *Neurology* 46:1206–1212, 1996, by permission of Little, Brown and Company, Inc.)

of response. There is danger in reassessing after too short an interval and in relying on subjective impressions of improvement.

▶ Although CIDP and its response to corticosteroids have been recognized for almost 40 years,[1] the range of its clinical presentation still confounds us. This paper illustrates the unusual features and relative resistance to treatment of 3 patients. Chronic inflammatory demyelinating polyneuropathy should be considered as a diagnosis in every patient with peripheral neuropathy, whether focal or generalized, and in patients with plexopathies.

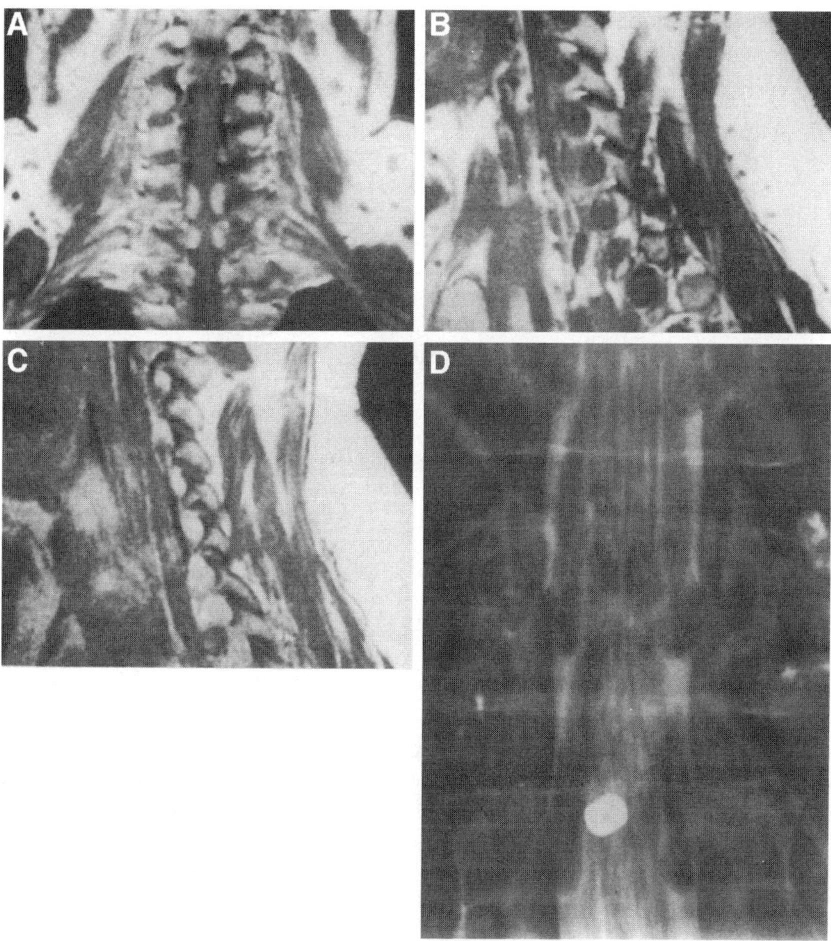

FIGURE 3.—Neuroimaging studies in 1 patient. **A:** Gadolinium-enhanced coronal sections through cervical spine show bilateral nerve root enhancement, with compression of the lower cervical cord by massively enlarged nerve roots. Sagittal sections through cervical spine 20 mm lateral to midline, without **(B)** and with **(C)** gadolinium, show enlarged enhancing cervical roots at all levels. **D:** Myelogram at L2–L4 level shows bilaterally enlarged nerve root profiles. (Courtesy of Midroni G, Dyck PJ: Chronic inflammatory demyelinating polyradiculopathy: Unusual clinical features and therapeutic responses. *Neurology* 46:1206–1212, 1996, by permission of Little, Brown and Company, Inc.)

Evidence of multifocal block and slowed nerve conduction support the diagnosis. Inflammation on distal sural nerve biopsy is relatively uncommon; the changes are usually simply of loss of myelinated fibers, axonal degeneration, and minor segmental demyelination.

A poor response of CIDP to immunotherapy may have several causes; some patients improve with one modality of treatment and are unaffected by another. If there is severe axonal loss by the time therapy is inititated, little recovery of lost function will occur. However, this paper emphasizes the fact

that prolonged, relatively low-grade immunotherapy may be needed to produce improvement in some cases.

W.G. Bradley, D.M., F.R.C.P.

Reference

1. Austin JH: Recurrent polyneuropathies and their corticosteroid treatment. *Brain* 81:157, 1958.

Peripheral Neurotoxicity Induced by Docetaxel
Hilkens PHE, Verweij J, Stoter G, et al (Dr Daniel den Hoed Cancer Ctr, Rotterdam, The Netherlands; Univ Hosp, Rotterdam, The Netherlands)
Neurology 46:104–108, 1996   1–7

Background.—Docetaxel is a new semisynthetic taxoid that works by the same mechanism as paclitaxel, but comes from a renewable source. It inhibits tubulin depolymerization and stabilizes microtubules through the promotion of microtubule assembly. Docetaxel is stronger than paclitaxel in vitro, and has shown antitumor activity against many types of solid tumors, such as ovarian carcinoma, breast cancer, melanoma, non–small-cell lung cancer, and small-cell lung cancer. Adverse effects include neu-tropenia, hypersensitivity reactions, and cumulative fluid retention syndrome. Neurotoxicity induced by docetaxel was evaluated in 4 multicenter phase II trials.

Methods.—There were 41 patients with metastatic or locally advanced cancer for which there was no other appropriate treatment. Patients were between 18 and 75 years of age. Docetaxel 100 mg/m^2 every 3 weeks was administered. Neuropathy was evaluated at baseline, after every 2 cycles, 2 weeks after the last dose, and then every 3 months by a standard neurologic examination and the Vibration Perception Threshold (VPT). The severity of neuropathy was scored through the use of Common Toxicity Criteria of the National Cancer Institute.

Results.—Most patients had mild neuropathy. However, 3 of 15 patients developed moderate neuropathy and 1 of 15 patients developed severe neuropathy at cumulative doses greater than 600 mg/m^2. No correlations were noted between the VPT and clinical sum scores, or between VPT and cumulative doses of docetaxel.

Conclusions.—A high percentage of patients treated with docetaxel developed a mild dose-dependent and predominantly sensory neuropathy. Higher doses of docetaxel may induce more severe and disabling neurop-athy. The VPT values are not a reliable indicator of docetaxel-induced neuropathy.

▶ The continued emergence of new anti-tumor agents has intensified the need for reliable methods to detect and monitor the onset and progression of iatrogenic peripheral neuropathy. Although not evident in this article, there is increased evidence that a pretreatment neuropathy predisposes to an earlier and more severe iatrogenic neuropathy and may lead to discontinuation of possibly life-extending treatment. As indicated, reliance on 1 modality of nerve function may give misleading results. Probably the best combination is a directed history and physical for neuropathic dysfunction, along with both vibration and thermal quantitative testing. Nerve conduction studies could then be performed for confirmation if needed. The detection of a pretreatment neuropathy may necessitate initial dosage modification and more frequent monitoring for iatrogenic neuropathy.

A.R. Berger, M.D.

Ethylene Oxide Neurotoxicity: A Cluster of 12 Nurses With Peripheral and Central Nervous System Toxicity

Brashear A, Unverzagt FW, Farber MO, et al (Indiana Univ, Indianapolis; Methodist Hosp, Indianapolis, Ind; Albert Einstein College of Medicine, New York)

Neurology 46:992–998, 1996

1–8

Objective.—Ethylene oxide, a commonly used sterilant gas, is neurotoxic. Little is known about the toxicity of a byproduct, ethylene chlorhydrin. A report of 12 technicians with rash, hand numbness and weakness, headache, and cognitive changes after a 5-month exposure to ethylene oxide and ethylene chlorhydrin from disposable surgical gowns was presented.

Methods.—Twelve female nurses and operating room technicians aged 25 to 52 years complained of symptoms 5 months after a manufacturer changed to a packaging procedure that allowed less evaporation of residual ethylene oxide from sterilized gowns.

Results.—All patients had rash. Nine patients had neuropathy on examination and 4 had neuropathy on conduction studies. Nerve conduction abnormalities suggested focal median nerve involvement on 2 patients, and focal slowing of ulnar conduction across the elbow in the other 2 patients. Ten patients had loss of protective sensations, 4 had an elevated vibratory sensory threshold, 3 had atrophy on a head MRI study, and 4 had mild cognitive impairment with neuropsychological testing. One patient had a sural nerve biopsy that showed accumulation of myelin debris and dense bodies in the cytoplasm of Schwann cells.

Conclusion.—The rash appeared several months before the onset of neurologic symptoms and may be a warning sign. This study suggests that other health professionals may be at risk from the neurotoxic effects of ethylene oxide.

▶ Focal neuropathies caused by overlying skin exposure to neurotoxins are exceedingly rare, if they occur at all. This is because surface exposure leads to hematologic dissemination, exposing all vulnerable structures to the toxin. I am doubtful that in the patients reported in this paper, focal median or ulnar entrapments developed de novo from ethylene oxide exposure. This is especially unlikely because these same patients did not manifest a generalized neuropathy, which one could postulate was the substrate upon which focal nerve entrapments could have developed. It is yet unclear whether focal neuropathies are more likely to develop in patients with toxic peripheral neuropathies or whether patients with pre-existing focal neuropathies are likely to have focal symptoms when exposed to a neurotoxin.

A.R. Berger, M.D.

Bell's Palsy Treatment With Acyclovir and Prednisone Compared With Prednisone Alone: A Double-Blind, Randomized, Controlled Trial

Adour KK, Ruboyianes JM, von Doersten PG, et al (Kaiser Permanente Med Ctr, Oakland, Calif; Kaiser Permanente Med Care Program, Oakland, Calif)
Ann Otol Rhinol Laryngol 105:371–378, 1996   1–9

Purpose.—A growing body of evidence suggests that Bell's palsy is caused by herpes simplex virus. Prednisone has proven beneficial in previous studies of this neuritis. The antiviral drug acyclovir, with or without prednisone, was evaluated for the treatment of Bell's palsy.

Methods.—The randomized, controlled, double-blind trial included 99 patients with Bell's palsy. Fifty-three patients received acyclovir, 400 mg 5 times daily, plus oral prednisone, whereas 46 received placebo plus prednisone. The results were assessed by the recovery profile and recovery

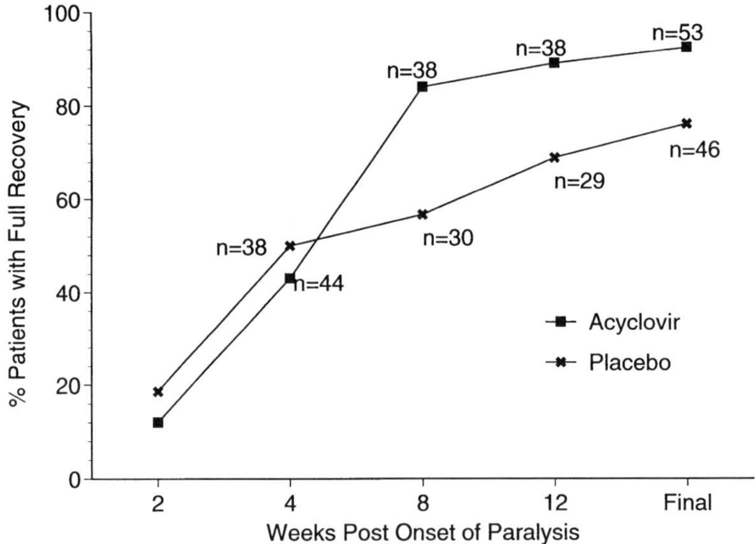

FIGURE 3.—Bell's palsy recovery rate in acyclovir-prednisone group vs. placebo-prednisone group as indicated by recovery profile of 10 in percentage of those appearing for examination 2, 4, 8, 12, and 16 (final) weeks after onset of paralysis. (Courtesy of Adour KK, Ruboyianes JM, von Doersten PG, et al: Bell's palsy treatment with acyclovir and prednisone compared with prednisone alone: A double-blind, randomized, controlled trial. *Ann Otol Rhinol Laryngol* 105:371–378, 1996.)

index and by electrical tests, including electroneurography and the maximal stimulation test.

Results.—Patients receiving acyclovir in addition to prednisone had better outcomes than those receiving placebo plus prednisone. The acyclovir-prednisone treatment was more effective in restoring volitional muscle motion to a recovery profile of 10 and in preventing partial nerve degeneration, as assessed by electrical tests (Fig 3). Both the recovery profile and recovery index were significantly better for the acyclovir-prednisone group. Taking acyclovir also reduced the incidence and severity of contracture with synkinesis, although this difference was not significant.

Conclusion.—The combination of acyclovir and prednisone represents a better treatment for Bell's palsy than prednisone alone. Including the antiviral drug enhances recovery and reduces neural degeneration. The findings strengthen the theory that Bell's palsy is caused by reactivated herpes simplex virus.

▶ Corticosteroid therapy has been proven to improve the degree of recovery from Bell's palsy. There is strong circumstantial evidence for the hypothesis that many cases of Bell's palsy are caused by herpes simplex infection. This double-blind, controlled trial of patients with Bell's palsy treated within 3 days of the onset of symptoms clearly demonstrates that acyclovir, 400 mg 5 times daily for 10 days produces significantly greater recovery than does placebo. All patients received prednisone, 1 mg/kg per day for 5 days with decreasing doses over the next 5 days.

The difference in the degree of recovery in the 2 groups appeared to be clinically significant (see Fig 3). There were relatively modest side effects. It appears that combination prednisone and acyclovir therapy is the treatment of choice for patients with Bell's palsy seen within 3 days of onset.

W.G. Bradley, D.M., F.R.C.P.

SOD1 Mutation Is Associated With Accumulation of Neurofilaments in Amyotrophic Lateral Sclerosis

Rouleau GA, Clark AW, Rooke K, et al (McGill Univ, Montreal; Univ of Calgary, Alberta, Canada; Univ of Rochester, NY)
Ann Neurol 39:128–131, 1996   1–10

Background.—Fifteen percent to 20% of patients with familial amyotrophic lateral sclerosis (FALS) have mutations in the Cu/Zn superoxide dismutase (SOD1) gene. Levels of neurofilament subunits have been found to be increased in transgenic mouse models of ALS, also suggesting that these proteins play a key role in the pathogenesis of the disease. The coexistence of an Ile[113] → Thr substitution in exon 4 of the SOD1 gene and marked neurofilamentous abnormality in the same patient with FALS was reported.

Case Report.—Woman, 65, with a mutation in SOD1 was investigated. De+ oxyribonucleic acid was extracted from a fragment of the cerebellum, and exon 4 of the SOD1 gene was amplified using polymerase chain reaction. Single-strand conformational analysis (SSCA) was performed, and the exon was sequenced. An aberrant band in exon 4 of the SOD1 gene was demonstrated on SSCA. Sequence analysis showed an Ile[113] $\rightarrow$ Thr substitution, which is a codon previously found to be mutated in other patients with FALS.

Conclusions.—This is the first patient with familial ALS reported to have an SOD1 mutation coexisting with a massive aberrant accumulation of neurofilaments. The current findings extend evidence for a pathogenetic link between oxidative damage and neurofilament accumulation.

▶ Several hypotheses continue to hold sway concerning the etiology of ALS. Mutations of the genes for SOD1 and of neurofilament proteins underlie the disease in a small number of patients with ALS, predominantly those that have familial ALS. Evidence for glutamate toxicity, and the ability of antiglutamate agents like riluzole to slow down the progression of the disease, support the excitoxic theory. The theory of free radical oxidative damage also has a considerable amount of experimental evidence to support it. The problem is to fit these various theories together, because it appears that we are dealing with one pathologic entity—ALS.

This paper by Rouleau and colleagues opens our eyes to the possibility that a defect in one biochemical system can produce changes in another. It is studies like this that will eventually help us put all the jigsaw puzzle pieces in place. This paper helps interlink at least 2 of the pieces of the puzzle, suggesting that the effect of mutations of the SOD1 gene may produce abnormalities of neurofilament proteins, leading to motor neuronal degeneration.

W.G. Bradley, D.M., F.R.C.P.

Physical Activity, Trauma, and ALS: A Case-Control Study
Strickland D, Smith SA, Dolliff G, et al (Univ of Nebraska, Omaha; Hennepin Faculty Assoc, Minneapolis; Univ of Minnesota, Minneapolis)
Acta Neurol Scand 94:45–50, 1996   1–11

Background.—Although the short-term effects of physical trauma have been well documented, chronic long-term outcomes are not well understood. Many researchers have studied the association of physical trauma with amyotrophic lateral sclerosis (ALS), but results have been conflicting. This relationship was further studied in a pilot case-control study.

Methods and Findings.—Twenty-five patients with ALS seen at a university muscle-disease clinic were selected and matched with 1 clinic patient with a different disease and with 1 community subject. The patients with ALS differed significantly from the control subjects in several respects. The patients with ALS had an odds ratio (OR) of 5.3 for head, neck, and back injury. Their OR for frequency of sweating in work or during leisure activity was 1.6. Their OR for earning a school letter for sports participation was 3.1. Other measures of trauma and activity were not statistically significantly different between groups but were consistent with the aforementioned findings.

Conclusions.—The occurrence of ALS is strongly associated with severe head, neck, and back injury and frequency of sweating in work and leisure activity. The current findings suggest that either trauma or vigorous exercise precipitates ALS, that trauma may be an early sign of disease, or that ALS may predispose to injury.

▶ There is a wealth of literature dealing with possible causes of ALS. Many of these papers are epidemiologic studies using the case-control methodology. A number of different statistically significant associations have been reported from these studies. It is interesting that positive associations in some studies are often not found in other studies that have different positive associations. The major problem with case-control studies is patients' memories and the intensity with which patients search their memory for a possible cause of this terrible disease from which they are suffering, ALS. We all have experienced patients who denied any surgical procedures, only to be seen to have scars all over their abdomen that they had "forgotten" during the questioning. Hence, patients with ALS may recall events, whereas case-controls may not. Strickland and colleagues try to control for this in a variety of ways, but this will always remain a weakness of such studies. The implication of an association between trauma and ALS is, of course, enormous in regard to medicolegal matters. Unfortunately, as good a case can be put forward for as against trauma causing ALS, and at this stage I regard the matter as being undecided.

W.G. Bradley, D.M., F.R.C.P.

Lack of Progression of Neurologic Deficit in Survivors of Paralytic Polio: A 5-Year Prospective Population-based Study
Windebank AJ, Litchy WJ, Daube JR, et al (Mayo Clinic and Mayo Found, Rochester, Minn)
Neurology 46:80–84, 1996
1–12

Background.—In the past 10 years, late progressive weakness and atrophy have been reported in survivors of paralytic polio. A second type of symptom cluster was described in 1987. It consisted of progressive muscle pain, weakness, and fatigue. The prevalence of this second entity is not known, but it is estimated to occur in about 70% of polio survivors. Polio survivors in Olmsted County, Minnesota were studied to gain more insight into the frequency and basis of these symptoms.

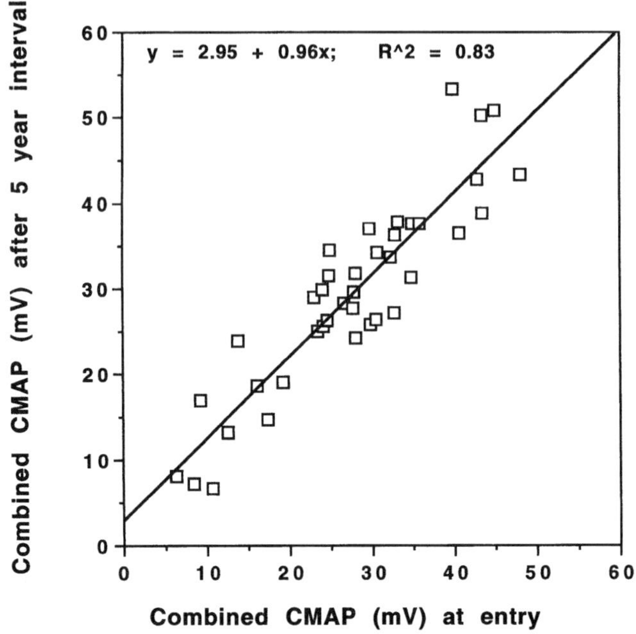

FIGURE 1.—Regression of summated compound muscle action potentials (CMAP) amplitudes (right and left thenar plus right and left extensor digitorum brevis muscles) at the second examination (5-year interval) compared with the summated CMAP amplitude at the first evaluation. The amplitudes are stable (slope = 0.96) and reproducible within individual subjects (r^2 = 0.83). (Courtesy of Windebank AJ, Litchy WJ, Daube JR, et al: Lack of progression of neurologic deficit in survivors of paralytic polio: A 5-year prospective population-based study. *Neurology* 46:80–84, 1996, by permission of Little, Brown, and Company Inc.)

Methods and Findings.—Fifty persons who had paralytic polio between 1935 and 1960 were included in the prospective, population-based cohort study. The individuals identified represented all 300 cases of paralytic polio in the county. Detailed quantitative clinical and electrophysiologic studies were done at study enrollment and after 5 years. Neuromuscular function in the cohort was stable, although 60% were symptomatic. The causes of symptoms were unrelated to the earlier polio in two-thirds of symptomatic patients. A mechanical disorder probably underlies the symptoms of the 20% with unexplained muscle pain, perception of weakness, and fatigue (Figs 1 and 2).

Conclusions.—This group of paralytic polio survivors had remarkably stable neuromuscular function. During the 5 years of observation, several attributes of neuromuscular function actually improved. The findings of muscle function testing raised the question of whether reinnervation still occurs 35 to 50 years after acute illness.

▶ The pendulum of opinion has swung wildly over the frequency of late deterioration in patients who previously suffered from paralytic poliomyelitis. The apogee was a postal survey of patients who suffered polio 30 or

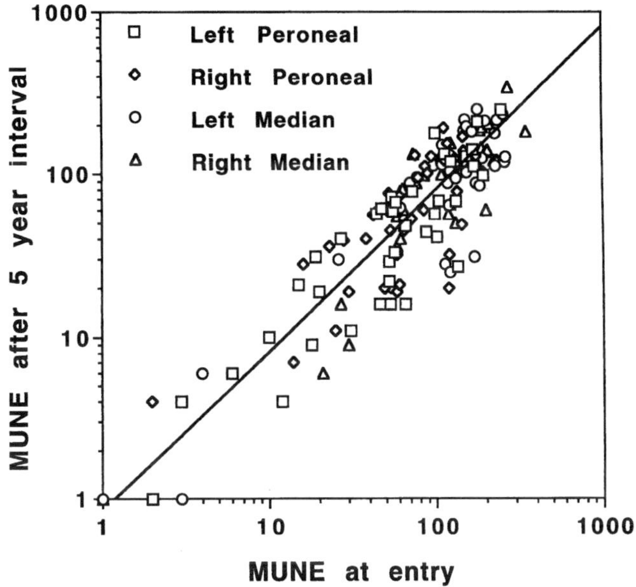

FIGURE 2.—Regression of motor unit number estimates (MUNE) at the second examination (5-year interval) compared with MUNE at the first evaluation. The peroneal nerve was stimulated at the fibular head recording over the extensor digitorum brevis muscle. The median nerve was stimulated at the elbow with recording over the abductor pollicis brevis muscle. (Courtesy of Windebank AJ, Litchy WJ, Daube JR, et al: Lack of progression of neurologic deficit in survivors of paralytic polio: A 5-year prospective population-based study. *Neurology* 46:80–84, 1996, by permission of Little, Brown, and Company Inc.)

more years previously in which it was shown that 85% suffered from a variety of postpolio symptoms. The perigee was the study by Windebank et al.[1] from the Mayo Clinic in which it was shown that only about a tenth of survivors suffered from the symptoms of fatigue, pain, and progressive weakness. This article reports an elegant and detailed follow-up study of 50 patients from the initial cohort from the Mayo, studied at 2 time points separated by 5 years. Symptoms that are believed to be part of the postpolio syndrome were present in 60% of the cohort, which might be taken to support the existence of the postpolio syndrome. However, detailed strength testing and electrophysiologic studies failed to show any evidence of major progression, and in fact some patients improved in the 5 year interval. They were able to interpret the symptoms as being due to a variety of other conditions in two-thirds of their patients. A similar observation was reported by Ivanyi et al[2] in a cohort of 43 patients with symptoms and 13 without, followed for about 6 years. In the symptomatic group, strength deteriorated in 6 muscle groups, and remained static or improved in 16 groups. In the asymptomatic group, strength deteriorated in 14 muscle groups and remained static or improved in 8. Another article by Grimby et al[3] demonstrated that motor units in muscles previously affected by polio are used at maximum effort for normal degrees of activity, have excellent capacity for force output, but have poor endurance. Nevertheless, Grimby et al.[4] have demonstrated progression of muscle weakness and wasting in a 4 year follow-up study of 18 subjects. What are we to conclude from this? Undoubtedly, patients with previous polio suffer from a higher frequency of neuromuscular symptoms than the general population. However, the causes are multifactorial, and the condition is likely to be nonprogressive in most of the patients. Hence, therapeutic nihilism should be abandoned. Many of these patients can be helped by rehabilitation and therapeutic control of processes that lead to pain, including muscular deconditioning. Physical therapy and graded endurance exercise programs can often be very beneficial.

W.G. Bradley, D.M., F.R.C.P.

References

1. Windebank AJ, Litchy WJ, Daube JR, et al: Late effects of paralytic poliomyelitis in Olmsted County, Minnesota. *Neurology* 451:501–507, 1995.
2. Ivanyi B, Nelemans PJ, de Jongh R, et al: Muscle strength in postpolio patients: A prospective follow-up study. *Muscle Nerve* 19:738–742, 1996.
3. Grimby L, Tollback A, Muller U, et al Fatigue of chronically overused motor units in prior polio patients. *Muscle Nerve* 19:728–737, 1996.
4. Grimby G, Kvist H, Grangard U, Reduction in thigh muscle cross-sectional area and strength in a 4-year follow-up in late polio. *Arch Phys Med Rehabil* 77:1044–1048, 1996.

2 Molecular Neurogenetics

The Inherited Ataxias and the New Genetics
Hammans SR (Southampton Gen Hosp, England)
J Neurol Neurosurg Psychiatry 61:327–332, 1996   2–1

Introduction.—Progress in genetic research has lent new insight into the molecular basis of inherited neurologic diseases. In the case of the inherited ataxias, genetic classifications are resolving long-standing diagnostic problems. The influence of recent genetic research on our understanding of the inherited ataxias previously considered "idiopathic" was reviewed.

Autosomal Recessive Ataxias.—Recent research has identified a gene on chromosome 9, designated *X25*, that is related to Friedreich's ataxia, the most common genetic ataxia. The available data suggest that this mutation interferes with transcription or RNA processing. The neuronal degeneration, cardiomyopathy, and increased diabetes risk seen in patients with Friedreich's ataxia may result from reduced levels of the *X25* gene product, fraxataxin, in the heart and spinal cord. Direct mutational analyses will determine the true range of disease associated with the Friedreich's ataxia genotype. So far, it seems likely that certain clinical variant's of Friedreich's ataxia are allelic variants as well. Fraxataxin gene mutational analysis should improve the diagnosis of patients with atypical Friedreich's ataxia, with important implications for prognosis and genetic counseling. Genetic research has also offered promising insight into certain rarer autosomal recessive ataxia, including early-onset cerebellar ataxia which is distinguished from Friedreich's ataxia by retained reflexes and ataxia with isolated vitamin E deficiency.

Autosomal Dominant Cerebellar Ataxias.—The autosomal dominant cerebellar ataxias (ADCAs) have always posed a diagnostic problem. The one with pigmentary macular dystrophy has been classified as ADCA type II, with other complicated ADCAs classified as type I. Types III and IV have been described as well. Linkage studies have shown that some families with ADCA have a disease locus designated SCA1 on chromosome 6p. This mutation is associated with a trinucleotide expansion and has characteristics in common with those seen in other trinucleotide repeat diseases. Another mutation, designated SCA3, has been linked to Machado-

TABLE 3.—Autosomal Dominant Cerebellar Ataxias: A Clinicogenetic Classification

Gene	Chromosome	Gene defect	Frequency*	Associated clinical features†
ADCA type I				
SCA1	6p22-p23	(CAG)n Normal: 6–39 Disease: 41–59	14/87, 5/19, 2/24, 3/29, 4/38 19/73, 13/120 Overall: 60/390 (15%)	Ophthalmoplegia, pyramidal and extrapyramidal signs, dementia, motor and sensory nerve involvement
SCA2	12q23-24·1	—	—	As SCA1 but more frequent hyporeflexia, supranuclear ophthalmoplegia
SCA3/MJD	14q32·1	(CAG)n Normal: 13–41 Disease: 62–80	7/24, 5/29, 19/38, 10/35 5/42, 28/120 Overall: 74/288 (26%)	As SCA1 but possibly with more frequent extrapyramidal signs (see text)
SCA4	16q24-ter	—	—	As SCA1 but with prominent sensory axonal neuropathy
SCA5	Cent 11	—	—	Benign relatively pure ataxia ? Harding type III
ADCA type II	3p12-21·1	—	—	Pigmentary macular dystrophy (see text)
DRPLA	12p	(CAG)n Normal: 8–35 Disease: 54–79	—	Myoclonus, chorea, epilepsy, dementia
Periodic ataxia				
EA-1	12p	KCNA1 mutations	—	Myokymia, brief attacks
EA-2	19p	—	—	Progressive ataxia, nystagmus, longer attacks

Note: Frequencies vary according to population and with the clinical characteristics of the families surveyed.
*Frequencies are expressed as a proportion of all autosomal dominant cerebellar ataxias (*ADCAs*) studied.
†The features of the ADCAs overlap.
(Courtesy of Hammans SR: The inherited ataxias and the new genetics. *J Neurol Neurosurg Psychiatry* 61:327–332, 1996.)

Joseph disease. Although there is no single feature differentiating these patients from other families with type I ADCA, evidence suggests that the different SCA loci do have differing phenotypes (Table 3). The difference may be noticeable only in group comparisons, as opposed to individual prediction of genotype. Most families with ADCA have neither of these loci; 3 further SCA loci have been mapped so far. Genetic studies are also providing insight into the mechanisms of ADCA types II and III, as well as the periodic ataxias.

Discussion.—Genetic research is providing new insights into the mechanisms and diagnosis of the inherited ataxias. The next step will be to study the functions of the proteins associated with the mutated genes, in the hope of treatment applications. Tests for mutations at the SCA1 and SCA3 loci, and for fraxataxin expansion, are already available and may be helpful diagnostically.

▶ For decades, eponyms glorified our predecessors but confused our colleagues. Genetics has come to the rescue. Seven dominant progressive ataxia genes have been localized, and all 3 thus far cloned are trinucleotide repeat mutations. Two periodic ataxia genes have been localized and 1, a potassium channel gene, has been cloned. Most recently, the Friedreich's trinucleotide repeat mutations were cloned. Studies in sporadic patients have not revealed mutations. Commercial genetic tests now available are the diagnostic tests of choice and permit more precise preventive genetic counseling. The molecular and cellular events are now being dissected and provide new hope that these diseases may soon be licked.

D.A. Stumpf, M.D., Ph.D.

Childhood Onset of Friedreich Ataxia: A Clinical and Genetic Study of 36 Cases
De Michele G, Di Maio L, Filla A, et al (Federico II Univ, Naples, Italy; Sanatrix Neurological Inst, Pozzilli, Italy)
Neuropediatrics 27:3–7, 1996   2–2

Background.—Friedreich ataxia (FA), the most common form of hereditary ataxia, is characterized by neurologic, skeletal, and cardiac abnormalities. The clinical variability of FA is too great for an autosomal recessive disease. Recently, an age of onset of 21–36 years and a milder course were reported in 1 group of patients whose disease was closely linked to the Friedreich ataxia locus (FRDA). Childhood onset of FA was studied in 36 patients.

Methods and Findings.—The genetic, clinical, and laboratory findings were investigated in 36 patients in whom FA onset occurred before the age of 10 years. Mean age of onset was 6.3 years. Most patients had dysmetria, dysarthria, Babinski's sign, pes cavus, scoliosis, and reduced vibration sense. Gait and stance ataxia as well as lower limb areflexia were constant. Compared with patients with later onset FA, the childhood onset group had a greater occurrence of diabetes (25%). Mean age at diabetes onset was 21 years. All the diabetic patients required insulin. In 71% of the patients, ECG showed abnormalities. Forty-three percent had echocardiographic evidence of hypertrophic cardiomyopathy. Linkage analysis was performed in 10 families. There was no recombination between the polymorphic markers of the 9q13-21.1 region and the disease locus with a peak lod score of 4.21 at a recombination fraction of 0.

Conclusions.—Childhood onset of FA represents 38% of total patients. Clinicians should consider this diagnosis in children with gait ataxia, poor coordination, skeletal deformities, areflexia, diabetes, and cardiomyopathy. Dysarthria and extensor plantar response are not always present early in the course of childhood-onset disease. Neurophysiologic and neuroradiologic evaluation may be useful in establishing the diagnosis. Assessing serum vitamin E levels appears to be worthwhile. This disorder may be treatable.

▶ The FA locus (FRDA) at chromosome 9q13-21.1 contains intronic GAA expansions, which lead to Friedreich disease. These authors expand the phenotypic variability resulting from such mutations by recognizing that onset occurred before age 10 in 38% of their patients. Other than age of onset, in an individual patient, there is no other feature distinct for typical Friedreich disease. It is not yet clear whether allelic mutations, degree of GAA expansion, modifier genes, or environmental factors produce earlier onset. The age range for onset of this disorder now extends from 2 to 24 years or more.

D.A. Stumpf, M.D., Ph.D.

CAG Trinucleotide RNA Repeats Interact With RNA-binding Proteins
McLaughlin BA, Spencer C, Eberwine J (Univ of Pennsylvania, Philadelphia)
Am J Hum Genet 59:561–569, 1996   2–3

Introduction.—An expanded CAG repeat is found in several neurologic diseases, including Huntington's disease (HD). There is an extended polyglutamine tract in the translated product of diseases in which the CAG repeat is in the mRNA-coding region. In mRNA, the CAG repeat normally ranges in size from 11 to 34 repeats; disease states are associated with more than 36 repeats. In ferritin and transferrin mRNAs, stem loop structures form and interact with proteins to regulate gene expression and are thought to be involved in regulating translation. The RNA-binding proteins transport mRNA from the nucleus to cytoplasm and may be important in regulating the subcellular cytoplasmic localization of mRNAs. The RNA-binding proteins are important mediators in the complex control of gene expression. The association of cytoplasmic proteins with normal length and extended CAG repeats is described.

Methods.—Gel shift and ultraviolet cross-linking assays were performed on cytosolic extracts of rat liver, hypothalamus, cortex, striatum, testes, spleen, and pituitary and on human cortex and striatum. Sites of neuronal degeneration in HD containing a 63-kD RNA-binding protein that specifically interacts with these CAG repeat sequences were used.

Results.—Protein-RNA interactions depended on the length of the CAG repeat. Longer repeats bound substantially more protein. Two CAG repeat–binding proteins were found to be present in human cortex and striatum; 1 comigrated with rat protein at 64 kD and the other migrated at 49 kD.

Discussion/Conclusion.—With HD used as an example, at least 3 models may explain the CAG repeat–associated disease pathogenesis: (1) RNA-binding protein interaction with CAG repeats of huntingtin mRNA may alter the amount of huntingtin protein produced, (2) the protein-RNA interaction may affect the subcellular distribution of the huntingtin mRNA, or (3) RNA-protein interaction may facilitate altered expression of other proteins. It is not known how a widely expressed gene product, such as in HD, can elicit specific cellular degeneration. It may be that the key feature of the degenerative process is not the presence of this protein, but the relative levels of expression of cellular mRNA in cells in which the huntingtin mRNA and 63-kD protein are coexpressed. Maybe a transgenic model of HD could explain this phenomenon.

▶ Neurology is exciting, in part because the complexity of the brain may reveal new insights about biology not evident in other systems. Such is the case with the trinucleotide repeat mutations, which provide a mechanism for astute clinicians' observations about anticipation. But they also represent novel mutations never before seen in biology. Current work is now unraveling unique pathophysiologic mechanisms. Trinucleotide repeats produce polyglutamate or polyserine regions in proteins. The former interact with other "associated proteins." The present article suggests a role of these associated proteins in mRNA transcription. Other hypothesized effects concern subcellular trafficking and localization of proteins. The necessity of at least a 2-molecule interaction may explain some phenotypic variation and the selective degeneration even with a widely expressed mutant protein.

D.A. Stumpf, M.D., Ph.D.

Longevity Assurance Genes: How Do They Influence Aging and Life Span?
Hodes RJ, McCormick AM, Pruzan M (Natl Inst on Aging, Bethesda, Md)
J Am Geriatr Soc 44:988–991, 1996   2–4

Introduction.—It is well known that the interaction of genes with various environmental factors and signals affects aging and longevity. Recent findings suggest that the life span of several animal species may be significantly increased by experimental manipulation of genetic or lifestyle considerations. It is not known which genes are involved in regulating the aging process, but the National Institute on Aging (NIA) has organized a multidisciplinary Longevity Assurance Gene (LAG) Interactive Network to address this issue. The LAGs are defined as "genes that promote longevity and extend the health span of a cell and/or organism, either alone or in combination with other genes." Findings of the LAG Interactive Network are reported.

Yeast.—Four genes have been identified in the modulation of longevity in yeast: LAG1, LAG2, RAS2, and PHB1. With the exception of LAG2, the other genes seem to be linked genetically and may function in a single pathway to regulate the replicative life span of yeast. In mammalian and human homologues of yeast, RAS2 and PHB1 have been identified and cloned. Analyzing the common pathway in which the LAG1, RAS2, and PHB1 genes function in years should advance knowledge of the biological functions of these genes and their role in regulating aging and longevity in yeast.

Drosophila.—Several genes are expressed differently in young and old fruit flies. A comparative analysis is being undertaken of the lifelong expression patterns of candidate genes. A candidate LAG named death-knell has been identified and is undergoing sequencing. Expression of this gene strongly correlated with longevity in Drosophila. Cloned genes are being prepared to facilitate the search for mammalian homologues and to help determine the function of this gene and its role in aging and longevity.

Caenarhabditis elegans.—Several genes involved in the regulation of nematode longevity have been recognized by the LAG Interactive Network. The LAG Interactive Network investigators are cloning these genes, 2 of which have been shown to encode signal transduction components that are conserved between nematodes and humans.

Mice.—Age-related changes in mice are being evaluated, and the fas gene in particular is undergoing extensive analysis. The fas gene may provide important information about the underlying causes of aging in the immune system.

Humans.—Cultured human cells serve as important models for analyzing the molecular genetic bases of aging and longevity of the individual cell. Numerous candidate genes are being investigated. The molecular genetic basis of Werner syndrome, a rare inherited disease characterized by premature aging and early onset of several diseases of old age, has given a potentially useful clue to the molecular genetic basis of certain aspects of human aging. The *WRN* gene and four different mutations of it have been identified in patients with Werner syndrome. This gene is a helicase, an enzyme that unwinds double-stranded DNA molecules in preparation for DNA replication, DNA repair, or expression of specific genes. Further investigation of the helicase *WRN* is under way.

Conclusion.—The NIA LAG initiative is doing exciting work. It may not be that years can be added to life, but the number of healthy years lived may be enhanced by this work. The positive impact of such findings can increase the well-being of older adults in a way that is sure to have an impact on related costs of medical and social support.

▶ The Fountain of Youth eluded Juan Ponce de León, but modern science may be getting close. Nematode mutants live 2 to 4 times longer, and calorie-restricted mice extend their survival. Through a mix of genetics and lifestyle, we might influence longevity, not by stamping out disease but by modulating the basic events underlying aging. What are they? Unknown—but the target of the NIA-sponsored LAG Interactive Network (LAGIN). Look for the cloning of these LAGs and definition of the effects of their gene products. Already implicated are SOD1 and free radicals, familiar themes to neurologists; signaling systems; and DNA repair systems, including the recently described mutations in humans with Werner syndrome. But hurry LAGIN! Some of us can't wait too long!

D.A. Stumpf, M.D., Ph.D.

Ataxia-Telangiectasia and the ATM Gene: Linking Neurodegeneration, Immunodeficency, and Cancer to Cell Cycle Checkpoints
Shiloh Y, Rotman G (Tel Aviv Univ, Israel)
J Clin Immunol 16:254–260, 1996   2–5

Background.—Ataxia-telangiectasia (A-T) is an autosomal recessive disease that progresses from cerebellar ataxia to general neuromotor dysfunction, with telangiectases appearing later on. Other findings are immunodeficiency, radiosensitivity, predisposition to cancer, and defective cell cycle checkpoints. The causative gene of A-T, designated *ATM*, was recently cloned and sequenced. The genetic mechanism of *ATM* was discussed.

The ATM Gene.—The *ATM* gene occupies 150 kb of genomic DNA and is transcribed onto a 13-kb transcript representing 66 exons. It belongs to a family of large proteins sharing the PI 3–kinase-like domain. Like proteins in various other organisms, the ATM protein plays a direct role in the cell cycle response to DNA damage. As part of a larger protein complex, the ATM protein would communicate a regulatory signal to other proteins in response to a certain type of DNA strand break. The signal slows the cell growth–regulating mechanisms to allow time for repair of the damaged DNA. When 1 of the signaling mechanisms is damaged, the result may be genome instability with increased programmed cell death, susceptibility to malignancy, or both. Although the immune and nervous systems are very different in their proliferation rates, both appear particularly sensitive to the lack of *ATM* function in A-T.

Discussion.—New knowledge regarding the *ATM* gene focuses attention on the importance of signal transduction initiated in the nucleus, as opposed to the external environment, for normal cellular growth. The clinical and cellular phenotype of A-T suggests that dysfunction of the systems for repair of DNA damage has particularly adverse effects on the immune and nervous systems.

▶ Ataxia-telangiectasia produces early developmental delays and ataxia; telangiectasia appears after several years. Most patients are neurologically disabled, but the deadly combination of progressive immune dysfunction and poor DNA repair results in neoplastic death for most patients. With a disease incidence of 1 in 40,000, the carrier state exists in 1 in 200. These carriers have an increased incidence of neoplasms, particularly breast cancer. The recently cloned causative gene, *ATM*, resembles PI 3-kinases involved in DNA repair and cell cycle control via nuclear signal transduction. Perhaps 4% of all breast cancer results from the *ATM* mutations; this is higher that the rate with *BRCA1* and *BRCA2*. This conclusion is tentative, however, and requires further study. See also Reference 1.

D.A. Stumpf, M.D., Ph.D.

Reference

1. Bishop DT, Hopper J: AT-tributable risks? *Nature Genet* 15:226, 1997.

3 Cerebral Vascular Disease

The Value of Intracranial Pressure Monitoring in Acute Hemispheric Stroke
Schwab S, Aschoff A, Spranger M, et al (Univ of Heidelberg, Germany)
Neurology 47:393–398, 1996   3–1

Objective.—Although increased intracranial pressure (ICP), resulting from severe head trauma and intracranial hemorrhage, is associated with poor outcome, there is no evidence that ICP monitoring improves the outcome in stroke patients. Results of a prospective study evaluating the clinical and neurologic course of stroke patients who were continuously monitored were presented.

Methods.—The ICP monitoring was performed on 48 patients (19 women) aged 17 to 68 years with acute middle cerebral artery stroke and evidence of acute, large hemispheric infarction. Monitoring devices included ICT/B Titan (n = 9), Spiegelberg pneumatic transducer (n = 34), and Epidyn Braun (n = 5). Epidural probes were placed ipsilaterally to the site of injury in all patients and also contralaterally in 7 patients. Patients were assessed at baseline using the Scandinavian Stroke Scale (SSS) and the Glasgow Coma Scale and after 4 weeks with the SSS and the Rankin Scale (RS). Activities of daily living were scored on the Barthel Index (BI). Computed tomography was performed at baseline and at least twice more during the hospitalization. Increased ICP was treated by osmotherapy, hyperventilation, THAM buffer, and barbiturates.

Results.—Only 9 patients survived. Of the 39 who died, 36 died after transtentorial herniation leading to brain death, including 1 who experienced severe epidural bleeding after removal of the monitoring probe. In the surviving patients, the SSS score had increased from 20.6 at baseline to 28.3 at 4 weeks and declined in nonsurvivors to 19.8; mean BI and RS scores for survivors at 4 weeks were 65 and 3, respectively.

Conclusion.—Medical interventions were ineffective in most patients. Whereas ICP monitoring was prognostic for patients with large hemispheric infarctions, it had no effect on outcome.

▶ I selected this article because this is a very common neurointensive care problem, and this is a well-reported series from an authoritative group, giving both the pros and the cons of ICP monitoring.

M.D. Ginsberg, M.D.

Adverse Effects of Pentobarbital on Cerebral Venous Oxygenation of Comatose Patients With Acute Traumatic Brain Swelling: Relationship to Outcome

Cruz J (Allegheny Univ of the Health Sciences, Philadelphia)
J Neurosurg 85:758–761, 1996   3–2

Background.—Pentobarbital sodium has been advocated as an alternative in the treatment of refractory intracranial hypertension. However, in previous studies, cerebral hemodynamic assessment, metabolic assessment, or both were not done.

Methods and Findings.—One hundred fifty-one comatose patients with acute traumatic brain swelling received pentobarbital sodium for the treatment of refractory intracranial hypertension. Global cerebrovenous oxygenation was assessed before and after IV administration. In 1 group of patients, the jugular oxyhemoglobin saturation (SjO_2) remained at or exceeded 45% after pentobarbital bolus, and in another group, the SjO_2 declined to less than 45%. These 2 groups were matched by predominant findings on CT scans of the head and by age, postresuscitation Glasgow Coma Scale scores, levels of total Hb content, SjO_2 intracranial pressure, and cerebral perfusion pressure before pentobarbital bolus. Patients with SjO_2 decreases to less than 45% had significantly worse outcomes than those whose SjO_2 was 45% or more, even though the 2 groups did not differ significantly in intracranial pressure and cerebral perfusion pressure after an IV bolus of pentobarbital.

Conclusions.—This is the first study to delineate 2 distinct patterns of cerebral venous oxygenation in response to pentobarbital injections in patients matched for several other parameters. This also is the first documentation of significant adverse effects of pentobarbital on cerebral venous oxygenation in patients with acute diffuse traumatic brain swelling.

▶ This provocative report in a large series of comatose patients with severe head–injuries with marked elevations of intracranial pressure (mean, 40–42 mm Hg), documents 2 types of responses to bolus pentobarbital therapy administered as part of a protocol to reduce intracranial pressure. Despite equivalent reductions of intracranial pressure in both groups (to mean values of 25–26 mm Hg), 1 group showed improved jugular bulb oxyhemoglobin saturation; the other group showed a deterioration. In the latter group,

Glasgow Coma Scale score failed to improve at 2 weeks, and only 31% of patients showed good long-term recovery or moderate disability; the former group showed marked improvement in coma score and a 70% incidence of good recovery or moderate disability. This remarkable result underscores the great importance of jugular venous oxygen saturation monitoring in patients with severe head injuries and emphasizes that pentobarbital therapy should not be used in the absence of such monitoring.

M.D. Ginsberg, M.D.

Body Temperature in Acute Stroke: Relation to Stroke Severity, Infarct Size, Mortality, and Outcome

Reith J, Jørgensen HS, Pedersen PM, et al (Bispebjerg Hosp, Copenhagen)
Lancet 347:422–425, 1996   3–3

Background.—Animal studies have demonstrated a strong correlation between body temperature and outcome after focal or global cerebral ischemia. The significance of body temperature in association with mortality and functional outcome was examined in a prospective clinical study.

Methods.—During a 2-year period, 390 consecutive patients admitted 6 hours or less after a stroke were studied. Body temperature was recorded on admission. The patients were evaluated with the Scandinavian Stroke Scale, which assesses neurologic deficits at admission, the next day, weekly during the hospital stay, and at discharge. The size of the infarct was

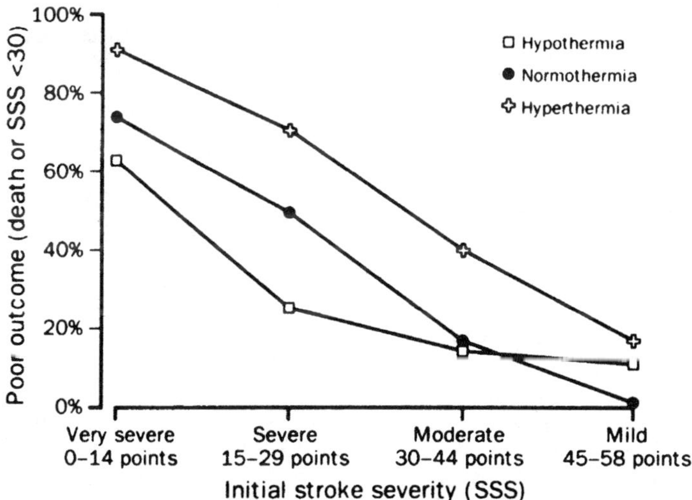

FIGURE.—Poor outcome as a function of initial stroke severity for patients with different body temperatures on admission. In the hypothermic group, initial stroke severity was very severe in 12 patients, severe in 7, moderate in 7, and mild in 18. Corresponding figures for the normothermia group were 33, 37, 73, and 106; for the hyperthermia group, the figures were 49, 20, 15, and 13. (Courtesy of Reith J, Jørgensen HS, Pedersen PM, et al: Body temperature in acute stroke: Relation to stroke severity, infarct size, mortality, and outcome. *Lancet* 347:422–425, copyright by The Lancet Ltd., 1996.)

determined with CT scanning. Multivariate linear and logistic analyses were performed to determine the significant predictors of initial stroke severity, infarct size, mortality, and neurologic outcome. The significance of body temperature was analyzed along with confounding and predictive factors: age, gender, stroke severity at admission, diabetes, atrial fibrillation, smoking, hypertension, ischemic heart disease, previous stroke, infections, leucocytosis, and comorbidity.

Results.—Body temperature had a significant, independent association with initial stroke severity, infarct size, mortality, and functional outcome. An increase of 1°C in body temperature was associated with an increase of 4 points in the Scandinavian Stroke Scale score at admission and at discharge, of 15 mm in infarct size, and of 80% in mortality (Fig).

Conclusions.—The associations between body temperature and initial stroke severity, infarct size, and outcome support experimental evidence of neuronal death caused by increased temperatures at and after the onset of stroke. Further study is needed to confirm a causal relationship, but these findings suggest that reducing body temperature could improve the outcome in stroke patients.

▶ Abundant animal data have shown that hypothermia confers neuroprotection in acute stroke, but the translation to the clinic has been slow. This article is remarkable for providing data that body temperature is related to initial stroke severity, infarct size, mortality, and outcome with a high degree of statistical significance. Articles such as this might provide the basis for a controlled study of hypothermia in stroke. This important article should be brought to the reader's attention.

M.D. Ginsberg, M.D.

Guidelines for Thrombolytic Therapy for Acute Stroke: A Supplement to the Guidelines for the Management of Patients With Acute Ischemic Stroke: A Statement for Healthcare Professionals From a Special Writing Group of the Stroke Council, American Heart Association
Adams HP Jr, Brott TG, Furlan AJ, et al (American Heart Assoc, Dallas)
Circulation 94:1167–1174, 1996
3–4

Introduction.—A panel of the American Heart Association wrote guidelines for the management of acute ischemic stroke in 1994. At that time, the panel predicted that its recommendations would change as results of ongoing clinical trials became available. The panel recommended that thrombolytic drugs not be administered to patients with acute ischemic stroke outside the clinical trial setting. Since the guidelines were published, results of clinical trials investigating the use of IV thrombolytic drugs have been reported and were described.

Studies of Intra-arterial Thrombolysis.—Intra-arterial thrombolysis can re-open arterial occlusions, but results vary. The rates of recanalization are lower for occlusions of the internal carotid artery or basilar artery than for occlusions of branches of the middle cerebral artery. There is no evidence that intra-arterial thrombolysis is superior or inferior to IV thrombolysis, that 1 thrombolytic drug is superior to another, or that the risk of hemorrhage is less with either intra-arterial or IV thrombolysis. It may be that concomitant administration of heparin influences the efficacy of intra-arterial thrombolysis, but this may increase the risk of bleeding. For now, further testing of intra-arterial thrombolysis should be considered investigational only and should be limited to the clinical trial setting. Only physicians who are experienced in neurointerventional techniques should perform intra-arterial thrombolysis in centers with neurologic expertise.

Management of Acute Ischemic Stroke Using Intravenous Thrombolysis.—Three trials of streptokinase were halted by safety committees because of high rates of acute mortality and intracranial bleeding: the Multicenter Acute Stroke Trial—Europe, the Australian Streptokinase Trial, and the Multicenter Acute Stroke Trial—Italy (Fig 1). The European Cooperative Acute Stroke Study reported inconclusive data about treatment with IV tissue plasminogen activator (r-TPA) (Fig 2). The National Institute of Neurological Disorders and Stroke r-TPA Stroke Study (NINDS study) showed improved stroke outcome after IV r-TPA (administered in a dose of 0.9 mg/kg up to a maximum of 90 mg—10% of the dose was administered in a bolus and the remainder was infused over a 1-hour period) within 3 hours of the onset of ischemic stroke.

Recommendations.—Intravenous r-TPA may be administered as described in the NINDS study for treatment within 3 hours of ischemic stroke and should be used with caution in patients with severe stroke. Its use beyond 3 hours of onset is not established, nor is it recommended when the time of stroke cannot be reliably ascertained. Intravenous streptokinase is not recommended outside the clinical investigation setting and is not recommended unless the diagnosis is established by a physician with expertise in the diagnosis of stroke and the brain CT scan is assessed by a physician expert in reading such scans. Thrombolytic therapy should not be administered to patients for any of the 13 reasons participants were excluded from the NINDS study. Without emergent ancillary care and the facilities to handle bleeding complications, thrombolytic therapy should not be administered. The risk of major bleeding should be discussed with the patient and family before treatment is initiated. The safety and efficacy of the use of r-TPA have not been established in neonates, infants, and children with acute ischemic stroke. With the understanding that a risk-benefit relationship has not been established, if r-TPA is given to a pediatric patient, the same guidelines should be followed as for adult patients. Neonates and infants should be treated only in exceptional circumstances because of the risk involved. It is recommended that patients who are taking warfarin or heparin or have prolongation of baseline clotting factors not be given r-PTA for the treatment of acute ischemic stroke. The use of aspirin before r-PTA does not exclude a patient from treatment. Patients who receive IV r-PTA should not be given aspirin, heparin, warfarin, ticlopidine, or other antithrombotic or antiplatelet aggregating drugs until 24 hours after treatment.

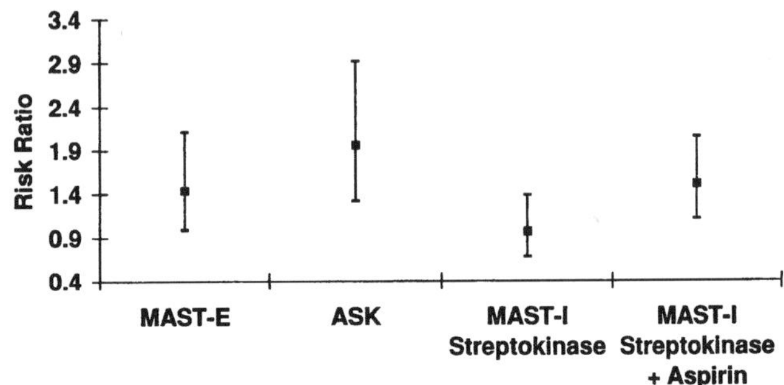

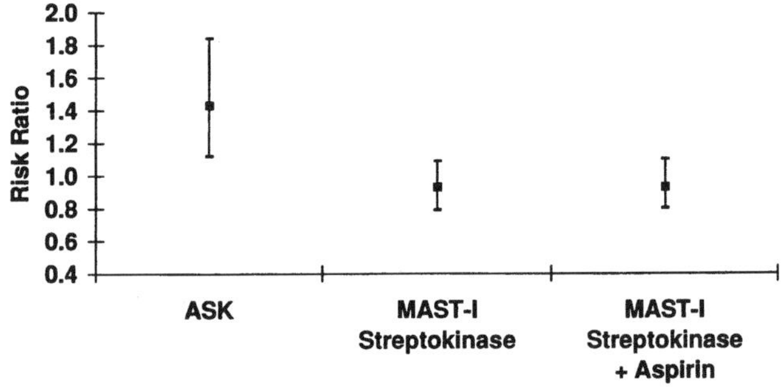

FIGURE 1.—Risk ratios for long-term mortality and death and disability among individuals given streptokinase for the treatment of acute ischemic stroke in the Multicenter Acute Stroke Trial—Europe (*MAST-E*), Australian Streptokinase Trial (*ASK*), and the Multicenter Acute Stroke Trial—Italy (*MAST-I*). Included are 95% confidence intervals. A risk ratio of less than 1.0 favors treatment with streptokinase. (Courtesy of Adams HP Jr, Brott TG, Furlan AJ, et al: Guidelines for thrombolytic therapy for acute stroke: A supplement to the guidelines for the management of patients with acute ischemic stroke: A Statement for Healthcare Professionals From a Special Writing Group of the Stroke Council, American Heart Association. *Circulation* 1996; 94:1167–1174. Reproduced with permission of *Circulation*, Copyright 1996, American Heart Association.)

Conclusion.—Reported are the results of trials investigating the use of thrombolytic therapy in the treatment of acute ischemic stroke. The guidelines presented are meant for neurologists, emergency physicians, primary care physicians, neurosurgeons, and vascular surgeons managing the treatment of patients seen within the first few hours after stroke.

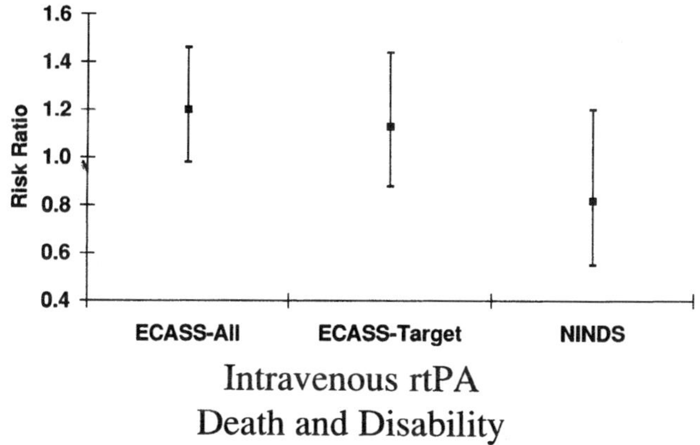

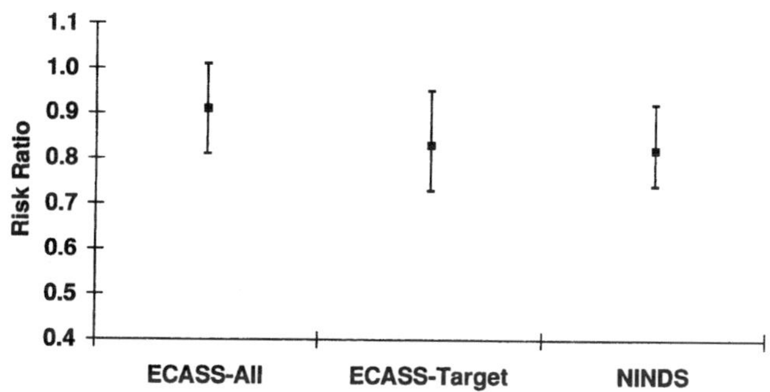

FIGURE 2.—Risk ratios for 30-day mortality and disability among individuals given IV recombinant tissue plasminogen activator (*rtPA*) for the treatment of acute ischemic stroke in the European Cooperative Acute Stroke Study (*ECASS*) and the National Institute of Neurological Disorders and Stroke study of r-TPA (*NINDS*). The ECASS study includes data collected from all randomly assigned patients (*All*) and the desired treatment group (*Target*). Included are 95% confidence intervals. A risk ratio of less than 1.0 favors treatment with rtPA. (Courtesy of Adams HP Jr, Brott TG, Furlan AJ, et al: Guidelines for thrombolytic therapy for acute stroke: A supplement to the guidelines for the management of patients with acute ischemic stroke: A Statement for Healthcare Professionals From a Special Writing Group of the Stroke Council, American Heart Association. *Circulation* 1996; 94:1167–1174. Reproduced with permission of *Circulation*, Copyright 1996, American Heart Association.)

▶ I chose this article because is is an absolutely vital up-to-date summary of a number of therapeutic trials and it gives the clinician-practitioner clear-cut guidelines as to how thrombolytics should be applied for stroke treatment. It is essential reading.

M.D. Ginsberg, M.D.

Practice Advisory: Thrombolytic Therapy for Acute Ischemic Stroke—Summary Statement

Report of the Quality Standards Subcommittee of the American Academy of Neurology (Minneapolis)

Neurology 47:835–839, 1996

3–5

Purpose.—In 1996, recombinant tissue plasminogen activator (rtPA) was approved for use in the treatment of acute ischemic stroke. The enthusiastic response to this treatment must be tempered by consideration of the possible adverse effects. The Quality Standards Subcommittee of the American Academy of Neurology offers research-based recommendations regarding thrombolytic therapy for acute ischemic stroke.

Recommendations.—The panel's recommendations were drawn mainly from 3 clinical trials of IV streptokinase for acute ischemic stroke and 2 trials of IV rtPA (Table 2). The data support the use of IV rtPA for administration within 3 hours of the onset of ischemic stroke. The recommended dosage is 0.9 mg of rtPA per kilogram, to a maximum of 90 mg, with 10% given as a bolus and the rest given by infusion over 90 minutes. The use of rtPA for stroke after 3 hours cannot be recommended. There are insufficient data to recommend IV streptokinase, outside of research settings. The diagnosis of stroke should be established by a physician with expertise in that area, with a supporting brain CT scan. Exclusion criteria for thrombolytic therapy must be observed, including anticoagulation. Thrombolysis should not be attempted unless the facilities to treat bleeding

TABLE 2.—Results of Recent Clinical Trials of IV rtPA in Treatment of Individuals With Acute Ischemic Stroke

	ECASS Intention-to-Treat (%)	ECASS Target Population (%)	NINDS (%)
30-day mortality			
rtPA	17.9	14.6	12.9
control	12.7	11.7	15.8
Symptomatic or parenchymal hemorrhage			
rtPA	19.8†	19.4†	6.4†
control	6.5	6.8	0.3
90-day mortality			
rtPA	22.4	19.4	17.4
control	15.8	14.8	20.6
90-day death and disability*			
rtPA	64.3	59.1‡	61†
control	70.7	70.8	74

*Disability as measured by Rankin Scale. In the NINDS Study, the Rankin Scale of 2 or greater (on a scale of 0 = normal to 6 = dead) was considered as disabled. In the ECASS Study, the Rankin Scale of 3 or greater was considered as disabled.

†*P* value = < 0.001 (Mantel-Haenszel test).

‡*P* value = 0.035 (Wilcoxon test).

Abbreviations: ECASS, European Cooperative Acute Stroke Study; NINDS, National Institute of Neurological Diseases and Stroke Acute Stroke Study.

(From The Quality Standards Subcommittee of the American Academy of Neurology: Practice advisory: Thrombolytic therapy for acute ischemic stroke—Summary Statement. *Neurology* 47:835–839, 1996. Courtesy of Adams HP, Brott T, Furlan A, et al: A supplement to the guidelines for the management of patients with acute ischemic stroke: Use of thrombolytic drugs. *Stroke,* in press. Reprinted from *Neurology* by permission of Little, Brown and Company Inc.)

complications are available, and the patient and the family must be apprised of the real risk of such complications.

Management of bleeding complications depends on several factors, including the location and size of the hematoma, the possibility of controlling the bleeding mechanically, and the risk that the patient will die or have neurologic deterioration. If the patient's neurologic condition does get worse, bleeding should be considered the likely cause until a CT scan is available. In case of life-threatening bleeding complications, stop the infusion of thrombolytic drug, take blood samples for coagulation testing, and obtain surgical consultation. Patients who have taken aspirin are candidates for rtPA treatment. Those taking warfarin or heparin or with prolonged clotting factors at baseline should not receive rtPA. There are insufficient data on the use of rtPA in patients taking antiplatelet drugs. Patients who have received rtPA should not take any of these drugs. The Panel recommends the ancillary management practices used in the National Institute of Neurological Diseases and Stroke Acute Stroke Study. There are no data on the use of thrombolytic therapy in pediatric age groups.

Discussion.—Although there are recommendations for thrombolytic therapy in the treatment of acute stroke, more research is needed to define the patient selection criteria, method of administration, and window of opportunity for effective treatment. The benefits of thrombolysis in lacunar stroke and larger infarcts must be re-evaluated as experience grows.

▶ Because of the rapidly accruing body of scientific literature concerning the use of thrombolytic agents in patients with acute ischemic stroke, there is an important need for summary statements critically reviewing the state of the art. This is the case with the present article, whose great utility is in summarizing the results of the European Cooperative Acute Stroke Study, known as ECASS, and the Stroke Study National Institute of Neurological Diseases and Stroke Acute/—the latter being the definitive therapeutic trial culminating in the clinical availability of tissue plasminogen activator for stroke. The report also summarizes the 3 recent clinical trials of IV streptokinase, calling attention to the excess in symptomatic hemorrhage and long-term mortality associated with that treatment. This report includes a highly useful table summarizing the emergency management of arterial hypertension in patients receiving thrombolytic therapy. This summary article is highly recommended to practicing clinicians.

M.D. Ginsberg, M.D.

Tissue Plasminogen Activator for Acute Ischemic Stroke
The National Institute of Neurological Disorders and Stroke rt-PA Stroke Study Group (Natl Inst of Neurological Disorders and Stroke, Bethesda, Md)
N Engl J Med 333:1581–1587, 1995   3–6

Background.—Initial trials of thrombolytic therapy for patients who had acute ischemic stroke were associated with high rates of intracerebral hemorrhage. These results prompted careful evaluation of the risks and benefits of recombinant human tissue plasminogen activator (t-PA) for cerebral arterial thrombolysis. Recent results have suggested that t-PA treatment is beneficial when given within 3 hours after the onset of stroke. The benefits of IV t-PA for patients with ischemic stroke were evaluated in a 2-part, randomized trial.

Methods.—The first part of the trial, which included 291 patients, sought to determine whether t-PA had clinical activity in patients with ischemic stroke. This outcome was defined as a 4-point improvement over baseline in the National Institutes of Health stroke scale (NIHSS) score, or by resolution of the neurologic deficit within 24 hours after onset of stroke. The second part of the study, which involved 333 patients, was designed to determine whether t-PA treatment had sustained clinical benefit at 3 months. The results were assessed by 4 outcome measures that addressed differing aspects of stroke recovery: the Barthel index, modified Rankin scale, Glasgow Coma Scale, and NIHSS. The results of the 2 parts were pooled and stratified to gain a complete picture of the effectiveness of t-PA.

Results.—In the first part of the study, the t-PA and placebo groups were not significantly different in the percentage of patients with neurologic improvement at 24 hours after onset of stroke. In the second part, however, patients who received t-PA had significant improvement on all 4 measures. The results of part 1 predicted long-term clinical benefit in part

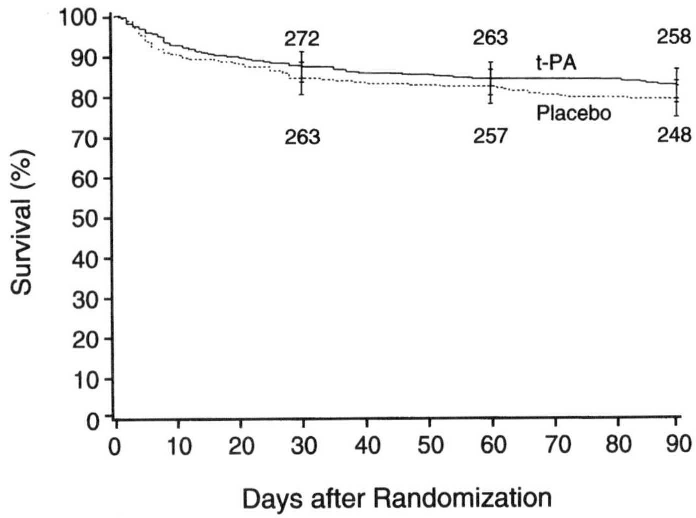

FIGURE 1.—Mean (±SE) survival at 3 months according to treatment. The combined results of parts 1 and 2 are shown. There were 312 patients in each group, and no patient had missing data on mortality. *Error bars* represent the standard errors of the point estimates of survival at 30, 60, and 90 days. The number of patients who survived at each interval is shown. (Courtesy of The National Institute of Neurological Disorders and Stroke rt-PA Stroke Study Group: Tissue plasminogen activator for acute ischemic stroke. *N Engl J Med* 333:1581–1587, 1995. Reprinted with permission of *The New England Journal of Medicine*, copyright 1995, Massachusetts Medical Society.)

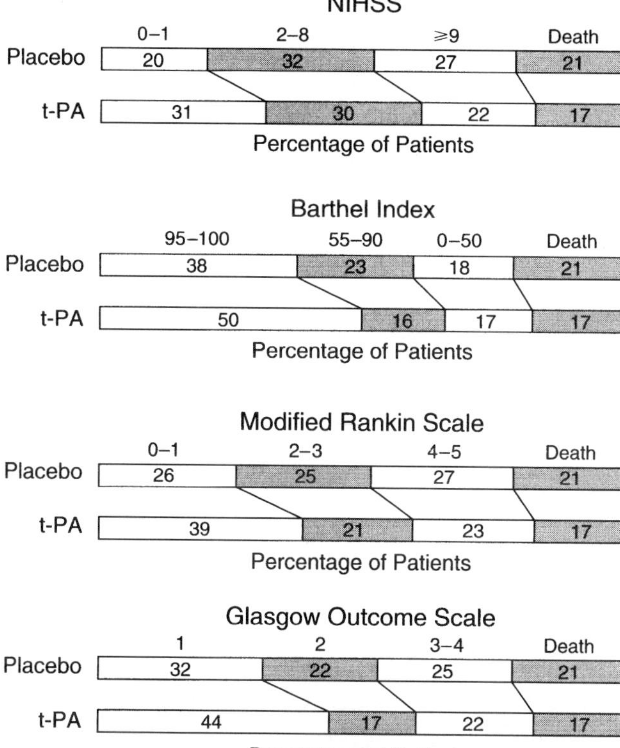

FIGURE 2.—Outcome at 3 months in part 2 of the study, according to treatment. Scores of 1 or less on the NIHSS, 95 or 100 on the Barthel index, 1 or less on the modified Rankin scale, and 1 on the Glasgow outcome scale were considered to indicate a favorable outcome. Values do not total 100% because of rounding. (Courtesy of The National Institute of Neurological Disorders and Stroke rt-PA Stroke Study Group: Tissue plasminogen activator for acute ischemic stroke. *N Engl J Med* 333:1581–1587, 1995. Reprinted with permission of *The New England Journal of Medicine*, copyright 1995, Massachusetts Medical Society.)

2, with a 1.7 global odds ratio for a favorable outcome. Patients in the t-PA group were 30% or more likely to be left with minimal or no disability at 3 months' follow-up (Figs 1 and 2). Six percent of patients in the t-PA group had symptomatic intracerebral hemorrhage within 36 hours after onset of stroke, compared with 0.6% of the placebo group (See Table 6). Three-month mortality rate was 17% and 21%, respectively.

Conclusions.—For patients who have acute ischemic stroke, giving IV t-PA within 3 hours after the onset of stroke appears to produce significantly better 3-month clinical outcomes than placebo. This benefit holds even though t-PA treatment carries a higher risk of symptomatic intracerebral hemorrhage. Outcomes are better with t-PA than with placebo, regardless of the type of stroke diagnosed at baseline.

TABLE 6.—Incidence of Intracranial Hemorrhage Within 36 Hours of Treatment for Stroke

Type of Intracranial Hemorrhage	t-PA	Placebo
	no. (%)	
Part 1	144	147
Symptomatic	8 (6)	0
Fatal*	4	0
Nonfatal	4	0
Asymptomatic	5 (3)	3 (2)
Part 2	168	165
Symptomatic	12 (7)	2 (1)
Fatal*	5	1
Nonfatal	7	1
Asymptomatic	9 (5)	6 (4)

*Values include all deaths attributed to hemorrhage.

(Courtesy of The National Institute of Neurological Disorders and Stroke rt-PA Stroke Study Group: Tissue plasminogen activator for acute ischemic stroke. *N Engl J Med* 333:1581–1587, 1995. Reprinted with permission of *The New England Journal of Medicine*, copyright 1995, Massachusetts Medical Society.)

▶ This study is the most important randomized control study of thrombolysis for acute ischemic stroke yet reported. The unique (and extremely crucial) aspect of the experimental design was the entry of patients within 3 hours of onset of stroke. The results are robust: Four different outcome measures were used, ranging from a crude global outcome score (the Glasgow) to an index of functional recovery (Barthel) to a detailed neurologic scale (NIHSS). On each of these measures, the percentage of patients in the best outcome category increased by 12–13 absolute percentage points. Although one may be disappointed by this modest improvement in outcome, its consistency across rating scales and its degree of statistical significance give great encouragement. In addition, patients who had either small-vessel or large-vessel occlusive disease, as well as those who had cardioembolic stroke, appeared to be equally improved. Notably, although symptomatic intracerebral hemorrhage soon after stroke onset occurred at 10 times the rate in treated patients, the mortality rate at 3 months was not affected by this phenomenon (nor was the quality of outcome), which suggests that this is a clinically tolerable degree of hemorrhagic transformation in this setting. Of great importance is the dose of t-PA used and the fact that patients with undue hypertension were excluded. The positive outcome of this study thus probably hinges on crucial variables: the early time to treatment, the moderate dose of t-PA used, and the avoidance of severely hypertensive patients. The design of this trial differs importantly from the ECASS Study, in which most patients were accrued 4–6 hours after onset of stroke and a significant degree of improvement was noted only in a "target-population" subset defined on the basis of CT criteria. The present NIH trial stands as a landmark.

M.D. Ginsberg, M.D.

Thrombolytic Therapy With Streptokinase in Acute Ischemic Stroke
Hommel M, for the Multicenter Acute Stroke Trial—Europe Study Group
(Centre Hospitalier de Grenoble, France)
N Engl J Med 335:145–150, 1996   3–7

Purpose.—Early thrombolytic therapy is believed to permit reperfusion of ischemic neurons and to enhance functional recovery in patients with acute ischemic stroke. At the same time, there is the possibility of thrombolysis-associated cerebral bleeding and reperfusion-associated injury. The efficacy and safety of thrombolysis with streptokinase for acute ischemic stroke were evaluated in a multicenter, double-blind, randomized controlled trial.

Methods.—The Multicenter Acute Stroke Trial—Europe included 310 patients at 48 French and British centers. All had moderate to severe acute ischemic stroke in the middle cerebral artery territory. Within 6 hours after the onset of stroke, the patients were treated with streptokinase, 1.5 million U over 1 hour, or placebo. Efficacy was evaluated by a binary criterion that comprised mortality and severe disability at 6 months. (A Rankin scale score of 3 or greater was considered to denote severe disability.) Safety was evaluated in terms of mortality at 10 days and cerebral hemorrhage.

Results.—Six-month evaluation showed that 79% of patients who received streptokinase and 81% of those who received placebo either had died or had severe disability. However, 10-day mortality was 34% in the streptokinase group vs. 18% in the placebo group. The excess deaths with streptokinase resulted from hemorrhagic transformation of ischemic cerebral infarcts. Forty-seven percent of the streptokinase-treated patients were dead at 6 months, compared with 38% of the placebo group. Recruitment for the trial was halted by the Data Monitoring Committee.

Conclusions.—Thrombolytic therapy with streptokinase increases mortality in patients with acute ischemic stroke. This is consistent with the results of most other trials of thrombolytic therapy for stroke; a meta-analysis of all of these trials is underway to see if there is any patient subgroup that can benefit from treatment. Streptokinase should not be a routine treatment for acute ischemic stroke.

▶ I selected this article because it is the definitive report of a randomized trial of thrombolysis with streptokinase for acute ischemic stroke. The important finding is that this study resulted in **increased** mortality, largely due to hemorrhage transformation of the infarct, in the treated patients. It represents the death knell for streptokinase, and certainly deserves notice.

M.D. Ginsberg, M.D.

Streptokinase for Acute Ischemic Stroke With Relationship to Time of Administration

Donnan GA, for the Australian Streptokinase (ASK) Trial Study Group (Austin and Repatriation Med Centre, Heidelberg, Australia; Royal Melbourne Hosp, Australia; Geelong Hosp, Australia; et al)
JAMA 276:961–966, 1996

3–8

Background.—Thrombolytic therapy has given promising results in the treatment of acute ischemic stroke. So far, the best results are achieved with tissue-type plasminogen activator, particularly when given within 3 hours after the onset of the stroke. Streptokinase is a less expensive agent that effectively reduces mortality after myocardial infarction. The effects of IV streptokinase on the morbidity and mortality of acute ischemic stroke were studied, including an analysis of the impact of time to administration.

Methods.—The randomized, double-blind, placebo-controlled study included 340 adult patients with moderate to severe strokes. The patients were treated at 40 centers across Australia. The patients were assigned to receive IV streptokinase, 1.5 million U, or placebo in 100 mL of normal saline infused over 1 hour. Morbidity and mortality were assessed at 3 months' follow-up. The effects of treatment were analyzed by intention-to-treat analysis, with a combined death and disability score as the primary end point. The effects of treatment before vs. after 3 hours of stroke onset were analyzed.

Results.—The risk of unfavorable outcomes was slightly but nonsignificantly increased in the streptokinase group (relative risk [RR], 1.08). Hematomas occurred in 13% of the streptokinase group vs. 3% in the placebo group. Patients treated more than 3 hours after the onset of stroke were more likely to have unfavorable outcomes (RR, 1.22). For patients treated with streptokinase within 3 hours, outcomes were significantly better; the RR of unfavorable outcome in this group was 0.66. For patients treated with streptokinase after 3 hours, the risk of death was significantly elevated (RR, 1.98).

Conclusions.—In patients with acute ischemic stroke, IV streptokinase treatment more than 3 hours after the onset of stroke may increase 3-month morbidity and mortality. The outcomes are significantly better when streptokinase is given within 3 hours but no better than with placebo. Early initiation of thrombolytic therapy appears to have a critical impact on the chances of treatment success.

▶ This important and timely trial assessed the possible efficacy of streptokinase administered IV within 4 hours of acute ischemic stroke. Unfortunately, streptokinase therapy was associated with a trend toward unfavorable outcome, particularly in those patients receiving the drug more than 3 hours after stroke onset. In contrast to tissue plasminogen activator, which has now been shown to confer significant benefit on patients receiving thrombolytic therapy within 3 hours of stroke onset, streptokinase, even when given within that time frame, showed no significant benefit over placebo.

This study further emphasizes the importance of timing of thrombolytic therapy, but in addition calls attention to important differences in efficacy among thrombolytic agents. Because of the excess of intracranial hematomas and deaths in the streptokinase group, this drug can no longer be included in the possible armentarium for acute stroke therapy.

M.D. Ginsberg, M.D.

Low-Molecular-Weight Heparin for the Treatment of Acute Ischemic Stroke

Kay R, Wong KS, Yu YL, et al (Prince of Wales Hosp, Hong Kong; Queen Mary Hosp,Hong Kong; Kwong Wah Hosp, Hong Kong)
N Engl J Med 333:1588–1593, 1995   3–9

Background.—Although the safety and efficacy of antithrombotic agents have been questioned, these agents are frequently used in patients who have acute ischemic stroke. Low–molecular weight heparin, which can be given only once or twice a day subcutaneously, may be more effective and safer than standard, unfractionated heparin.

Methods.—Three hundred twelve patients with ischemic stroke were included in a double-blind, placebo-controlled comparison of 2 dosages of low–molecular weight heparin and placebo. Within 48 hours of onset of symptoms, patients were randomly assigned to receive high-dose nadroparin, low-dose nadroparin, or placebo treatments subcutaneously. Treatment duration was 10 days. The main outcome measure was death or dependence in activities of daily living 6 months after treatment initiation.

Findings.—Data on 306 patients were evaluable at 6 months. Death or dependence at 6 months was documented in 45% of patients given high-dose nadroparin, 52% given low-dose nadroparin, and 65% given placebo (Fig 1). A significant dose-dependent effect was noted in favor of active treatment.

Conclusions.—Low–molecular weight heparin improved 6-month outcomes in this series of patients with ischemic stroke when begun within 48 hours of symptom onset. Additional research is needed to establish optimal dosage and treatment duration.

▶ This carefully conducted, placebo-controlled, double-blind study assessed the efficacy of low–molecular weight heparin in patients with ischemic stroke who were randomly assigned to treatment within 48 hours of symptom onset. Results were evaluated with an activities-of-daily-living outcome measure at 6 months. Patients with CT evidence of hemorrhage, transient ischemic attack; or hypertension were excluded. Early death and complication rates were similar across treatment and placebo groups. Of note is that the treatment was safe, even at the highest dose, as there was no difference among groups in rates of hemorrhagic transformation of the

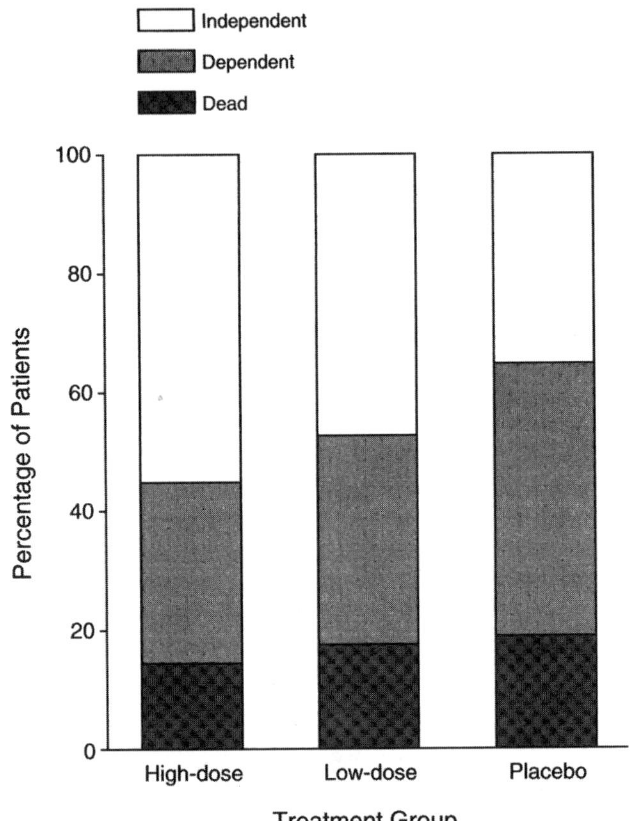

FIGURE 1.—Outcomes of patients in each treatment group 6 months after randomization. There was a significant dose-dependent reduction in the risk of death or dependency at 6 months among the patients treated with low–molecular weight heparin (chi square for trend, 8.066; $P = 0.005$.) (Courtesy of Kay R, Wong KS, Yu YL, et al: Low-molecular-weight heparin for the treatment of acute ischemic stroke. *N Engl J Med* 333:1588–1593, 1995. Reprinted with permission of *The New England Journal of Medicine*, copyright 1995, Massachusetts Medical Society.)

infarct or other complications. The authors suggest that, for every 5 patients treated at the dose of 4,100 antifactor Xa IU twice daily for 10 days, 1 death and 1 case of dependency may be avoided. The benefit-to-risk ratio of this treatment, therefore, would appear to commend itself for more widespread clinical application.

M.D. Ginsberg, M.D.

Implementation of an Acute Stroke Program Decreases Hospitalization Costs and Length of Stay
Wentworth DA, Atkinson RP (Mercy Gen Hosp, Sacramento, Calif)
Stroke 27:1040–1043, 1996   3–10

Background.—Disability after stroke results in enormous social and financial costs. In the first 90 days after ischemic stroke, initial hospitalization and doctor fees amount to a significant proportion (57%) of the total cost of health care. An acute stroke program was instituted at a large community hospital with the goals of monitoring care, improving its quality, and decreasing initial hospital time through management of patients in a consistent, systematic, and efficient manner.

Methods.—Standing orders for acute stroke were developed, with a critical path determined by these orders and the expected length of stay. Rehabilitation was begun early in the hospital stay by a multidisciplinary team that also monitored patient progress and length of stay and provided discharge placement. Data were collected through retrospective chart review over a 4-year period.

Results.—The initial length of hospital stay for 414 Medicare patients declined steadily from 7.0 to 4.6 days over the 4-year period. The total hospital charges decreased from $14,076 to $10,740 per patient for a total savings of $453,000 per year. The mortality rate in the last 6 months of the study (1994) was 4.6%. The patients were discharged to nursing homes (32.6%), acute rehabilitation centers (16.9%), and their own homes (46.5%).

Discussion.—Implementation of the stroke program allowed for decreased length of stay for Medicare acute stroke patients and financial savings for the hospital. The outcome 3–6 months after discharge must now be studied to determine the level of function, type of placement, and patient satisfaction with the hospital care received.

▶ Although this is a retrospective chart review, the findings should evoke animated discussion on the part of those who favor acute stroke programs. The reduction in length of stay and in hospital charges is impressive.

M.D. Ginsberg, M.D.

European Stroke Prevention Study 2: Dipyridamole and Acetylsalicylic Acid in the Secondary Prevention of Stroke
Diener HC, Cunha L, Forbes C, et al (Univ of Essen, Germany; Hospitais da Universidade de Coimbra, Portugal; Ninewells Hosp and Med School, Dundee, Scotland; et al)
J Neurol Sci 143:1–13, 1996   3–11

Background.—The European Stroke Prevention Study, first published in 1987, showed that combined treatment with dipyridamole and acetylsalicylic acid (ASA) reduced secondary stroke by 38% compared with placebo in patients with prior stroke or transient ischemic attack (TIA). This was a markedly greater reduction than achieved with ASA alone. The second European Stroke Prevention Study determined the efficacy of dipyridamole and ASA alone for preventing secondary stroke, whether combined treatment is better than each agent alone, and whether low-dose ASA (50 mg daily) eliminates the propensity to induce bleeding.

Methods.—Data were obtained from 6,602 patients. The primary endpoints were stroke, death, and the combination of stroke or death. Secondary endpoints were TIA and other vascular events. Treatment and follow-up was continued for 2 years.

Findings.—In a factorial analysis, ASA and dipyridamole alone significantly reduced the risk of stroke and stroke or death combined. Compared with placebo, stroke risk was reduced by 18% with ASA alone, 16% with dipyridamole alone, and 37% with combined treatment. The risk of stroke

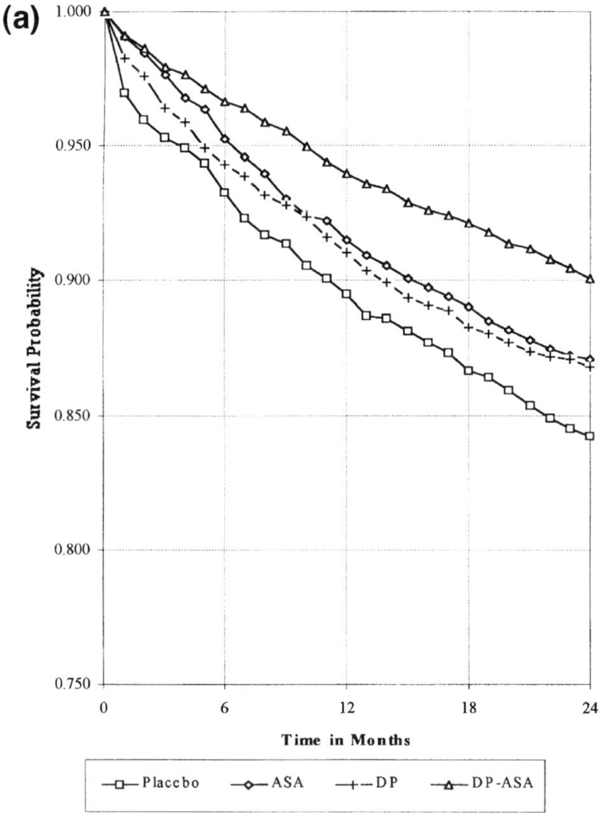

(*Continued*)

FIGURE 1 (cont.)

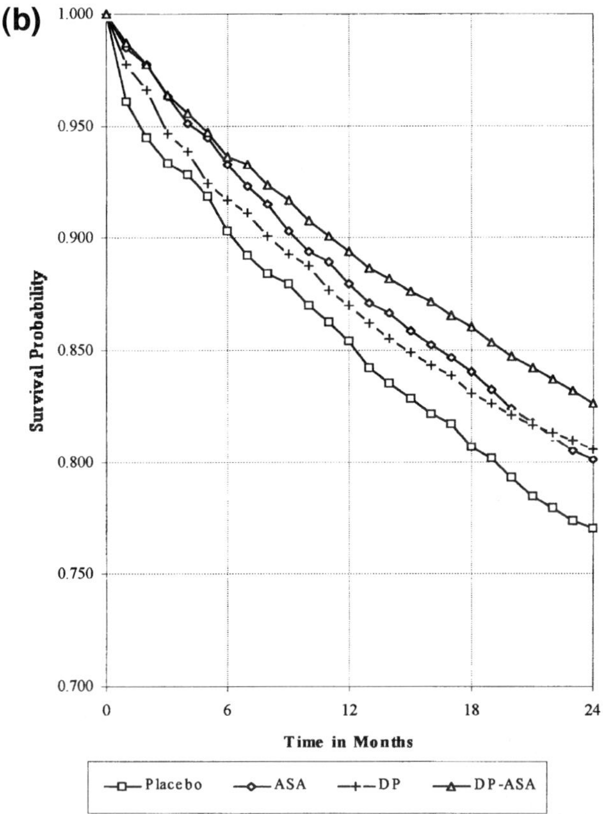

FIGURE 1.—End point–free survival curves for the end points (A) stroke, and (B) stroke or death in patients with prior stroke or transient ischemic attack treated with acetylsalicylic acid (*ASA*), dipyridamole (*DP*), the 2 combined (*DP-ASA*), or placebo. (Courtesy of Diener HC, Cunha L, Forbes C, et al: European stroke prevention study 2: Dipyridamole and acetylsalicylic acid in the secondary prevention of stroke. *J Neurol Sci* 143:1–13, 1996.)

or death was decreased by 13%, 15%, and 24% with ASA alone, dipyridamole alone, and combined treatment, respectively. Treatment did not significantly affect death rate alone. Dipyridamole and ASA also significantly prevented TIA. Compared with placebo, combined treatment reduced the risk by 36%. The most common adverse event was headache, which occurred more often in patients receiving dipyridamole. Patients receiving ASA had significantly more common instances of all-site bleeding and GI bleeding (Fig 1).

Conclusions.—The efficacy of ASA, 25 mg twice daily, and modified-release dipyridamole, 200 mg twice daily, is equal in the secondary prevention of ischemic stroke and TIA. When prescribed together, the protective effects are additive. Combined treatment is significantly more effective than either agent alone. Low-dose ASA does not eliminate the propensity for induced bleeding.

▶ This randomized, double-blind study is important for several reasons. First, the authors have shown that low-dose ASA alone (50 mg) given to patients with prior stroke or TIA, is beneficial in reducing the risk of future stroke or combined stroke and death. This evidence that lower-dose ASA is effective in secondary stroke prevention will come as welcome news to clinicians, despite the fact that even this dose is not free of hemorrhagic complications.

Secondly, this study supports an independent beneficial effect of dipyridamole (in modified-release form)—an agent for which a beneficial effect could not be established in 2 large previous studies (including the American-Canadian Cooperative Stroke Study of 1983), possibly because of a lack of sufficient statistical power. Thirdly, the combination of the 2 agents showed a substantially greater protective effect (risk reduction for combined outcome, 36%) than the agents given singly.

The odds ratio for active treatment with the dipyridamole-ASA combination in stroke prevention was 0.59 (95% confidence interval, 0.48–0.73—an impressive degree of efficacy). The absence of statistical interaction between the 2 agents is consistent with their acting via different mechanisms (thromboxane inhibition for ASA, and raising antiplatelet levels of cyclic adenosine monophosphate and guanosine monophosphate for dipyridamole). This study is expected to have a positive impact in clinical practice.

M.D. Ginsberg, M.D.

Differential Effect of Aspirin Versus Warfarin on Clinical Stroke Types in Patients With Atrial Fibrillation
Miller VT, and the Stroke Prevention in Atrial Fibrillation Investigators (Natl Inst of Neurological Disorders and Stroke, Bethesda, Md)
Neurology 46:238–240, 1996   3–12

Background.—Aspirin has been found to have a differential effect on the prevention of certain clinical types of ischemic stroke. In the Stroke Prevention in Atrial Fibrillation I (SPAF I) study, aspirin prevented noncardioembolic (non-CE) strokes more effectively than CE strokes compared with placebo. The SPAF II study compared the efficacy and safety of aspirin with that of warfarin in patients with atrial fibrillation.

Methods.—A total of 1,100 patients with atrial fibrillation received either 325 mg of aspirin daily or warfarin adjusted to maintain the International Normalized Ratio at 2 to 4.5. Primary end points were ischemic strokes or systemic emboli.

Findings.—Sixty-three ischemic strokes occurred in 63 patients. At the time of the event, 14 were not taking a study medication, so only 49 strokes were analyzed. Warfarin was found to be significantly better than aspirin in preventing CE strokes as well as strokes of uncertain pathophysiology. The 2 agents were equally effective in preventing non-CE strokes.

Conclusions.—Patients with atrial fibrillation at particular risk for CE stroke apparently benefit most from warfarin treatment. It is hoped that the current data will increase interest in defining more reliable clinical markers of pathophysiologic stroke mechanisms and better elucidate the pharmacologic activity of antithrombotic treatments.

▶ This further analysis of the SPAF II data shows that warfarin is more effective than aspirin in the prevention of CE strokes, but apparently not different from aspirin in the prevention of non-CE strokes. It is a clinically useful summary of a large important clinical database and deserves attention.

M.D. Ginsberg, M.D.

Stroke Severity in Atrial Fibrillation: The Framingham Study
Lin H-J, Wolf PA, Kelly-Hayes M, et al (Boston Univ; Natl Heart, Lung, and Blood Inst, Framingham, Mass)
Stroke 27:1760–1764, 1996   3–13

Objective.—Individuals with atrial fibrillation (AF) are at a four- to five-fold increased risk of stroke. The clinical evidence suggests that AF-related strokes are more severe or more likely to be fatal than other strokes. However, there are few supporting data from prospective, epidemiologic studies. Follow-up data on the Framingham Study cohort were analyzed to assess the effects of AF on the severity, mortality, and disability of stroke.

Methods.—Forty-year follow-up data of 5,070 adults identified 501 initial ischemic strokes, including 103 in patients with AF. The severity of each stroke was rated as none, mild, moderate, severe, or fatal. After 1981, standardized serial assessments were done using the Barthel index at 3, 6, and 12 months after the stroke. This part of the study included 150 strokes, 30 AF-related.

Results.—The AF-associated strokes were more severe, although this difference was not significant after stratification for age. The 30-day mortality was 25% in the AF group vs. 14% in the non-AF group. The adjusted odds ratio of 30-day mortality for patients with AF-related stroke was 1.84. The serial assessments showed that patients with AF-related stroke had worse survival and were more likely to have recurrent strokes over 1 year of follow-up. The mean Barthel score in the acute period was 30 in the AF group vs. 59 in the non-AF group. The Barthel score remained significantly lower in AF patients through 12 months of follow-up.

Conclusions.—The clinical impression that AF-related ischemic strokes are more severe than non–AF-related strokes is supported by this study. Patients who had a stroke and AF are nearly twice as likely to die of their stroke. They are also more likely to have recurrent strokes and more likely to be left with severe functional deficits. The occurrence of stroke in a patient with AF may be the first manifestation of embolism. These patients need primary preventive strategies to reduce the morbidity and mortality of stroke.

▶ For decades, the Framingham Study has provided absolutely essential longitudinal information on cardiovascular disease and stroke in a cohort of over 5,000 individuals followed up for as long as 40 years. The observations here echo those of the Copenhagen Stroke Study—namely, a nearly twofold increase in mortality in stroke associated with AF, more frequent stroke recurrence, and more severe functional deficits in patients surviving stroke. This study emphasizes the importance of primary prevention of stroke in this very high-risk population.

M.D. Ginsberg, M.D.

Pregnancy and the Risk of Stroke

Kittner SJ, Stern BJ, Feeser BR, et al (Univ of Maryland, Baltimore; Emory Univ, Atlanta, Ga; Johns Hopkins Univ, Baltimore, Md; et al)
N Engl J Med 335:768–774, 1996   3–14

Introduction.—Despite the widespread belief that pregnancy is related to an increased risk of stroke, few supporting data are available. The 1 population-based study performed to date has found no such link. The risk of cerebral infarction and intracerebral hemorrhage during and in the weeks after pregnancy was assessed in a large, population-based study.

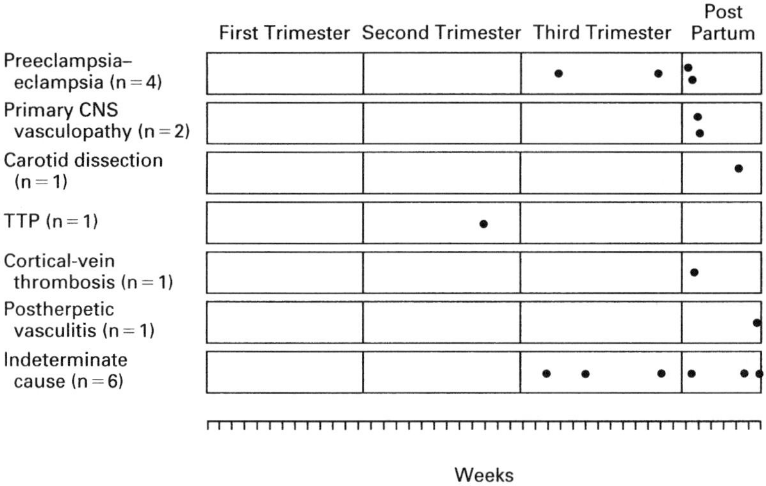

FIGURE 1.—Timing of cerebral infarction during pregnancy or after delivery, according to cause. *Abbreviations: CNS*, central nervous system; *TTP*, thrombotic thrombocytopenic purpura. One stroke that occurred after an abortion is not included. (Courtesy of Kittner SJ, Stern BJ, Feeser BR, et al: Pregnancy and the risk of stroke. *N Engl J Med* 335:768–774, 1996. Reprinted permission of *The New England Journal of Medicine*, Copyright 1996 by Massachusetts Medical Society.)

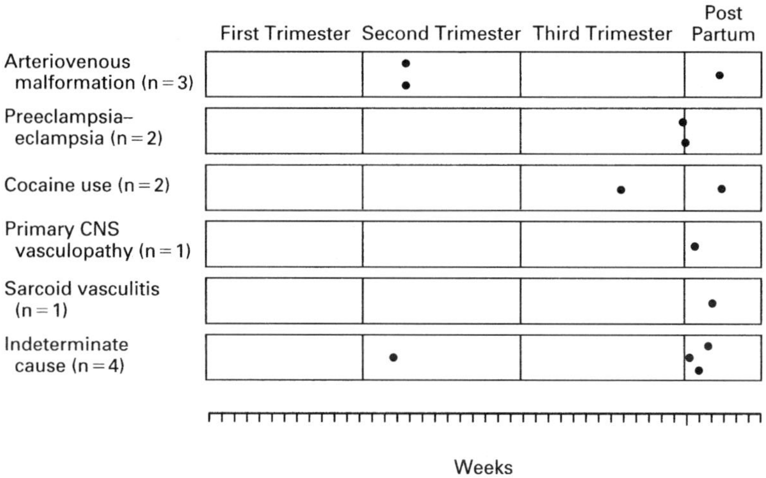

FIGURE 2.—Timing of intracerebral hemorrhage during pregnancy or after delivery, according to cause. *Abbreviations: CNS*, central nervous system; *TTP*, thrombotic thrombocytopenic purpura. (Courtesy of Kittner SJ, Stern BJ, Feeser BR, et al: Pregnancy and the risk of stroke. *N Engl J Med* 335:768–774, 1996. Reprinted permission of *The New England Journal of Medicine*, Copyright 1996 by Massachusetts Medical Society.)

Methods.—Data were drawn from The Baltimore-Washington Cooperative Young Stroke Study, a hospital-based registry designed to study the causes and incidence of stroke among young adults. The registry was used to identify all women aged 15 to 44 years in the study region with a discharge diagnosis consistent with cerebral infarction or intracerebral hemorrhage. Each case was reviewed to determine whether the patient was pregnant at the time of the stroke or within the 6 previous weeks. Women with a recent live birth, still birth, or spontaneous or induced abortion were included.

Results.—The registry included data on 17 pregnancy-related cerebral infarctions and 14 pregnancy-related intracerebral hemorrhages in about 8 million woman-weeks of exposure. Most of these strokes were of indeterminate cause (Figs 1 and 2). During the same time, 175 women had non–pregnancy-related cerebral hemorrhages and 48 had non–pregnancy-related intracerebral hemorrhages. The age- and race-related relative risk of cerebral infarction was 0.7 during pregnancy. After a live birth or stillbirth, this risk increased to 8.7. The adjusted relative risk of intracerebral hemorrhage increased from 2.5 during pregnancy to 28.3 during the postpartum period. The total adjusted relative risk of stroke during or within 6 weeks after pregnancy was 2.4. The excess stroke risk was 8.1 strokes per 100,000 pregnancies.

Conclusion.—Women are at significantly increased risk of stroke, especially intracerebral hemorrhage, during the postpartum period. Stroke risk is not significantly elevated during pregnancy but it is increased in the 6 weeks after delivery. The risk estimates derived from this study are probably on the conservative side.

▶ Stroke figures prominently among the neurologic complications of pregnancy and the postpartum period. This is a careful population analysis of stroke in women of childbearing age, which establishes that the 6–week period after delivery is a time of increased risk for both cerebral infarction and intracerebral hemorrhage. This risk is apparently not present during the pregnancy itself. This carefully executed study bears scrutiny.

M.D. Ginsberg, M.D.

Clinical Spectrum of CADASIL: A Study of 7 Families
Chabriat H, Vahedi K, Iba-Zizen MT, et al (Hôpital Saint-Antoine, Paris; Hôpital des Quinze-Vingts, Paris; INSERM U25, Paris; et al)
Lancet 346:934–939, 1995   3–15

Background.—Cerebral autosomal dominant arteriopathy with subcortical infarcts and leukoencephalopathy (CADASIL) is an inherited arterial brain disease that results in stroke and dementia. Recently, CADASIL was mapped to chromosome 19. The clinical and neuroimaging features in members of 7 large affected families with linkage to the CADASIL locus were reported.

Methods and Findings.—One hundred forty-eight members of affected families underwent MRI and genetic linkage analysis. Forty-five members had clinical disease. Eighty-four percent had recurrent subcortical ischemic events; 31%, progressive or stepwise subcortical dementia with pseudobulbar palsy; 22%, migraine with aura; and 20%, mood disorders with severe depressive episodes. In all symptomatic members, signal abnormalities on MRI were prominent, with hyperintense lesions on T2–weighted images in the subcortical white matter and basal ganglia. These findings were also noted in 19 asymptomatic members. Mean age at onset of symptoms was 45 years. Attacks of migraine with aura occurred earlier in life than did ischemic events. Mean age at death was 64.5 years. The MR data suggest that the penetrance of CADASIL is completed between 30 and 40 years. All 7 families studied had strong linkage to the CADASIL locus on genetic analysis, which suggests genetic homogeneity (Fig 3).

Conclusions.—The diagnosis of CADASIL should be considered in patients who have recurrent small subcortical infarcts resulting in dementia, as well as in patients who have transient ischemic attacks, migraine with aura, or severe mood disturbances when MRI shows prominent signal abnormalities in the subcortical white matter and basal ganglia. Individuals who belong to the family of such patients must also undergo clinical and MR assessment. Genetic linkage analysis confirms the diagnosis of CADASIL.

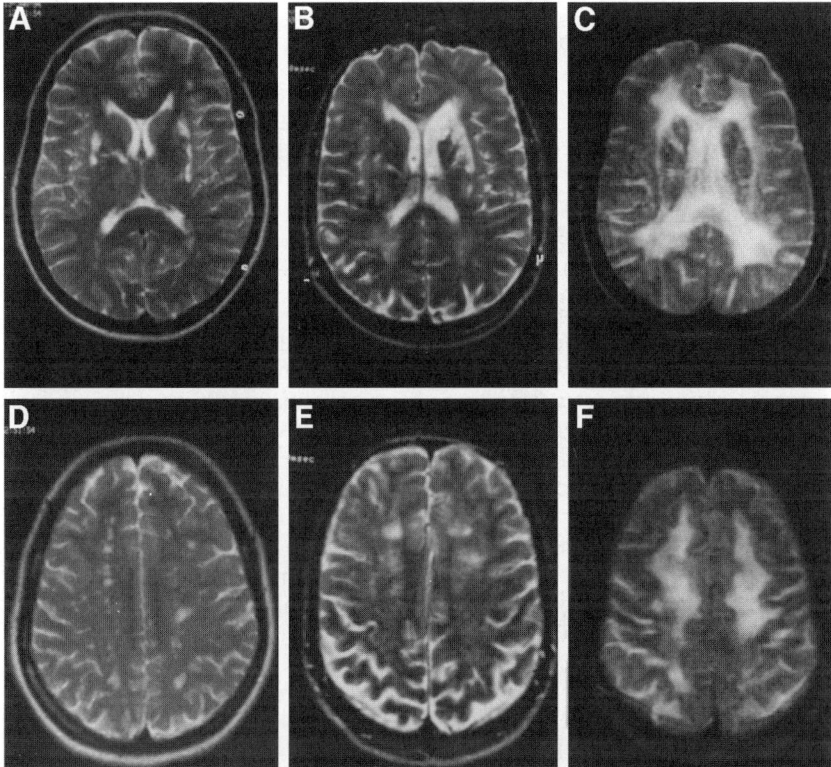

FIGURE 3.—Magnetic resonance T2–weighted images. **A and B,** a patient, aged 39 years, who had 5 transient ischemic attacks. (2 episodes of left hemianopia, 3 episodes of dysphasia), 1 stroke (a right-sided pure motor deficit), and 2 attacks of migraine with typical ophthalmic aura since the age of 33. **C and D,** a man, aged 43 years, with a normal neurologic examination who had severe manic episodes followed by major depression of melancholic type as defined by *Diagnostic and Statistical Manual of Mental Disorders,* ed 3, and recorded by a standardized interview. **E and F,** a woman, aged 56 years, who had 2 strokes (2 episodes of dysarthria with gait imbalance) before a progressive dementia with pseudobulbar palsy and bladder incontinence after 53 years of age. Hyperintense lesions were observed in the lobar white matter (centrum semi-ovale), in the periventricular white matter (near the frontal and occipital horns), in the external capsule and in basal ganglias in these 3 symptomatic patients at MRI examination. (Courtesy of Chabriat H, Vahedi K, Iba-Zizen MT, et al: Clinical spectrum of CADASIL: A study of 7 families. *Lancet* 346:934–939, copyright by The Lancet Ltd., 1995.)

▶ In this valuable article, the authors have studied a rather large number of individuals with this unusual genetic form of cerebrovascular disease. The clinical presentations of CADASIL, including recurrent infarction leading to dementia as well as migraine and mood disturbances, are well described. Hyperintense lesions of the lobar and periventricular white matter on T2–weighted MRI are impressive, and MRI abnormalities may occur in asymptomatic patients. Genetically, the disease appears to be rather homogeneous, and diagnosis can be confirmed by linkage analysis. The authors conclude, with probable correctness, that the disease has been largely undiagnosed heretofore. The article thus does a valuable service in bringing this condition to the reader's attention.

M.D. Ginsberg, M.D.

Basilar Artery Blood Flow During Head Rotation in Vertebrobasilar Ischemia
Petersen B, von Maravic M, Zeller JA, et al (Ernst Moritz Arndt Univ Greifswald, Germany; Univ of Lübeck, Germany)
Acta Neurol Scand 94:294–301, 1996   3–16

Introduction.—Previous studies have suggested that the close anatomical contact between the vertebral arteries (VAs) and the cervical spine may place the posterior circulation at risk of ischemia. However, the clinical importance of physiologic compression of the VA during head rotation is open to debate. Transcranial Doppler ultrasonography was used to examine the effects of head rotation on basilar artery (BA) blood flow.

Methods.—The study included 46 patients with vertebrobasilar ischemia and 40 controls. Each underwent assessment of BA blood flow using transcranial pulsed-wave Doppler ultrasonography with a 2–MHZ probe. Measurements were made with the head in neutral position and then in an extreme but tolerable position of rotation. Blood flow was measured in both BAs.

Results.—The controls showed no difference in BA blood flow velocity in neutral vs. rotated position. This suggested that a greater than 20% reduction in BA blood flow should be regarded as an abnormal finding. Seven percent of the patients with vertebrobasilar ischemia had no BA blood flow detected by transcranial Doppler ultrasonography. In the rest, the effect of head rotation on BA blood flow velocity was strongly affected by the condition of the VA. A significant reduction in BA blood flow was seen only in patients with atherosclerotic lesions or hypoplasia of the VA. Of 11 patients with unilateral VA, 2 had significant reductions (27% and 31%) in BA blood flow, although neither was symptomatic. There were 9 patients with bilateral VA, 5 of whom had at least a 30% reduction in BA blood flow during rotation. The mean reduction was 52%. Four of these 5 patients experienced vertigo, diplopia, or other clinical symptoms during head rotation.

Conclusion.—For some patients with vertebrobasilar ischemia and lesions of the VA, head rotation can produce clinically significant reductions in BA blood flow. Older patients with more atherosclerotic lesions may have reduced blood flow with only moderate head rotation. Not all patients with VA lesions have this reduction of BA blood flow, suggesting that individual vascular mechanisms play a major role in compensating for mechanical compression of the VA.

▶ This study represents an important application of transcranial Doppler technology to study blood flow velocity in the BA during head rotation. It confirms the clinical impression that patients with VA lesions, particularly when bilateral, undergo quite significant reductions in blood flow through the BA with head rotation, and in a sizeable proportion of bilateral cases, clinical symptoms develop during the maneuver itsself. Although there is considerable interpatient variation, this report underscores the importance of eliciting a history of head position–related symptoms in patients with posterior fossa ischemia and of cautioning patients against such maneuvers.

M.D. Ginsberg, M.D.

Long-term Prognosis and the Effect of Carotid Endarterectomy in Patients With Recurrent Ipsilateral Ischemic Events

Paddock-Eliasziw LM, for the North American Symptomatic Carotid Endarterectomy Trial Group (John P Robarts Research Inst, London, Ont, Canada)
Neurology 47:1158–1162, 1996   3–17

Background.—Research has demonstrated the benefit of carotid endarterectomy (CE) for patients with symptoms of transient ischemic attack (TIA) or nondisabling stroke associated with an angiographically severe carotid stenosis. The urgency for CE and its benefits will depend on the anticipated level of stroke risk. The long-term prognosis and effect of CE

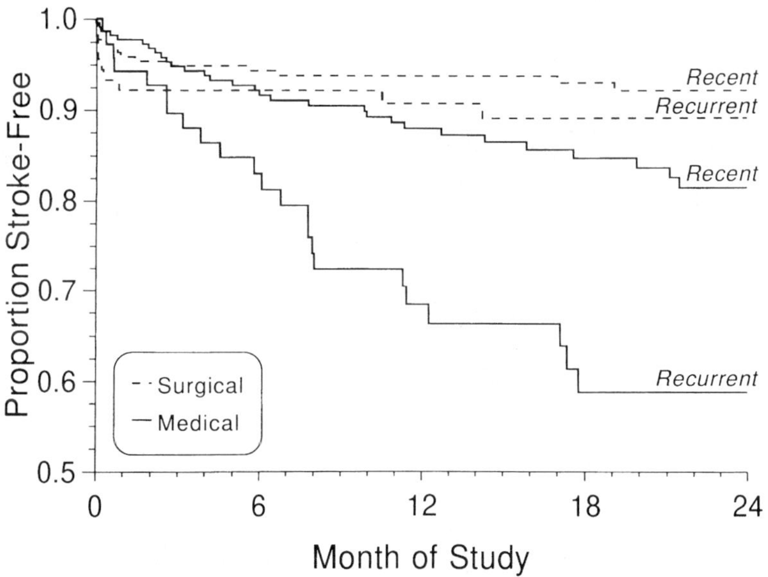

FIGURE 1.—Kaplan-Meier curves for ipsilateral strokes. The risk of ipsilateral stroke at 2 years for medically treated patients was 18.6% in the recent group and 41.2% in the recurrent group. For surgically treated patients, the risks were 7.8% and 10.8% for the recent and recurrent groups, respectively. (Reprinted from *Neurology*, courtesy of Paddock-Eliasziw LM, for the North American Symptomatic Carotid Endarterectomy Trial Group. 47:1158–1162, 1996, by permission of Little, Brown and Company Inc.)

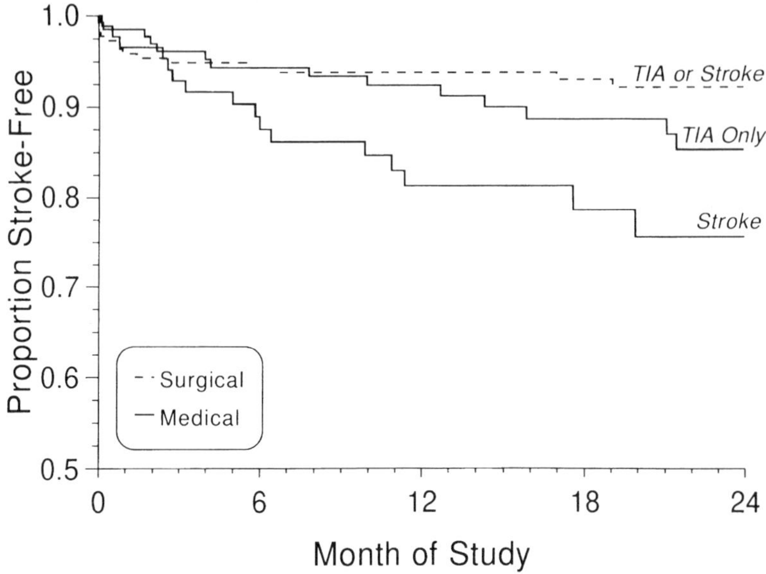

FIGURE 2.—Kaplan-Meier curves for ipsilateral strokes in the recent group. The risk of ipsilateral stroke at 2 years for medically treated patients was 14.7% if they had only transient ischemic attacks (*TIAs*) and 24.4% if 1 of recent events was a stroke. For surgically treated patients, the risk was 7.8%. Only 1 line appears for the surgically treated patients because the data remained in aggregate form. (Reprinted from *Neurology*, courtesy of Paddock-Eliasziw LM, for the North American Symptomatic Carotid Endarterectomy Trial Group. 47:1158–1162, 1996, by permission of Little, Brown and Company Inc.)

in patients with recurrent ischemic events referable to a severely stenotic carotid artery who are prone to a greater risk of stroke, were investigated.

Methods.—Six hundred eight patients with an ischemic event referable to a 70% to 99% carotid artery stenosis were studied. Four hundred forty-four patients had onset of new symptoms within 6 months of the presenting event. The remaining 164 patients had had 1 or more ischemic events within the 6 months preceding their presenting event and 1 or more events within the previous 7–12 months.

Findings.—Two-year Kaplan-Meier risk estimates of ipsilateral stroke for medically treated patients were 18.6% in the new-onset group and 41.2% in the recurrent group. These risks were 7.8% and 10.8%, respectively, after CE (Figs 1 and 2).

Conclusion.—Carotid endarterectomy must be urgently considered for patients with 70% to 99% carotid artery stenosis and recurrent ipsilateral ischemic events extending back more than 6 months. The risk of stroke in these patients is twice that of newly symptomatic patients.

▶ This important analysis of data from the North American Symptomatic Carotid Endarterectomy Trial Group study highlights the urgent need to carry out carotid endarterectomy in patients with high-grade (70% to 99%) carotid artery stenosis whose ipsilateral ischemic events extend back in time for more than 6 months (as this subgroup) if treated nonsurgically. These patients have over a twofold greater risk of ipsilateral stroke in the ensuing 2 years, compared with medically treated patients whose symptoms began only within the previous 6 months.

Surgical therapy in the recurrent group lowers the risk of stroke almost fourfold, compared with an approximately 2.5–fold reduction in the recently symptomatic group. These are vitally important observations for clinicians involved in the management of patients with ischemic stroke.

M.D. Ginsberg, M.D.

Early Hemorrhage Growth in Patients With Intracerebral Hemorrhage
Brott T, Broderick J, Kothari R, et al (Univ of Cincinnati, Ohio; Univ of Michigan, Ann Arbor; MetroHealth Med Ctr, Cleveland, Ohio)
Stroke 28:1–5, 1997   3–18

Background.—Traditionally, the bleeding of intracerebral hemorrhage (ICH) has been thought to be complete within a few minutes after it starts. Recent studies using repeated CT scans have suggested that the volume of parenchymal hemorrhage may increase over time. This prospective study examined the early growth of ICH and its association with early neurologic deterioration.

Methods.—The observational study included 103 patients with primary spontaneous ICH. All were studied beginning within 3 hours after onset. The patients underwent neurologic evaluation and CT scanning at 3 time points: baseline, 1 hour after baseline, and 20 hours after baseline. The study sought to determine what percentage of patients had continued cerebral bleeding during the period studied. It also looked at associated factors, functional outcomes, and the link between early hemorrhage growth and neurologic deterioration.

Results.—Twenty-six percent of patients had more than a one third increase in the volume of parenchymal hemorrhage from baseline to 1 hour. Furthermore, 12% had significant growth between 1 and 20 hours. There was a significant association between continued hemorrhage from baseline to 1 hour and clinical deterioration on the Glasgow Coma Scale and the National Institutes of Health Stroke Scale. None of the clinical or CT factors evaluated was able to predict growth of parenchymal hemorrhage.

Conclusion.—Many patients with ICH have substantial early hemorrhage growth demonstrable on CT. This finding is linked to neurologic deterioration. Randomized trials are needed to see whether very early surgery can prevent early neurologic deterioration and improve long-term outcomes for patients with ICH.

▶ This study of 103 patients with spontaneous primary ICH was conducted within the context of the Greater Cincinnatti–Northern Kentucky Stroke Network—an exemplary consortium of university and community hospitals which contributed enormously to the success of the recently published National Institute of Neurological Disorders and Stroke thrombolytic trial in acute ischemic stroke. In the study abstracted here, the authors have shown that enlargement of the volume of parenchymal hemmorhage occurs in over one quarter of patients between baseline and 1–hour CT scans and in about one eighth of additional patients between 1 and 20 hours. Nearly half of the patients with hemorrhage growth deteriorated during the first 20 hours but, interestingly, so did one third of the patients without hemorrhage growth.

These findings stand in contrast to a now decades-old study of this problem in which chromium-labelled red cells were injected into patients with acute ICH and the absence of radioactivity at subsequent necropsy was used to infer that hemorrhage was largely completed by admission.[1] The present study, using modern CT techniques, prompts a revision of this concept.

M.D. Ginsberg, M.D.

Reference

1. Herbstein D., Schaumburg H: Hypertensive intracerebral hematoma: An investigation of the initial hemorrhage and rebleeding using Cr 51–labeled erythrocytes. *Arch Neurol* 30:412–414, 1974.

Low Total Serum Cholesterol and Intracerebral Hemorrhagic Stroke: Is the Association Confined to Elderly Men? The Kaiser Permanente Medical Care Program
Iribarren C, Jacobs DR Jr, Sadler M, et al (Univ of Minnesota, Minneapolis; Kaiser Permanente Division of Research, Oakland, Calif)
Stroke 27:1993–1998, 1996
3–19

Introduction.—Previous studies have shown that people with low total serum cholesterol levels have higher rates of intracerebral hemorrhagic (ICH) stroke than people with high serum cholesterol levels. There is evidence that low cholesterol may affect the arteriosclerotic process in intracerebral penetrating arterioles. A large, well-defined, ethnically diverse population was used to test the effect of serum cholesterol level on the incidence of ICH stroke.

Methods.—The study population consisted of 61,756 health plan enrollees in the San Francisco–Oakland metropolitan area. Fifty-four percent of the subjects were women and 63% were white. At the start of the analysis in 1976, all subjects were 40 to 89 years of age and free of cardiovascular disease. Follow-up data were used to determine the incidence of combined nonfatal and fatal ICH stroke. The stroke data were compared against serum cholesterol measurements made at checkups between 1977 and 1985. The effects of serum cholesterol on ICH stroke risk were assessed, including the possible influence of age or hypertension.

Results.—Follow-up averaged 11 years. During this time, there were 386 ICH stroke events. Of 201 events in men, 201 were fatal; of 185 events in women, 185 were fatal. Men over 65 years of age with serum cholesterol levels below the sex-specific tenth percentile had nearly a 3 times higher risk of ICH (relative risk, 2.7). The tenth percentile for serum cholesterol level in this age/sex group was 178 mg/dL. The risk of ICH also tended to be higher for elderly women with very low cholesterol levels, but a chance effect could not be ruled out. In younger age groups, there was no relationship between serum cholesterol and ICH risk. In neither sex was there any relationship between serum cholesterol and hypertension.

Conclusion.—Elderly men with very low serum cholesterol levels are at elevated risk of ICH stroke. This relationship is not apparent in younger subjects and may not apply to elderly women. The findings suggest that the best way to prevent morbidity and mortality from ICH stroke is to focus on such modifiable risk factors as hypertension, alcohol abuse, and smoking.

▶ This study is important because of the very large cohort (more than 60,000 health plan participants) studied for the relationship between serum cholesterol level and the occurrence of ICH. The significant finding is that a very low cholesterol level (below the sex-specific tenth percentile, or 178 mg/dL in men) is associated with significantly increased risk only in men aged 65 years or older; it is not a risk factor in younger men or in women (small numbers precluded conclusions regarding elderly women). Intriguingly, there was no statistical interaction between low serum cholesterol and hypertension—perhaps a counterintuitive finding given the known predisposing influence of chronic hypertension on ICH. This field could well profit from basic experimental studies designed to assess cerebrovascular stability and integrity as a function of serum cholesterol level.

M.D. Ginsberg, M.D.

Vascular Events During Follow-up in Patients With Aortic Arch Atherosclerosis
Mitusch R, Doherty C, Wucherpfennig H, et al (Univ of Lübeck, Germany; Univ of Greifswald, Germany)
Stroke 28:36–39, 1997   3–20

Background.—Although aortic arch atherosclerosis has been associated with vascular events, few follow-up data exist. Patients with moderate to severe aortic arch atherosclerosis detected by transesophageal echocardiography were followed up prospectively.

Methods.—One hundred eighty-three patients were included. One hundred thirty-six had raised plaques, with a thickness of less than 5 mm, and 47 complex plaques with a thickness of 5 mm or more or plaques with mobile components. The mean follow-up was 16 months.

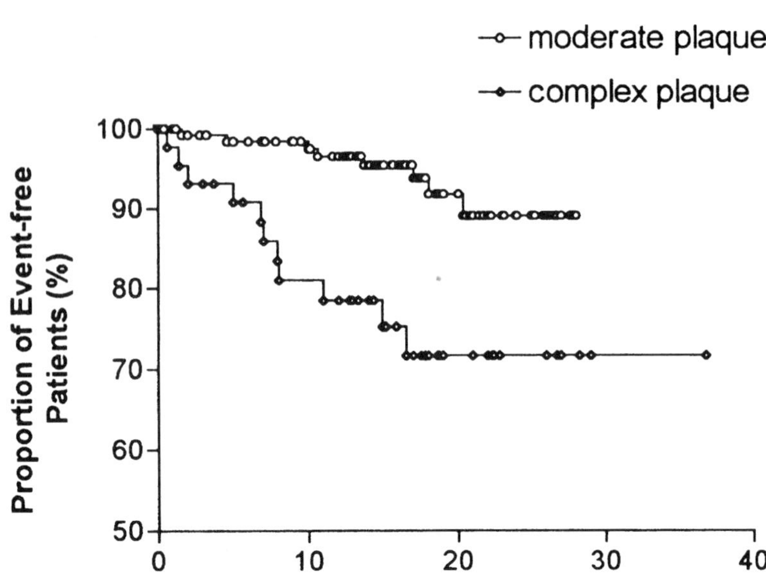

FIGURE.—Survival curves for vascular events in patients with moderate atherosclerosis (plaque thickness less than 5 mm) and patients with complex atherosclerosis (plaque thickness greater than or equal to 5 mm or mobile components) in the aortic arch. Kaplan-Meier analysis revealed a significant difference between the 2 groups of patients ($P < 0.01$. (Courtesy of Mitusch R, Doherty C, Wucherpfennig H, et al: Vascular events during follow-up in patients with aortic arch atherosclerosis. *Stroke* 28:36–39, 1997. Reproduced with permission *Stroke* Copyright 1997 American Heart Association.)

Findings.—Fifteen patients experienced vascular events with a presumed embolic origin during follow-up. The incidence in patients with raised plaques and in those with complex plaques was 4.1 and 13.7 per 100 person-years, respectively. According to a Kaplan-Meir survival analysis, the rate of vascular events was significantly higher in patients with complex plaques (Fig). In a Cox proportional hazards analysis, independent predictors of vascular events were complex plaques, coronary artery disease, and a history of previous embolism.

Conclusions.—Patients with complex aortic arch atherosclerosis may be at greater risk for subsequent vascular events. Such complex disease includes protruding plaques and plaque-related mobile masses.

▶ This is a follow-up study of 183 patients previously shown to have atherosclerosis of the aortic arch with raised plaques by transesophageal echocardiography. The authors have shown a 3.3–fold higher incidence of vascular events of presumed embolic origin in patients with complex plaques (i.e., protruding lesions or plaque-related mobile masses), compared with patients with raised plaques. Aortic arch atherosclerosis in this study carried a 4.3–fold increased risk of new embolic events. The Kaplan-Meier analysis of patients with complex plaques in this study suggests, ominously, that about 30% of patients with complex plaques will have a vascular event within 2 to 3 years of detection. These statistics are of concern and suggest the need for effective stroke prophylaxis in this high-risk group.

M.D. Ginsberg, M.D.

4 Neuro-Rehabilitation

What Role Do Neurologists Play in Determining the Costs and Outcomes of Stroke Patients?
Mitchell JB, Ballard DJ, Whisnant JP, et al (Health Economics Research Inc, Waltham, Mass; Emory Univ, Atlanta, Ga; Mayo Clinic, Rochester, Minn; et al)
Stroke 27:1937–1943, 1996
4–1

Background.—Among physicians, subspecialists appear to be greater users of tests and procedures, even after adjustment for patient mix, rising concern over the large number of specialists in the United States, and the costs associated with increased service intensity. Little information is available, however, describing whether treatment of stroke varies by physician specialty. The costs and outcomes of acute stroke were thus compared as to physician specialty, particularly neurologist vs. nonneurologist status.

Methods.—Medicare records were examined for a random sample of 38,612 patients aged 65 years and older admitted for cerebral infarction during a 9-month period. The physician billing for routine hospital visits on the first 7 days of the patient's hospitalization was considered the attending physician.

Results.—When stroke patients were treated by neurologists, expense was significantly greater; however, 90-day mortality rates were significantly lower (Table 2). Adjustment for patient age, co-morbidity, hospital teaching status, and other characteristics did not alter these results. Neurologists were more likely than were other attending physicians to order diagnostic cerebrovascular tests, to discharge patients to inpatient rehabilitation facilities, or to prescribe warfarin.

Discussion.—Stroke patients treated by neurologists appear to have better outcomes, although the treatment is costlier. The differences in outcome noted between neurologists and other physicians might be attributable to clinical characteristics used in triage that are not reflected in the medicare data, or the neurologists might be better at identifying the mechanism of stroke.

TABLE 2.—Costs and Outcomes for Stroke Patients by Specialty of Attending Physician

	Neurologists	Internists	FPs	Combinations	Other Specialists
Costs, $					
Hospitalization	7218	5972‡	5096‡	7527†	5977‡
Inpatient physician services	1453	1104‡	886‡	1671†	1123‡
Post-acute care	7248	5988‡	5856‡	7579	6116‡
Total episode	15 919	13 065‡	11 838‡	16 777‡	13 216‡
Outcomes, %					
90-day mortality	16.1	23.3‡	25.3‡	19.4‡	24.9‡
Discharge destination*	...	...‡	...‡	...‡	...‡
Rehabilitation facility	21.9	16.0	13.0	23.3	16.5
SNF/nursing home	22.2	33.1	39.6	28.0	32.5
Home	55.9	50.9	47.4	48.7	51.0

Note: Source: 20% sample of patients admitted for cerebral infarction from January 1 to September 30, 1991.
*Based on patients discharged alive only. Columns total 100%.
†$P = 0.05$, significantly different from neurologists.
‡$P = 0.01$, significantly different from neurologists.
(Reprinted with permission, from Mitchell JB, Ballard DJ, Whisnant JP, et al: What role do neurologists play in determining the costs and outcomes of stroke patients? *Stroke* 27:1937–1943, 1996. Copyright 1996 American Heart Association.)

Clinical Significance.—Outcome for stroke patients appears better when they are treated by a neurologist. Given current pressures to substitute generalists for specialists, this topic warrants further consideration.

▶ This article presents objective data indicating that outcomes are better for stroke patients cared for by neurologists rather than by internists or family practitioners. The differences are not trivial; the death rate is 60% higher for patients cared for by nonneurologists. The cost of care by neurologists (total episode $15,919) was 20% to 35% higher than for other physicians, but a higher percentage of patients went home (56% vs 47% to 51%) and fewer to nursing homes (22% vs. 33% to 40%), with the rest going to rehabilitation facilities. These data suggest that care of stroke patients by neurologists saves lives and improves quality of life of the survivors, while costing little or nothing more or even saving health care dollars in the longer run.

J. Blass, M.D.

Hospital Services for Stroke Care: A European Perspective

Beech R, for the European Study of Stroke Care (United Med and Dental Schools of Guy's and St Thomas's Hosps, London)
Stroke 27:1958–1964, 1996

4–2

Objective.—Stroke is a major public health problem in Europe in terms of economics as well as morbidity and mortality. Studies have shown significant variation in stroke outcomes across Europe, suggesting important variations in care delivery. Analyzing these variations may provide useful insights into the cost-effective allocation of resources for stroke care. The care and outcomes of European stroke patients were analyzed in a multicenter study.

Methods.—The study included data about stroke care from 9 hospitals in 6 European countries. The analysis included information about patient baseline characteristics, clinical status, and inpatient service utilization. Variations in the amount and types of services provided were analyzed, including the extent to which these services were affected by case mix.

Results.—The analysis revealed significant differences in several areas related to stroke care. Length of stay varied widely among hospitals, with a mean of 11–39 days and a median of 8–21 days. As few as 30% of patients admitted for stroke underwent brain imaging studies at some hospitals, compared with 98% at others. The percentage of patients undergoing neurosurgery ranges from 0% to 31%. The hospitals were also compared for the percentage of patients receiving certain services for which they had an identified "need." The range was 44% to 90% for physical therapy, 0% to 65% for occupational therapy, and 0% to 59% for speech therapy. The hospitals did vary significantly in their case mix, including patient age, level of consciousness, presence of incontinence, and prestroke Rankin Scale score. However, these variations could not account for the differences in services provided.

Conclusion.—There is wide variation in the care provided to stroke patients at various European centers. Differences in case mix cannot account for all of the difference in care. Future studies will determine whether the differences in care result in differences in outcome. The authors hope to identify ways of improving the quality, effectiveness, and cost effectiveness of care for European stroke patients.

▶ This comparative review of outcome from stroke shows large differences among European countries, all of which have nationalized health services. Thus, 4% of patients died in the hospital studied in Hamburg, Germany, whereas 19% or more died in the hospital studied in Italy and the 2 hospitals studied in England. The differences could not be attributed to different degrees of illness at admission. The authors point out that "... the current overall pattern of care cannot be either effective or cost-effective. There is likely to be overprovision of ineffective services in some centers and under-provision of effective services in others.

J. Blass, M.D.

Predicting Disability in Stroke—A Critical Review of the Literature
Kwakkel G, Wagenaar RC, Kollen BJ, et al (Vrije Universiteit, Amsterdam, Sophia Hosp, Zwolle, The Netherlands)
Age Ageing 25:479–489, 1996   4–3

Introduction.—Independence in activities of daily life is eventually regained in 58% of patients who survive a first stroke, with 82% being able to walk independently. Within the first 2 months, most functional recovery occurs, and little further functional recovery occurs after 6 months. Accurate and reliable predictors of functional recovery are needed for stroke management. Stroke outcome can be affected by more than 50 demographic, radiologic, neurophysiologic, and neurologic determinants, and the accuracy of predictions varies from 40% to 70%. To identify studies that met sound methodological principles of prognosis for outcome after stroke, research articles were analyzed.

Methods.—A literature review was conducted using a computer-aided search of published prognostic studies. The 78 studies found were tested for several factors, including adherence to control for dropouts during period observations, statistical testing of presumed relation between dependent and independent variables, sufficient sample size, reliability and validity of measurement instruments to assess dependent and independent variables, inclusion of an inception cohort, and adequate and uniform end point of observation.

Results.—Of the 78 studies, only 3 satisfied 9 of the 11 criteria, and 10 studies satisfied 8 of the 11 criteria. The variables that predicted functional recovery after stroke included age, urinary continence, previous stroke, disorientation in time and place, consciousness at onset, sitting balance, severity of paralysis, admission activities of daily life score, metabolic rate of glucose outside the infarct area in patients with hypertension, and the level of social support.

Conclusion.—Future studies need to address flaws in internal and statistical validity. A new statistical technique such as growth curve analysis would help model the time course of when activities of daily life can be resumed.

▶ This attempt at a meta-analysis of predictors of disability in stroke comes to 2 conclusions. Most of the 78 studies reviewed by the authors did not measure up to their criteria for epidemiologically valid studies. Meta-analysis of the "valid" studies confirmed the widely accepted predictors of age and previous stroke outcome was related to manifestations of severity of brain damage, urinary incontinence, consciousness at outset, disorientation to time and place, severity of paralysis, sitting balance, admission activities of daily living score, level of social support, and metabolic rate of glucose utilization (CMR_{glu}) outside the infarct area. The authors suggest that future studies of predictors of outcome in stroke should follow higher epidemiologic and statistical standards. Whether such studies would come up with new and clinically useful information is an interesting question.

J. Blass, M.D.

Prolonged Muscular Flaccidity After Stroke: Morphological and Functional Brain Alterations
Pantano P, Formisano R, Ricci M, et al (Univ of Rome 'La Sapienza'; IRCCS, Rome)
Brain 118:1329–1338, 1995   4–4

Background.—After a stroke, patients may experience muscular flaccidity, but it is unclear why this muscular flaccidity evolves into spasticity in many patients, but persists in others. Prolonged muscular flaccidity (PMF) is more common in older patients, patients with massive lesions, or those with severe paralysis. If the hypoperfusion of the cerebellum represents a true dysfunction of the cerebellar hemisphere ipsilateral to paretic limbs, then it may be a factor in prolonged flaccidity. Prolonged muscular flaccidity may result from cerebral blood flow (CBF) abnormalities in structures involved in motor control and responsible for crossed cerebellar diaschisis. The correlation between PMF and size and location of infarct or functional CBF abnormalities in intact areas of the brain was studied, as well as the relationship between PMF and severity of motor deficit.

Methods.—Computed tomography and MRI scans, plus CBF single photon emission CT (SPECT) studies, were obtained in 42 consecutive patients in the postacute phase of stroke. Patients were divided into 2 groups: 24 patients with PMF (mean age 61.9 years), and 18 patients with muscular spasticity (mean age 63.1 years). Motor deficit was measured using Adams' scale (0 = normal, 28 =hemiplegia). Results of scans were correlated with clinical findings at a mean of 3 months after stroke.

Results.—Greater motor deficit was seen in patients with PMF, but the mean structural volume of ischemic lesions was similar for both groups of

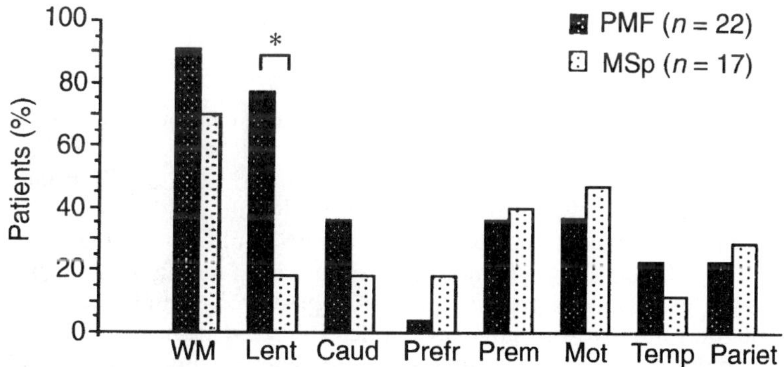

FIGURE 1.—Percentage of stroke patients with either prolonged muscular flaccidity or muscular spasticity showing CT/MRI damage in various anatomical brain structures. *Note:* The thalamus, supplementary motor area, occipital cortex, and cerebellum were spared in all patients. *Significantly different ($P < 0.001, \chi^2$) between patients with prolonged muscular flaccidity and muscular spasticity. *Abbreviations: PMF,* prolonged muscular flaccidity; *MSp,* muscular spasticity; *WM,* white matter (internal capsule/corona radiata); *Lent,* lentiform nucleus; *Caud,* caudate nucleus; *Prefr,* prefrontal cortex; *Prem,* premotor cortex; *Mot,* primary motor cortex; *Temp,* temporal cortex; *Pariet,* Parietal cortex. (Courtesy of Pantano P, Formisano R, Ricci M, et al: Prolonged muscular flaccidity after stroke: Morphological and functional brain alterations. *Brain* 118:1329–1338, 1995, by permission of Oxford University Press.)

patients. In patients with PMF, there was a significantly higher incidence of structural involvement of the lentiform nucleus (Fig 1). In patients with PMF, there was significantly lower relative perfusion in the lentiform nucleus, thalamus, and contralateral cerebellar hemisphere. In a subgroup of patients with subcortical structural lesions only, there was significantly lower relative perfusion in the ipsilateral frontal association regions.

Conclusions.—The structural damage to the lentiform nucleus may explain the prolonged flaccidity in these patients. However, the thalamus, cerebellum, or other brain regions that are structurally intact, but functionally impaired, may also be involved. In patients with a subcortical infarct only, the prefrontal cortex, premotor area, and supplementary motor area were also impaired. Limitations of this study include a lack of cerebral metabolic data because of the use of SPECT, the assumption that changes in CBF represent abnormalities in neuronal function, and that cerebrovascular patients are a heterogeneous group in terms of clinical presentation and morphological characteristics of cerebral lesions.

▶ This Italian study is an example of the classical approach of anatomic-clinical correlations in neurology. The modern twist is that the data were gathered not at autopsy but during life, by anatomic (CT/MRI) and functional (SPECT) imaging. As with neuropathologic-clinical correlations, further studies from other institutions will be needed to test the validity of the authors' interpretation—in this instance, that damage to the lentiform nucleus is a major cause of post-stroke flaccidity.

J. Blass, M.D.

Poststroke Rehabilitation in Older Americans: The Medicare Experience
Lee AJ, Huber J, Stason WB (Ctr for Health Economics Research, Waltham, Mass; Harvard School of Public Health, Cambridge, Mass)
Med Care 34:811–825, 1996   4–5

Background.—Stroke is the third most common cause of death and the major cause of disability in adults in the United States. Rehabilitation programs are conducted in general hospitals, inpatient rehabilitation hospitals and subunits, skilled nursing facilities, home health agencies, and outpatient facilities. The needs of the patient should be the main factor determining the setting of rehabilitation services. There is little information on the practice and per-patient cost of poststroke rehabilitation, and most of the information that is available is derived from the fewer than 20% of patients who receive inpatient care. The use and cost of rehabilitative services by survivors of stroke were examined during a 6-month period.

Methods.—Data were collected from the National Claims History data file from the Health Care Financing Administration. Information was obtained for rehabilitative services rendered during a 6-month period to a

20% sample of Medicare patients aged 65 and older in acute care hospitals after stroke. The use and cost of rehabilitative services were estimated. Average service use rates were determined across all stroke patients in a census division and in the 30 largest metropolitan statistical areas.

Results.—About 60% of the cost of rehabilitation after stroke is incurred in acute care facilities (Fig 1). Analysis of Medicare claims showed that 73% of the survivors of stroke receive institutional or ambulatory rehabilitative care in the first 6 months after stroke. The literature stressed the minority of patients and showed that 16.5% of patients receive inpatient rehabilitative care. Medicare analysis showed that rehabilitative care after stroke varies greatly among geographic areas. These differences indicate that there are large geographically related differences in the cost of rehabilitation of these patients.

Discussion.—These findings show that in the United States, the distribution of poststroke rehabilitative services is uneven. The differences cannot be attributed to uncontrolled demographic, clinical, environmental, or regional factors. In some areas, survivors of stroke are receiving too few or too many services. Further research should address who benefits

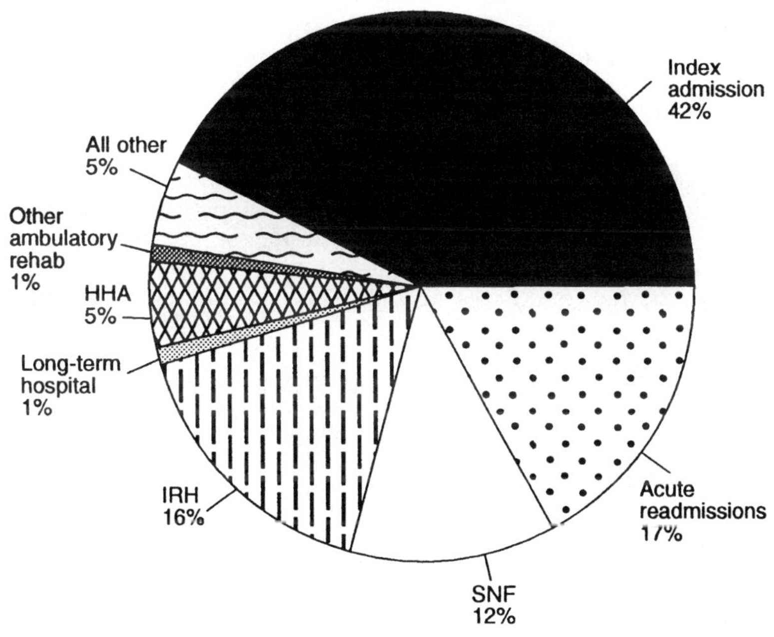

FIGURE 1.—Distribution of poststroke Medicare costs (excludes those who died during the index admission) from the Center for Health Economics Research analysis of Medicare National Claims History Data, 1991. *Abbreviations: HHA,* home health agency; *IRH,* inpatient rehabilitation hospital; *SNF,* skilled nursing facility. (Courtesy of Lee AJ, Huber J, Stason WB: Poststroke rehabilitation in older Americans: The Medicare experience. *Med Care* 34:811–825, 1996.)

from rehabilitation and in what setting, whether differences in patient outcome justify differences in cost, and whether the use of alternative treatment settings is clinically appropriate.

▶ Customary practices in all branches of medicine and surgery are being put to the test of effectiveness in terms of both patient outcomes and cost. Stroke rehabilitation is no exception. This study, based on Medicare data from over 30,000 patients, indicates that practices in stroke rehabilitation vary widely in different parts of the country, with attendant variation in cost. Furthermore, the published literature emphasizes outcomes in the 16.5% of stroke patients who have been cared for in specialized rehabilitation hospitals rather than the 56% of patients who receive poststroke rehabilitation in other settings. Clearly, further research on stroke rehabilitation is urgently needed to *prospectively* identify the patients with stroke who benefit from specific types of rehabilitation and to determine the most cost-effective means to provide such care.

J. Blass, M.D.

Effects of Fluoxetine and Maprotiline on Functional Recovery in Post-stroke Hemiplegic Patients Undergoing Rehabilitation Therapy
Dam M, Tonin P, de Boni A, et al (Univ of Verona, Italy; Hosp San Camillo, Venice, Italy; Univ of Padua, Italy)
Stroke 27:1211–1214, 1996   4–6

Background.—Depression after stroke occurs in 20% to 60% of patients and is associated with poor outcome. Such patients are often given antidepressants to improve their quality of life and participation in rehabilitation programs. Noradrenergic drugs help recovery in lesioned animals, but serotonergic drugs do not. This suggests that these different

TABLE 3.—Functional Recovery in Poststroke Hemiplegic Patients
Undergoing Rehabilitation Therapy

Treatment Group	Before Therapy	After Therapy
Placebo (n = 16)		
HSS Gait score	5.8±0.4	4.6±1.3*
BI score	35.0±10.8	54.1±21.1*
Fluoxetine (n = 16)		
HSS Gait score	5.9±0.5	3.8±0.9*†
BI score	38.4±11.2	61.9±13.0*†
Maprotiline (n = 14)		
HSS Gait score	5.7±0.7	4.8±1.5*
BI score	36.4±17.8	47.9±15.5*

Note: Values are means ± SD.
*Significantly different from the mean score before therapy $P \leq 0.05$).
†Significantly different from the corresponding mean value of the group treated with maprotiline ($P \leq 0.05$).
(Courtesy of Dam M, Tonin P, de Boni A, et al: Effects of fluoxetine and maprotiline on functional recovery in poststroke hemiplegic patients undergoing rehabilitation therapy. *Stroke* 1996; 27:1211–1214. Reproduced with permission of *Stroke*, Copyright 1996, American Heart Association.)

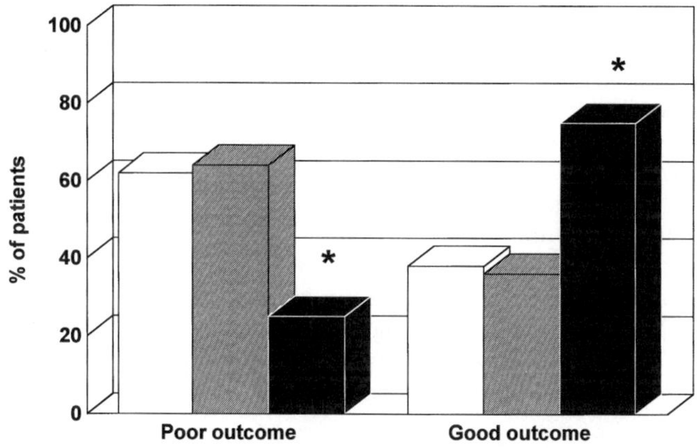

FIGURE 1.—Percentage of patients treated with placebo (*white bars*), maprotiline (*gray bars*), and fluoxetine (*black bars*) classified by cluster analysis in the poor (HSS Gait mean score, 5.4 ± 0.7; BI score, 39.8 ± 9.1) and good (HSS Gait mean score, 3.4 ± 0.6; BI score, 70 ± 10.8) outcome groups. *Significantly different from groups treated with placebo and maprotiline ($P< 0.05$). (Courtesy of Dam M, Tonin P, de Boni A, et al: Effects of fluoxetine and maprotiline on functional recovery in poststroke hemiplegic patients undergoing rehabilitation therapy. *Stroke* 1996; 27:1211–1214. Reproduced with permission of *Stroke*, Copyright 1996, American Heart Association.)

classes of antidepressants may affect the restorative processes in humans differently. The effect of fluoxetine, a serotonin reuptake blocker, and maprotiline, a norepinephrine uptake blocker, on the motor and functional recovery of patients after stroke was investigated.

Methods.—Fifty-two patients were unable to walk at 1–6 months after sustaining a stroke. Patients were divided into 3 groups and given fluoxetine, 20 mg/day, maprotiline, 150 mg/day, or placebo for 3 months in conjunction with physical therapy. Fluoxetine and maprotiline have little or no anticholinergic activity. Neurologic impairment and autonomy in daily activities were assessed.

Results.—The 3 different treatments improved walking and daily activities to different degrees. The greatest improvements were in patients treated with fluoxetine (Table 3). The smallest improvements were in patients treated with maprotiline. Significantly more patients treated with fluoxetine had a good recovery than those given maprotiline or placebo (Fig 1). There was no relation between these drug effects and their effectiveness in treating depressive symptoms.

Conclusions.—Fluoxetine and maprotiline may have different effects on the functional outcome of patients after stroke. It is unclear whether fluoxetine stimulates recovery or maprotiline hinders recovery. More research is needed on serotonergic antidepressants and their potential ability to help survivors of stroke in physical therapy recover.

▶ Selective serotonin reuptake inhibitors (SSRIs) were introduced as antidepressants, but the variety of conditions that are no longer classified as "depressive equivalents" for which the SSRIs are reportedly beneficial argue that these medications can more usefully be regarded as treating relative central serotonin deficiency. This placebo-controlled study of hemiplegic patients suggests that although all patient groups improved, the patients treated with fluoxetine (an SSRI) or maprotiline (a norepinephrine reuptake inhibitor) improved more than those receiving placebo, both in terms of motor function and depression. The data suggest that there is an element of relative serotonergic and relative adrenergic insufficiency in many patients with hemiplegia. Whether the effects of fluoxetine and maprotiline are looked on as treatment of an "unrecognized depression" or treatment of a neurochemical imbalance is essentially a matter of choice. Previous studies by others have also implied that treatment with "antidepressants" can improve rehabilitation after stroke, and more definitive studies to determine which patients benefit from this intervention are needed.

J. Blass, M.D.

Spinal Cord Injury, Exercise and Quality of Life
Noreau L, Shephard RJ (Laval Univ, Quebec City, Quebec, Canada; Univ of Toronto; Brock Univ, St Catharines Ontario, Canada)
Sports Med 20:226–250, 1995   4–7

Introduction.—In the last 30 years, the number of individuals with spinal cord injury (SCI) has increased. Individuals between 16 and 30 years of age account for more than 60% of new cases. The goal of rehabilitation is to improve the individual's level of independent living and quality of life.

Secondary Impairments.—Spinal cord injury also leads to the development of secondary impairments. For example, the maximal heart rate may be 115 to 120 beats per minute in individuals with quadriplegia because of deficits in sympathetic outflow. The loss of the use of abdominal and intercostal muscles can limit peak respiratory function. Problems with bladder or bowel function can also occur.

Benefits of Exercise on Secondary Impairments.—The benefits of exercise are most evident at the physiologic level. Exercise affects cardiovascular and pulmonary function, musculoskeletal impairments, metabolic disturbances, and other impairments such as pressure sores and urinary tract infections. However, the peak physiologic responses can vary tremendously between and within levels of injury (Fig 3). A summary of 13 cardiorespiratory studies reported a 20% average increase in maximum oxygen uptake after training for 4 to 20 weeks. Spinal cord injury also changes the breathing pattern and pulmonary capacity, especially in those with cervical lesions. In individuals with high level lesions, forced vital capacity, forced expiratory volume, and maximal breathing capacity are lowered. There are no conclusive studies that show pulmonary function limits exercise after SCI. Studies are needed to determine if exercise can prevent pulmonary complications in individuals with SCI.

Psychological Components.—The main problems of individuals with SCI are often psychological; anger, denial, and depression are common.

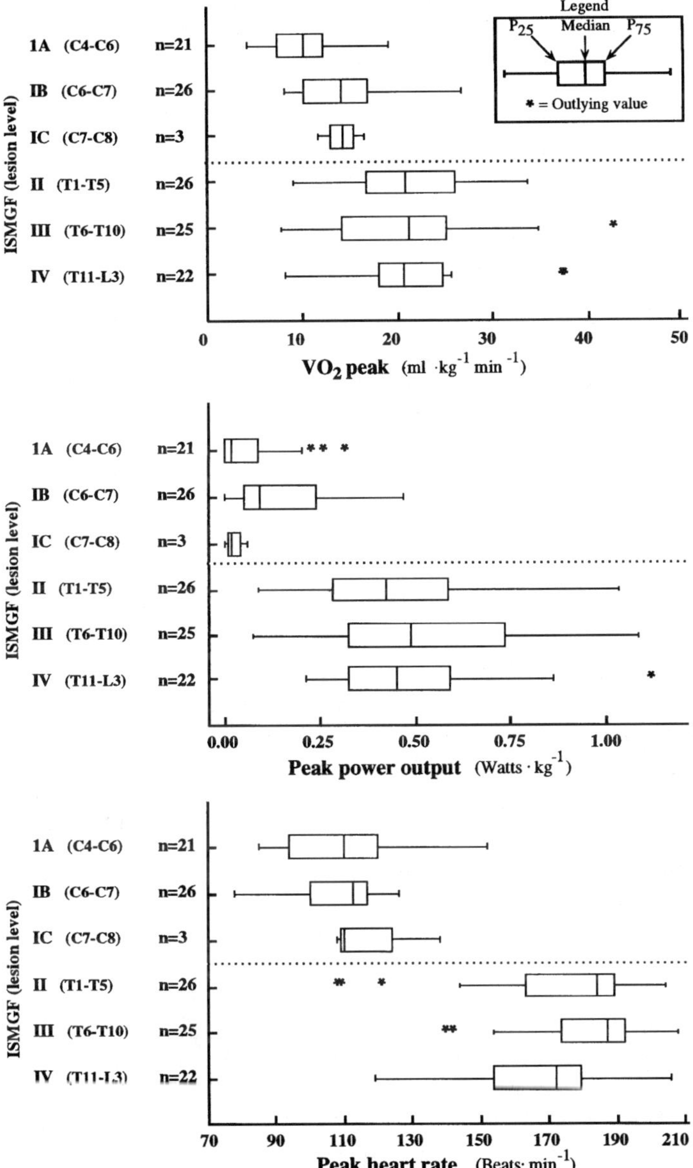

FIGURE 3.—Distribution of peak physiological response to wheelchair exercise in a group of 123 individuals with spinal cord injury. Data are presented according to the International Stoke-Mandeville Games Federation classification. *Boxes* illustrate the median with 25th and 75th percentiles for the given lesion level. *Asterisk*, outlying value. *Abbreviation:* VO_{2max}, maximum oxygen uptake. (Courtesy of Noreau L, Shephard RJ: Spinal cord injury, exercise, and quality of life. *Sports Med* 20:226–250, 1995.)

Studies have shown that wheelchair athletes tend to have below average scores on tension, depression, anger, fatigue, and confusion subscales, and very high scores on the vigor subscale. Comparative studies have shown that wheelchair athletes score lower on the depression subscale and higher on the vigor subscale than inactive individuals with SCI. Wheelchair athletes also have greater self-satisfaction, stronger self-image, fewer suicidal tendencies, and a more independent attitude than individuals with SCI who do not exercise.

Conclusions.—Rehabilitation is important to the lives of all individuals with SCI. The benefits can be seen at a psychological as well as the physiologic level. The degree of improvement in quality of life varies with the objectives of the individual. Because the physiologic strain of daily living cannot generally maintain an adequate level of cardiorespiratory fitness, high aerobic activities should be included in any program to improve the fitness level of individuals with SCI.

▶ The life expectancy of patients with SCI has approached normal, and further improvements in care will have to focus on quality-of-life issues. This laudable review from Canada describes the state of the art in this important area. Unfortunately, it emphasizes again how hard it is to disentangle quality-of-life measurements from prior, sometimes unrecognized assumptions. For instance, patients rated on whether or not they say they are satisfied involves the assumption that stated feelings are true feelings, i.e., dependent on Benthamite rather than Freudian psychology. It remains unclear whether wheelchair athletics make people with SCI feel better, or prior personality factors lead people with SCI who are generally more "up-beat" to participate in wheelchair athletics.

J. Blass, M.D.

Chronic Intrathecal Delivery of Baclofen by a Programmable Pump for the Treatment of Severe Spasticity

Ordia JI, Fischer E, Adamski E, et al (Boston Univ)
J Neurosurg 85:452–457, 1996

4–8

Background.—Spasticity is one of the most troublesome problems in patients with upper motor neuron lesions. Baclofen, the most widely used antispasmodic agent, often results in tolerance when given orally, and higher oral doses produce adverse CNS effects. The efficacy, safety, and cost-effectiveness of long-term intrathecal baclofen delivered in a programmable pump in patients with severe toxicity were investigated.

Methods.—Sixty-six patients were screened for the study. All had severe spasticity of spinal cord origin that was refractory to oral baclofen or had intolerable side effects associated with oral baclofen. The first 9 patients were included in a double-blind, randomized, placebo-controlled study to determine their response to a bolus dose of intrathecal baclofen. The rest of the patients participated in an open-label study with no placebo. The pump was implanted in 59 patients.

Findings.—The mean Ashworth score for rigidity declined from 4.3 before pump implantation to 1.4 after intrathecal baclofen treatment. The mean spasm frequency score declined from 3.6 to 0.5. In some patients, activities of daily living, sleep, and skin integrity were improved, and pain was eradicated. Six patients reported constipation. Dosage reductions were needed in 3 ambulatory patients because of muscular hypotonia; in another 3 because of areflexic bladder and urinary retention; and in 1 because of nausea, dizziness, and drowsiness. Fifteen patients had catheter-related problems. One pump was explanted because of infection in the pump pocket, and another after it eroded through the skin. None of the pumps failed. The mean length of subsequent hospitalizations was decreased with intrathecal baclofen.

Conclusions.—Long-term intrathecal baclofen delivered in an implanted programmable pump is effective in the treatment of severe intractable spasticity of spinal origin. The most common adverse effects are drowsiness, dizziness, constipation, and muscular hypotonia. This method of administration also makes treatment cost-effective.

▶ Baclofen is the drug of choice for treatment of the problems of spinal spasticity and, to a lesser extent, spasticity of supraspinal origin. However, intrathecal baclofen is clearly more effective than oral baclofen, with fewer systemic side effects. This study is an important survey of 59 patients receiving intrathecal baclofen by an implanted pump. Complications were relatively few, and the procedure was clearly beneficial to the patients. The study is interesting in that it includes a cost benefit analysis; it is important to remember that the patient's benefit is not included in that cost benefit analysis!

W.G. Bradley, D.M., F.R.C.P.

Effects of Intrathecal Baclofen on Chronic Spinal Cord Injury Pain
Loubser PG, Akman NM (Inst for Rehabilitation and Research, Houston; Baylor College of Medicine, Houston; Inuonu Univ, Malaya, Turkey)
J Pain Symptom Manage 12:241–247, 1996   4–9

Purpose.—Chronic pain can be a difficult, disabling problem for patients with spinal cord injury (SCI). Previous reports have shown the efficacy of intrathecal baclofen for the management of spasticity in patients with SCI and other neurologic disorders. This drug's effects on pain, which often accompanies spasticity, are unknown. The effects of intrathecal baclofen on pain in patients with SCI—who were primarily being treated for spasticity—were evaluated.

Methods.—The study included 16 patients with SCI who were scheduled for intrathecal baclofen pump implantation. All patients had severe spasticity that responded to temporary intrathecal baclofen infusion. The

TABLE 3.—Musculoskeletal Pain Response to Intrathecal Baclofen

Patient	Response	VAS^0	VAS^6	VAS^{12}	ΔVAS^6	ΔVAS^{12}	Medication status
2	Reduction	6.2	1.8	2.2	−4.4	−4.0	NC
3	NC	4.9	4.6	4.5	−0.3	−0.4	continued NSAID
4	Reduction	7.3	4.2	3.9	−3.1	−3.4	NC
5	Reduction	6.6	1.4	1.6	−5.2	−5.0	NC
7	Reduction	5.7	1.6	1.3	−4.1	−4.4	NC
8	Reduction	7.1	0.9	0.9	−6.2	−6.2	discontinued NSAID

Abbreviations: NC, no change; *NSAID*, nonsteroidal anti-inflammatory agent; *VAS*, visual analogue scale; VAS^0, baseline VAS score (cm); VAS^6, VAS score (cm) at 6 months; VAS^{12}, VAS score (cm) at 12 months; ΔVAS^6, change (cm) in VAS score at 6 months; ΔVAS^{12}, change (cm) in VAS score at 12 months.

(Reprinted by permission of Elsevier Science, Inc., from Effects of intrathecal baclofen on chronic spinal cord injury pain, by Loubser PG, Akman NM, *Journal of Pain and Symptom Management*, Vol. 12 No. 4, pp. 241–247, Copyright 1996 by the U.S. Cancer Pain Relief Committee.)

patients' pain was assessed in detail before and 6 and 12 months after pump implantation. The pain was divided into neurogenic and musculo-skeletal components and analyzed for changes in nature, quality, and severity. Analgesic use was evaluated as well.

Results.—Twelve of the 16 patients had chronic pain before pump implantation. The pain was neurogenic in 6 patients, musculoskeletal in 3, and mixed in 3. At follow-up, just 2 (22%) of the patients with neurogenic pain had a change in pain severity. In both of these patients, the pain got worse. In contrast, a significant improvement in musculoskeletal pain was observed in 5 (83%) of patients with this type of pain (Table 3). This improvement occurred along with a reduction in spasticity. Pump implantation had no effect on oral analgesic use.

Conclusions.—In patients with SCI and severe spasticity, intrathecal baclofen treatment can reduce associated musculoskeletal pain. However, it has no effect on chronic neurogenic pain. Higher doses of intrathecal baclofen might be more effective in reducing pain but could have excessive effects on spasticity.

▶ Intrathecal baclofen has been used to relieve spasticity in a variety of neurologic disorders, and this study examines the effect of this modality on the relief of pain. The number of patients studied is small, but the results appear clear-cut: intrathecal baclofen reduces the musculoskeletal pain associated with spasticity with little or no effect on neurogenic pain of CNS origin. This intuitively reasonable finding needs replication in larger numbers of patients, but the available data can help guide clinicians in choosing patients most likely to benefit from intrathecal administration of baclofen.

J. Blass, M.D.

Botulinum Toxin A in the Treatment of Spasticity: Functional Implications and Patient Selection

Pierson SH, Katz DI, Tarsy D (Braintree Hosp, Mass; Boston Univ; Harvard Med School, Boston)
Arch Phys Med Rehabil 77:717–721, 1996   4–10

Background.—Botulinum toxin A is effective in treating focal dystonia and may also be effective in treating spasticity. Prior studies have addressed the safety of botulinum toxin A and its effects on muscle tone, hygiene, and pain. These studies did not use functional improvement as an outcome measure or indication for treatment and did not relate functional improvement to reduced spasticity. The effect of botulinum toxin A on functional measures in patients with spasticity was studied retrospectively.

Methods.—Thirty-nine patients who had 40 limbs with spasticity were selected for treatment based on their potential for functional improvement. The mean patient age was 43 years. Two to 3 doses of 100 U of botulinum toxin A in 1 mL of saline were injected into target muscles.

Results.—Treatment goals were reduction of tone, better tolerance and fit of bracing, pain relief, and improved motor function, hygiene, and positioning. The mean dose per limb of botulinum toxin A was 180 U, and the mean number of muscles injected per limb was 2. Objective or subjective improvement was noted in 29 patients. The mean improvement on the Ashworth Scale was 1 point. The mean gain in active range of motion was 17.0 degrees, and the mean gain in passive range of motion was 18.4 degrees. In 14 of 22 patients, brace tolerance improved, and 10 of 13 patients experienced pain relief (Table 5). No adverse effects were reported. The duration of effect was similar in patients with dystonia.

Conclusions.—Botulinum toxin A is effective in treating spasticity. It improved tone and function and reduced pain in these patients. The objective improvements observed were statistically significant. The benefit was independent of site and cause of injury. Focal spasticity and a functional treatment goal are important factors in selecting patients for treatment with botulinum toxin A.

▶ This observational study supports the use of botulinum toxin to treat spasticity. Firmer conclusions will require replications, including the use of placebo injections. A comparison of botulinum toxin and saline injections

TABLE 5.—Subjective Improvement

	UE	LE	Total
Patient Self-Report of Functional Improvement	*n* = 23 17 (74%)	*n* = 17 10 (59%)	*n* = 10 27 (67%)
Patient Self Report of Pain	*n* = 7	*n* = 6	*n* = 13
Pain Improvement	6 (86%)	4 (67%)	10 (77%)

Abbreviations: UE, upper extremity; *LE*, lower extremity.
(Courtesy of Pierson SH, Katz DI, Tarsy D: Botulinum toxin A in the treatment of spasticity: Functional implications and patient selection. *Arch Phys Med Rehabil* 77:717–721, 1996.)

could be done in a time-limited study so that no patient would be denied the (still putative) beneficial effects of botulinum toxin. The need for placebo controls is not trivial. The act of injecting the spastic muscle, perhaps even with sterile saline or sterile water, may itself prove beneficial. If so, a cheaper and even safer means of treating spasticity would have been found.

J. Blass, M.D.

The Effect of Urapidil on Neurogenic Bladder: A Placebo Controlled Double-blind Study

Yasuda K, Yamanishi T, Kawabe K, et al (Chiba Univ, Japan; Tokyo Med and Dental Univ)
J Urol 156:1125–1130, 1996   4–11

Background.—Recent studies of the role of the sympathetic nervous system in the lower urinary tract have shown that α-adrenoceptors are present in the bladder base, posterior urethra, and prostate. α-Blockers improve urinary flow rates and residual urine in individuals with voiding dysfunction from benign prostatic hyperplasia. Urapidil is a new α-blocker that has been shown to be effective for hypertension and voiding dysfunction resulting from benign prostatic hyperplasia. The effect of urapidil on neurogenic voiding dysfunction was previously evaluated in a pressure-flow study. Because a significant decrease was noted only for pressure at maximum flow rate and minimum urethral resistance, minimum urethral resistance is considered the most important urodynamic parameter to evaluate the efficacy of α-blockers on voiding dysfunction in individuals with neurogenic bladder dysfunction. A prospective, double-blind trial was conducted to study the safety and efficacy of a new α-blocker in patients with neurogenic bladder dysfunction.

Methods.—Evaluations were made in 136 patients with a neurogenic bladder. Patients were assigned to 1 of 3 groups: group 1 received placebo; group 2 received urapidil, 15 mg twice per day for 4 weeks; and group 3 received urapidil, 15 mg twice per day for 2 weeks, then 30 mg twice per day for 2 weeks. Urodynamic evaluations included uroflowmetry, cystometrography, external urethral sphincter electromyography, and pressure-flow study.

Results.—In group 3 only, urinary frequencies decreased significantly. In all groups, obstructive symptom scores decreased significantly. There was no significant difference in subjective symptoms among the groups. In groups 2 and 3, significant improvement was noted in average and maximum flow rates and residual urine. Cystometric parameters did not significantly change in any group. In group 3 only, the pressure at maximum flow rate and minimum urethral resistance decreased significantly. The improvement in urodynamic assessment in group 3 was significant when compared with the improvement in group 1. Symptomatic and urodynamic improvement was similar in men and women and among patients with different underlying diseases. Three patients had adverse effects, but none were severe.

Conclusions.—In these patients with a neurogenic bladder, urapidil improved voiding dysfunction and decreased urethral resistance in a dose-dependent manner. There were no significant differences among the study groups, in contrast to a previous report that showed significant differences among study groups.

▶ This careful clinical trial reports that treatment with a new α-blocker, urapidil, improves voiding dysfunction in patients with neurogenic bladder while decreasing urethral resistance in a dose-related fashion. This observation is in accord with previous studies that indicated that other α-blockers were effective in the treatment of neurogenic bladder. The sample was adequately large (96 participants) and the design appropriate, although a more detailed description of the statistical methods used would be of interest in a study with so many multiple comparisons. Although no single therapeutic trial establishes a treatment, the data in this paper are convincing.

J. Blass, M.D.

5 Infectious Neurological Disorders

AIDS Dementia Complex in the Italian National AIDS Registry: Temporal Trends (1987–93) and Differential Incidence According to Mode of Transmission of HIV-1 Infection
Chiesi A, Seeber AC, Dally LG, et al (Istituto Superiore di Sanità, Rome)
J Neurol Sci 144:107–113, 1996   5–1

Purpose.—AIDS dementia complex (ADC), or HIV-1 associated cognitive/motor complex, is a common late complication of AIDS. Reported estimates of its prevalence and incidence vary substantially. Factors affect-

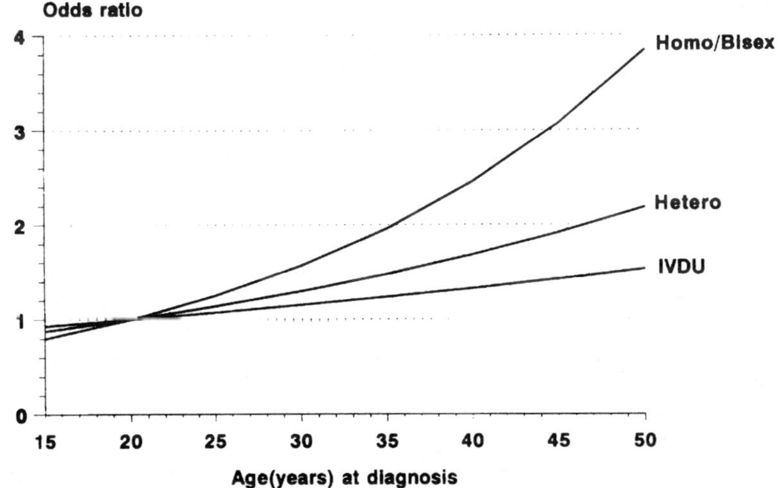

FIGURE 3.—Estimated risk of AIDS dementia complex at AIDS diagnosis, relative to 20–year-old patients. *Abbreviations: Homo/Bisex*, homosexual/bisexual; *Hetero*, heterosexual; *IVDU*, IV drug users. (Courtesy of Chiesi A, Seeber AC, Dally LG, et al: AIDS dementia complex in the Italian National AIDS Registry: Temporal trends (1987–93) and differential incidence according to mode of transmission of HIV-1 infection. *J Neurol Sci* 144:107–113, 1996.)

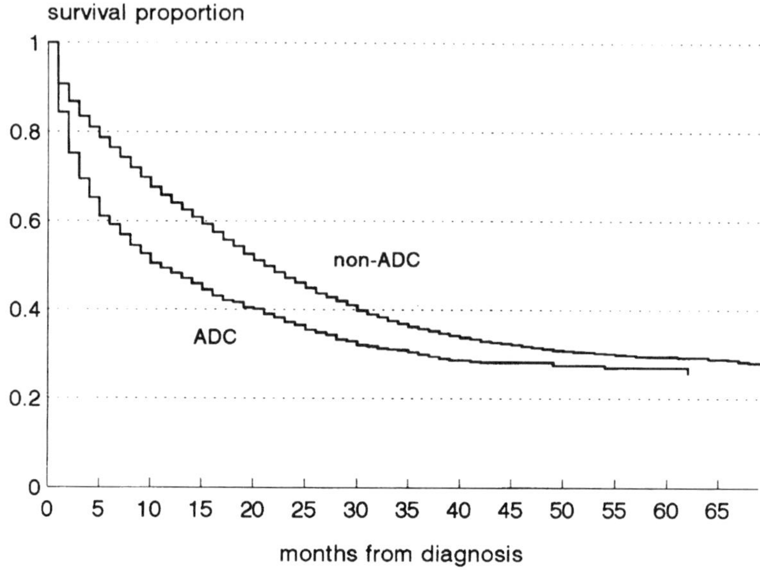

FIGURE 5.—Estimated survival curves for AIDS dementia complex (*ADC*) and non-ADC patients. (Courtesy of Chiesi A, Seeber AC, Dally LG, et al: AIDS dementia complex in the Italian National AIDS Registry: Temporal trends (1987–93) and differential incidence according to mode of transmission of HIV-1 infection. *J Neurol Sci* 144:107–113, 1996.)

ing the occurrence of ADC and its response to antiretroviral therapy are also unclear. Data from an Italian AIDS registry were analyzed to define trends in incidence.

Methods.—The study included 16,813 patients reported to the Italian National AIDS Registry (NAR) from 1987 to 1993. Data were drawn from case notification forms completed by the physician at the time of diagnosis. Multiple logistic regression, with adjustment for month of diagnosis, was performed to identify factors associated with the risk of having ADC at the time of AIDS diagnosis.

Results.—AIDS dementia complex was present at diagnosis—as the only manifestation or together with other AIDS-defining conditions—in 8% of patients reported to the registry. The rate of ADC at presentation was 9% in IV drug users, compared with 6% in heterosexual patients and 5% in heterosexual or bisexual men. A quadratic trend in the monthly proportion of ADC cases was apparent; this trend peaked in March 1990 and declined thereafter. On multiple logistic regression, risk of ADC was consistently highest for IV drug users and lowest for homosexual/bisexual men. This difference was somewhat lessened by advancing age, which itself was a risk factor in the heterosexual and homosexual/bisexual risk groups (Fig 3). The risk of ADC was unaffected by CD4+ cell count. The median survival was 11 months for patients with ADC at the time of AIDS diagnosis, compared with 21 months for patients without ADC (Fig 5).

Conclusion.—This Italian study finds that ADC is present at the time of AIDS diagnosis in about 8% of patients. The risk is greater in IV drug users than in other risk groups and rises with advancing age. Monthly reported cases have been on the decline since 1990, possibly reflecting the influence of zidovudine.

▶ Two important observations are derived from this study of a large cohort of patients with AIDS. First, in this population, ADC was frequent at the time of diagnosis of AIDS and often heralded the diagnosis of AIDS. More than 8% of patients had ADC as an AIDS-defining diagnosis. In this study, the percentage of patients with ADC at the time of AIDS diagnosis was significantly higher than the 3% derived from the Multicenter AIDS Cohort Study in the United States. Second, the authors found ADC in higher percentages among parenteral drug abusers than among other "at risk" populations. This contrasts with other studies that have failed to demonstrate a significant risk for cognitive decline in HIV-infected parenteral drug abusers when compared with a suitable control population.

J.R. Berger, M.D.

The Effect on Human Immunodeficiency Virus Type 1 RNA Levels in Cerebrospinal Fluid After Initiation of Zidovudine or Didanosine

Gisslén M, Norkrans G, Svennerholm B, et al (Göteborg Univ, Sweden)
J Infect Dis 175:434–437, 1997   5–2

Objective.—Central nervous system involvement is an early event in HIV-1 infection. Elevated levels of neopterin and β_2-microglobulin are found in the CSF before HIV disease becomes symptomatic. There is a need for some efficient anti-HIV treatment directed against CNS infection. The effects of antiretroviral treatment on the HIV-1 RNA load in CSF were studied.

Methods.—The analysis included 16 patients with HIV-1 infection who were starting antiretroviral monotherapy. They were studied during a total of 21 treatment periods: 13 with zidovudine and 8 with didanosine. Before treatment and for 3 to 13 months after the start of treatment, levels of HIV-1 RNA, neopterin, and β_2-microglobulin in the CSF were measured. Associations between these measurements were evaluated.

Results.—Zidovudine treatment was associated with a mean 1.05 $\log_{10}$ decrease in HIV-1 RNA levels in the CSF, a reduction of 91%. This was accompanied by a 57% reduction in neopterin level and a 33% reduction in β_2-microglobulin level. In contrast, none of the 3 variables changed during treatment with didanosine. The alteration in HIV-1 RNA level was significantly correlated with changes in neopterin and β_2-microglobulin levels. Zidovudine produced a significantly greater reduction of HIV-1 RNA in CSF than in serum.

Conclusion.—Zidovudine, but not didanosine, significantly reduces the HIV-1 viral load in the CNS. Zidovudine should be an important part of antiretroviral therapy for long-term neuroprotection. The finding of no correlation between changes in serum and CSF HIV-1 RNA levels supports the notion that there is no major exchange of free HIV between serum and CSF.

▶ This study convincingly shows that zidovudine therapy effectively reduces the HIV burden in the CNS. Zidovudine has been previously shown to improve cognitive function in both children and adults with HIV encephalopathy. Conventional wisdom dictates that the reduction in CNS viral load and the associated reduction in the release of inflammatory cytokines are likely to be causally related to this improvement. The authors' suggestion that zidovudine is likely to be useful in long-term neuroprotection in AIDS will require additional investigation. A natural selection of the zidovudine-resistant strains of HIV over time will undoubtedly diminish its efficacy in this capacity.

J.R. Berger, M.D.

Abnormal Cerebral Glucose Metabolism in HIV-1 Seropositive Subjects With and Without Dementia
Rottenberg DA, Sidtis JJ, Strother SC, et al (Minneapolis VA Med Ctr; Univ of Minnesota, Minneapolis)
J Nucl Med 37:1133–1141, 1996   5–3

Background.—In previous research, the authors reported relative basal ganglia hypermetabolism in patients with AIDS dementia complex (ADC). These findings were extended in the current study, and clinically useful metabolic indices of CNS involvement in HIV-positive patients were developed.

Methods.—Twenty-one HIV-positive patients, including 11 with AIDS, underwent [fluorine-18]-uorodeoxyglucose positron emission tomography (FDG-PET) scanning. Follow-up scans were obtained at 6 months in 12 patients and at 12 months in 4 patients. The control group consisted of 43 age-matched heterosexual volunteers. Scans were done with arterial blood sampling and analyzed using the Scaled Subprofile Model with principal component analysis.

Findings.—Two major disease-related metabolic components were identified in the combined-group FDG-PET data set. The first was a nonspecific indicator of cerebral dysfunction, which was significantly associated with age, cerebral atrophy, and ADC stage. The second was the striatum, which was heavily weighted (relatively hypermetabolic) and seemed to provide a disease-specific measure of early CNS involvement.

Conclusions.—In HIV-positive patients with or without AIDS or ADC, FDG-PET scans provide quantitative measures of abnormal functional connectivity. These measures apparently track the progression of CNS involvement in patients with subclinical neurologic or neuropsychological dysfunction.

▶ These investigators have expanded their initial observations regarding the alterations of cerebral metabolism in HIV-infected individuals as determined by PET scanning. They have once again shown that hypermetabolism in the basal ganglia provides an early clue to the presence of CNS disease. This interesting observation conforms to the predominantly subcortical nature of HIV dementia and the parkinsonian manifestations that attend advanced disease. As the neurochemical alterations that arise in the basal ganglia in the face of HIV dementia become better characterized, potential therapies, other than those directed against the virus, are conceivable.

J.R. Berger, M.D.

Human Immunodeficiency Virus Type 1–related Transient Neurological Deficits
Brew BJ, Miller J (St Vincent's Hosp, Sydney, Australia)
Am J Med 101:257–261, 1996   5–4

Introduction.—In some patients with HIV-1 infection, transient neurologic deficit (TND) will develop. In about half of these cases, no infective or neoplastic cause of the TND can be identified. This group of patients has not been sufficiently studied, nor has the relation between TND and AIDS dementia complex (ADC). The frequency and clinical characteristics of TND in patients with HIV-1 infection were prospectively analyzed.

Methods.—The study included all patients with HIV-1 and unexplained TND seen at a tertiary referral center over a 3–year period. Those with an accompanying opportunistic infection, neoplasm, neurosyphilis, or seizure were excluded. The patients' clinical characteristics were analyzed, including the relationship between TND and ADC. The frequency of TND in hospitalized patients with HIV-1 infection was compared with that of hospitalized patients without HIV-1 infection, and with the frequency of thromboembolic events in the same group of HIV-positive patients.

Results.—Twenty-seven patients (mean age, 39 years) met the study criteria. Their mean CD4+ cell count was 130/µL. Clinically, the TND was associated with hemiparesis and hemianesthesia in 85% of the patients and with dysphasia in 67%. Fifteen patients had ADC before TND, including 7 with stage 1 TND and 8 with stage 2 TND. In another 3 patients, ADC developed within 18 months after TND. Seventy percent of patients had anticardiolipin antibodies and 53% had low protein S levels; these findings were more frequent than in patients with similarly advanced HIV-1 disease but no neurologic abnormalities. The frequency of TND was 0.8% among hospitalized patients with HIV-1 and 0.4% among hospitalized patients without HIV-1, a nonsignificant difference. In the same group of HIV-infected patients, the frequency of thromboembolic events was 0.9%.

Conclusions.—Transient neurologic deficit is a possible complication of HIV-1 infection. These episodes are commonly associated with ADC. The patients may have elevated concentrations of anticardiolipin antibodies and low protein S levels. The meaning of these associations, and the efficacy of antiretroviral therapy for TND, remains to be determined.

▶ Brew and Miller studied 27 HIV-infected patients with TND characterized chiefly by brief episodes of hemiparesis and hemisensory loss. This disorder was observed in less than 1% of all patients admitted to the AIDS medicine unit in Sydney, essentially identical to the number of patients in that unit admitted for nonneurologic thromboembolic disease. Of interest, in 18 (67%) of the 27 patients with TND HIV dementia was found or ultimately developed, suggesting that TND is a marker for HIV dementia. The authors speculate that vascular etiology is possible because of the associated elevation of anticardiolipin antibodies and low protein S levels in this population. However, in only 2 of the 27 patients did cerebral infarction develop. The etiology of this occasionally observed phenomenon remains a conundrum, and a focal seizure or migrainous phenomenon still needs to be considered, as the authors correctly assert.

J.R. Berger, M.D.

Acute Lumbosacral Polyradiculopathy Due to Cytomegalovirus in Advanced HIV Disease: CSF Findings in 17 Patients
Miller RF, Fox JD, Thomas P, et al (Middlesex Hosp, London; Westminster Hosp Health Care Trust, London)
J Neurol Neurosurg Psychiatry 61:456–460, 1996   5–5

Introduction.—In patients with advanced HIV disease, acute lumbosacral polyradiculopathy is an uncommon but distinctive neurologic syndrome. There is subacute onset of bilateral lower motor neuron leg weakness, which may progress to flaccid paraparesis with pain and paresthesia of the legs and perineum, sphincter dysfunction, and areflexia. Reporting findings include abnormalities in CSF, most often a pleocytosis with a polymorphonuclear leukocyte preponderance. Cerebrospinal fluid findings from patients infected with HIV who had acute lumbosacral polyradiculopathy were studied.

Methods.—For 17 HIV-infected patients with cytomegalovirus (CMV)-associated acute lumbosacral polyradiculopathy, the records were reviewed retrospectively. Cerebrospinal fluid protein and glucose concentrations were determined, as was the presence or absence of pleocytosis, malignant cells, bacteria, mycobacteria, and fungi.

Results.—Nine of 17 patients had leocytosis noted in the CSF with a cell count of 28–1,142/mm³ (median, 150). A polymorphonuclear leukocyte preponderance was seen in 7 patients. In 13 patients, protein concentrations were moderately or considerably raised in the CSF. In 5 patients, the CSF plasma glucose ratios were less than or equal to 50%. Normal or near normal protein values, no pleocytosis, and normal CSF plasma glucose was seen in 2 patients.

Conclusions.—There is a variance in the abnormalities in CSF in CMV associated acute lumbosacral polyradiculopathy. A typical polymorphonuclear preponderant pleocytosis was found in only 50% of patients. A demonstration of polymorphonuclear preponderant pleocytosis should not be the only factor in diagnosing this condition. So that specific anti-CMV treatment may be instituted, there should be identification of CMV DNA in CSF and the exclusion of other opportunistic infections and lymphoma.

▶ A high index of suspicion for CMV lumbosacral polyradiculopathy must be held for the patient with AIDS seen with unilateral or bilateral lower limb weakness, asymmetric areflexia, leg and perineal pain and paresthesias, and sphincter disturbances. A preponderance of polymorphonuclear cells in the CSF has been incorrectly considered by some authors to be a sine qua non for the diagnosis of CMV infection of the nervous system in HIV infection, particularly acute lumbosacral polyradiculopathy.

Miller and colleagues show in their cohort of 17 patients with acute lumbosacral polyradiculopathy complicating HIV infection that only 9 had a cell count of more than 5 /mm^3 in their CSF. Furthermore, CSF polymorphonuclear cells were observed in only 9 patients (range, 40% to 100%); all but 1 had white blood cell counts greater than 5/mm^3. If polymorphonuclear cells are observed in the CSF, the diagnosis of CMV needs to be strongly considered. However, CMV may exist in the absence of pleocytosis or polymorphonucelar preponderance. The authors also emphasize the importance of polymerase chain reaction for establishing the diagnosis of CMV. One simply cannot rely on viral cultures to confirm the diagnosis.

J.R. Berger, M.D.

Creutzfeldt-Jakob Disease in Austria

Hainfellner JA, Jellinger K, Diringer H, et al (Univ of Vienna; Hosp Lainz, Vienna; Univ of Graz, Austria)
J Neurol Neurosurg Psychiatry 61:139–142, 1996   5–6

Background.—Creutzfeldt-Jakob disease (CJD) is the most common, widespread transmissible spongiform encephalopathy in humans. The worldwide incidence of this disease is about 1 per million per year. The epidemiologic, clinical, and neuropathologic characteristics of neuropathologically diagnosed and immunocytochemically confirmed CJD cases in Austria were investigated.

Methods and Findings.—Seventy-nine Austrians were diagnosed as having CJD between 1969 and 1995. The annual incidence has increased significantly, from a mean of 0.18 per million between 1969 and 1985 to 0.67 per million between 1986 and 1994. Until 1989, there was also a significant increase in the percentage of patients with CJD who were older than 70 years at death. After 1989, the percentage declined. No regional clustering, familial occurrence, or recognized iatrogenic risk was documented. Ages at death were distributed symmetrically around the median of 64 years. The median disease duration was 4 months. Seventy-six percent of the patients died within 6 months of disease onset. Eighty-six percent of the patients retrospectively met clinical criteria of probable or possible CJD. Neuropathologic assessment showed the classic triad of spongiform change, astrogliosis, and neuronal loss in most patients. In 2 patients, no unequivocal tissue changes were observed, but anti–prion protein immunocytochemistry revealed prion protein deposits in these patients.

Conclusions.—The recent increase in the incidence of CJD in Austria probably reflects an increased awareness and diagnosis of CJD (rather than a real increase). These findings do not support a relation between a rise in the incidence of sporadic CJD and bovine spongiform encephalopathy.

▶ A consistent increase in the numbers of patients with pathologically proved CJD in Austria between 1969 and 1996 was observed by Budka and colleagues.[1] Using only the neuropathologically confirmed cases, the incidence was estimated at 1.25 per million in 1995. The authors conclude, probably correctly, that this increase (similar to one noted in south Florida between 1985 and 1995) was not related to bovine spongiform encephalopathy. The study would have been enhanced with better clinical description of the cases, particularly for the 2 women, aged 27 and 30 years. Relying on only neuropathologically confirmed cases likely results in a significant underestimate of the true incidence of this disease.

J.R. Berger, M.D.

Reference

1. Berger JR, Landy H, Sardo J, et al: Creutzfeldt-Jakob disease. *Neurology* 44:A260, (Suppl 2), 1994.

A New Variant of Creutzfeldt-Jakob Disease in the UK
Will RG, Ironside JW, Zeidler M, et al (Western Gen Hosp, Edinburgh, Scotland; London School of Hygiene and Tropical Medicine; Hopital de la Salpetriere, Paris; et al)
Lancet 347:921–925, 1996   5–7

Introduction.—A British epidemic of bovine spongiform encephalopathy (BSE) in cattle prompted a surveillance study of Creutzfeldt-Jakob disease (CJD) that began in 1990. This study sought to identify any links between BSE in cattle and CJD in humans. Ten cases of CJD with an unusual neuropathologic and clinical profile were identified in the course of that trial.

Methods.—Most cases of CJD were directly referred to the CJD surveillance unit by neurologists and neuropathologists. For each referred case, the clinical records were analyzed and information on possible risk factors for CJD was obtained by a questionnaire administered to the patient's family. Seventy percent of suspected cases of CJD underwent neuropathologic examination. The findings were compared with those of recent surveys of CJD in other European countries.

Results.—Of 207 cases identified, 10 had distinctive neuropathologic findings. The most striking feature in these cases was the extensive distribution of prion protein plaques, many of which resembled kuru-type plaques. They had a dense eosinophilic center and pale periphery and were surrounded by an area of spongiform change. The median age of patients was 29 years. All patients had an unusual clinical course with behavioral change as an early event. Only 2 had impaired memory as part of the initial clinical picture, although all went on to have progressive dementia. The typical electroencephalogram findings of CJD were absent in all cases. No patients who fit this pattern were identified from French, German, Italian, or Dutch surveillance studies performed in the 1990s.

Conclusions.—A new British variant of CJD is identified. This cluster of cases could be causally linked to the epidemic of BSE in cattle, but there is insufficient information to confirm such a link. More data about the current and past clinical and neuropathologic findings of CJD in the United Kingdom and elsewhere are needed. If there is such a relationship, human exposure to the BSE agent was probably greatest during the late 1980s, before a ban on the use of specified bovine offal was implemented.

▶ This is a key reference to the debate about whether a possibly zoonotic form of prion disease associated with BSE ("mad cow disease") may have broken out in the United Kingdom. This is only 1 of several reports of a CJD-like disorder that has unusually occurred in very young individuals that some claim may have been contracted by ingestion of products derived from animals with BSE. At the time of this writing, there was no conclusive evidence for a link between BSE and CJD in very young individuals.

R. Kuljis, M.D.

Human T-cell Lymphotropic Virus Type II–associated Myelopathy: Clinical and Immunologic Profiles
Lehky TJ, Flerlage N, Katz D, et al (NIH, Bethesda, Md; Univ of Maryland, Baltimore; VAMC Washington, DC; et al)
Ann Neurol 40:714–723, 1996

5–8

Introduction.—In several distinct geographic populations of the world, such as Ameridian tribes in North and South America and isolated tribes in Mongolia and North Africa, human T-cell lymphotropic virus type II (HTLV-II) is endemic. In the United States and Europe, the virus has been isolated in IV drug users, and it can be transmitted by shared contaminated needles, blood transfusions, breast milk, and sexual contact. The association of the virus with disease is not well understood and there are sparse

TABLE 1.—Characteristics of Patients With Human T-cell Lymphotropic Virus Type II

Patient No.	Age (yr)/ Sex	Origin	Disease	Duration	EDSS*	MRI Head	MRI Spine	CSF WBC	CSF Protein	CSF IgG Index	CSF OCB
		Clinical Characteristics of HTLV-II Patients				Laboratory Characteristics of HTLV-II Patients					
1	53/M	Black,† Indian‡	Spastic para- plegia	5	8.0	T2 wm§	T2 wm‖	4	79	0.52	+/−¶
2	46/M	Black,† Indian‡	Spastic quadri- paresis	4	7.5	T2 wm§	T2 wm§	16	57	0.56	+
3	34/F	Black,† Indian‡	Spastic quadri- paresis	4	9.0	T2 wm§	C-spine swelling	6	73	0.58	−
4	70/M	Black†	Spastic quadri- paresis	12	8.0	††	‡‡	2	ND**	ND**	+

*Expanded Disability Scale.
†Black.
‡Amerindian (Cherokee or Blackfoot).
§White matter (*wm*) lesions on T2-weighted MRI images.
‖White matter lesion on T2-weighted MRI images with some gadolinium enhancement. Thoracic cord atrophy also noted.
¶Oligoclonal bands positive initially; follow-up studies negative.
**Not done; traumatic tap.
††Computed tomography, head showing mild atrophy consistent with age, no lesions.
‡‡Complete myelogram showing thoracic cord atrophy.
Abbreviations: HTLV-II, human T-cell lymphotropic virus type II; *WBC,* white blood cells; *OCB,* oligoclonal bands.
(Courtesy of Lehky TJ, Flerlage N, Katz D, et al: Human T-cell lymphotropic virus type II–associated myelopathy: Clinical and immunologic profiles. Reprinted from *Annals of Neurology* Vol. 40, pp 714–723, 1996, by permission of Little, Brown and Company Inc.)

data. To determine clinical and immunologic findings, 4 patients with HTLV-II seropositive and spastic paraparesis were studied.

Patients and Methods.—Three patients were of Amerindian descent, and all were black. All patients were seronegative for HIV. They had MRI and CSF studies. Spontaneous lymphoproliferation was compared with HTLV-I–associated myelopathy/tropical spastic paraparesis. One patient had a spinal cord biopsy.

Results.—In less than 5 years, the patients progressed to a nonambulatory state. White matter disease in the cerebrum and spinal cord were found in MRI studies obtained from 3 of the patients (Table 1). Antibodies to human HTLV-II were found in the CSF and serum. Polymerase chain reaction analysis of peripheral blood lymphocytes was used to confirm the presence of proviral HTLV-II. Some HTLV RNA was found within a lesion in 1 patient who had a spinal cord biopsy. Spontaneous lymphoproliferation of peripheral blood lymphocytes was seen in 2 patients who had immunologic studies; however, they were decreased relative to patients infected with HTLV-I.

Conclusion.—These patients infected with HTLV-II have clinical and immunologic findings that resemble those found in HTLV-I–associated myelopathy/tropical spastic paraparesis.

▶ Human T-cell lymphotropic virus type II does not appear as prevalent as HTLV-I in the United States and is largely confined to the population of parenteral drug abusers, although it is seen in some members of Amerindian tribes in North and South America. This study by Lehky and colleagues conclusively shows that HTLV-II, like the related virus HTLV-I, which is responsible for HTLV-I–asociated myelopathy tropical spastic paraparesis, also may cause a myelopathy. The similarities and differences between the myelopathies resulting from HTLV-I and HTLV-II will require additional studies of larger numbers of cases. However, the presence of a detectable sensory level on physical examination and spinal cord abnormalities detected by MRI in some of these patients are unusual features for HTLV-I–associated myelopathy/tropical spastic paraparesis.

Before observations of Lehky et al., the evidence for the association between HTLV-II and myelopathy had been chiefly anecdotal, with the first case report of a tropical spastic paraparesis–like illness in association with HTLV-II reported by my colleagues and me in 1991. To date, the number of cases of HTLV II associated myelopathy remains quite small, and it is unlikely that the risk for the development of this complication is as high as that seen with HTLV-I.

J.R. Berger, M.D.

Interferon-Alpha Is Effective in HTLV-I-Associated Myelopathy: A Multicenter, Randomized, Double-Blind, Controlled Trial

Izumo S, Goto I, Itoyama Y, et al (Kagoshima Univ, Japan; Kyushu Univ, Japan; Oita Med Univ, Japan; et al)
Neurology 46:1016–1021, 1996

5–9

Background.—In carriers of human T-lymphotropic virus type 1 (HTLV-I), progressive spastic paraparesis is termed HTLV-I−associated myelopathy/tropical spastic paraparesis (HAM/TSP). Studies have reported immunologic processes in the pathogenesis of HAM/TSP. The treatment effects of prednisolone, plasma exchange, and interferon-α have been studied, but none of the studies were blinded. The effect of natural interferon-α in patients with HTLV-I in a multi-center, double-blind, randomized study was studied.

Methods.—There were 48 patients with HAM/TSP between 20 and 75 years of age. Human lymphoblastoid interferon 0.3 MU, 1.0 MU, or 3.0 MU was administered for 28 days. Motor dysfunction, urinary disturbance, and other physical and neurological signs and symptoms were evaluated at baseline, 2 weeks and 4 weeks after start of therapy, and 4 weeks after treatment was completed.

Results.—The percentages of patients who had a good or excellent response to treatment at 4 weeks after start and 4 weeks after treatment was completed were 7.1% and 8.3% in patients given 0.3 MU, 23.5% and 26.7% in patients given 1.0 MU, and 66.7% and 61.5% in patients given 3.0 MU. The frequency of adverse effects was similar for all groups. Some patients given 1.0 MU and 3.0 MU had abnormal laboratory data, but most of these patients were able to continue their treatment schedule.

Discussion.—Human lymphoblastoid interferon-α 3.0 MU for 4 weeks can be safely used to treat patients with HAM/TSP. The response rate seen in this trial was better than the response rate in a prior study of oral prednisolone. In these patients, motor dysfunction and many other neurological signs and symptoms improved. Interferon-α may reduce the increased HTLV-I load in patients with HTLV-I−associated myelopathy. The reduction of this increased HTLV-I load and regulation of abnormal immune responses may be the most appropriate treatment of HAM/TSP.

▶ The treatment of patients with HAM/TSP is a frustrating experience. Corticosteroids, danazol, interferon-α, and plasma exhange have been reported to be of benefit. Izumo and colleagues performed a double-blinded, controlled trial with interferon-α that showed efficacy with the higher doses of 3.0 MU every day for 4 weeks. However, the design of their study extended observations to 2 months after the initiation of the therapy. In my experience, it has not been unusual to witness an initial improvement that is persistent up to 6 or more months with any form of therapy, only to observe a progressive decline in function thereafter. Additionally, the pace of the illness seems to vary significantly from patient to patient. For instance, those individuals who have acquired the infection as a consequence of blood transfusion appear to have shorter latencies to its development and more aggressive courses. Others seem to have fairly benign courses. The study of this group of Japanese investigators is a welcome addition to the literature on the therapy of HAM/TSP and future studies of the duration of the efficacy of interferon-α are warranted.

J.R. Berger, M.D.

The Role of Laboratory Investigation in the Diagnosis and Management of Patients With Suspected Herpes Simplex Encephalitis: A Consensus Report

Cleator GM, for the EU Concerted Action on Virus Meningitis and Encephalitis (Universita di Roma "La Sapienza"; Ospedale San Raffaele, Milan, Italy; Instituto de Salud Carlos III, Madrid; et al)
J Neurol Neurosurg Psychiatry 61:339–345, 1996   5–10

Background.—Herpes simplex encephalitis (HSE) is a common and serious problem in immunocompetent adults. The presentation of HSE varies, but it is rapidly progressive without treatment. A specific, effective treatment is available in the form of acyclovir, making specific and rapid diagnosis essential. The role of the virology laboratory in the diagnosis of HSE was reviewed.

Laboratory Diagnosis of HSE.—The diagnosis of HSE should be considered in any patient with evidence of acute encephalitis. Although imaging studies, electroencephalogram recordings, and CSF analysis are helpful, they cannot establish an etiologic diagnosis of HSE. Previous studies have shown that the polymerase chain reaction can reliably detect herpes simplex virus (HSV) type 1 or 2 in the CSF. It is the procedure of choice for early etiologic diagnosis of HSE. The polymerase chain reaction can be combined with detection of a specific intrathecal antibody response to HSV for reliable diagnosis and monitoring of patients with HSE. These techniques also can identify atypical manifestations of nervous system HSV infection. They also can be used to evaluate patients with relapsed encephalitis after a first episode of HSE. Once the diagnosis of HSE is made, the patient should immediately receive acyclovir, 10 mg/per kilogram every 8 hours for 10 days.

Discussion.—The virology laboratory plays a key role in the diagnosis of HSE. There is a diagnostic algorithm for patients with suspected HSE (Fig). Polymerase chain reaction can make an early diagnosis of HSE, usually up to 10 days after symptom onset. The diagnosis is supported by the subsequent finding of intrathecal antibody production. Although questions remain about the efficacy of acyclovir treatment, there is no doubt that a prompt etiologic diagnosis and immediate acyclovir therapy provide the best possible clinical outcomes for patients with HSE.

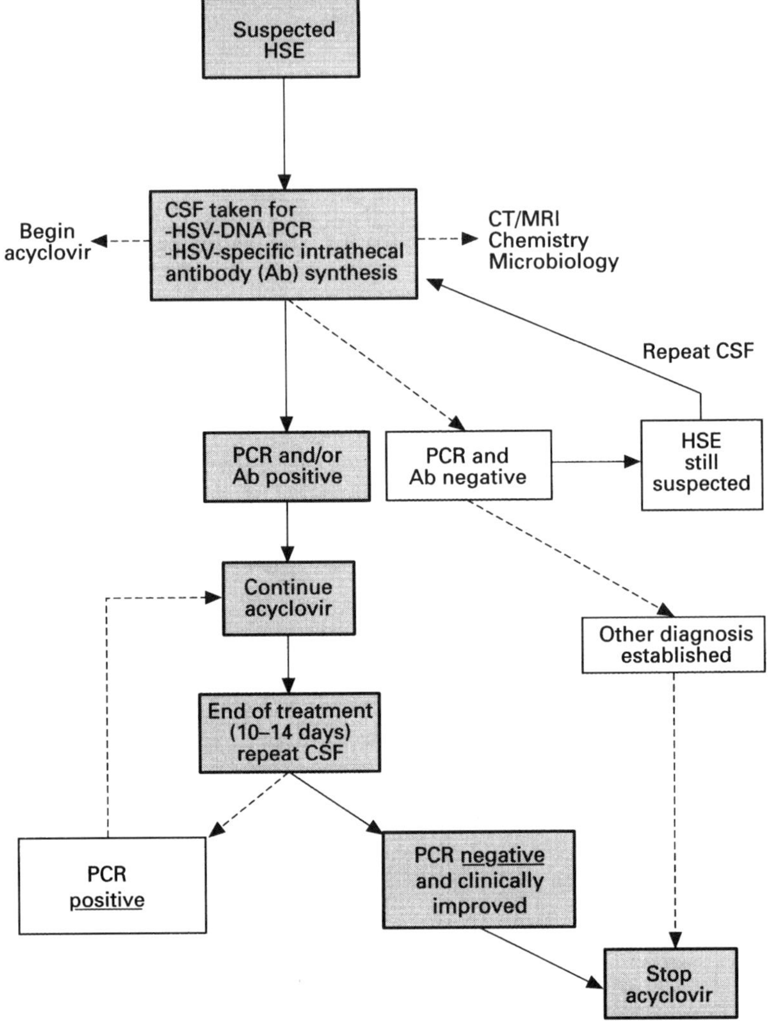

FIGURE.—Diagnostic algorithm for management of patients with suspected herpes simplex encephalitis. Because patients may be seen with raised intracranial pressure, immediate lumbar puncture may not be possible. In these circumstances, start of acyclovir treatment before lumbar puncture is warranted. *Abbreviation: PCR,* polymerase chain reaction. (Courtesy of Cleator GM, for the EU concerted action on virus meningitis and encephalitis: The role of laboratory investigation in the diagnosis and management of patients with suspected herpes simplex encephalitis: A consensus report. *J Neurol Neurosurg Psychiatry* 61:339–345, 1996.)

▶ As the authors express in this consensus statement, before the introduction of polymerase chain reaction, the definitive means of identification of HSV encephalitis was brain biopsy. Twenty years ago, Whitley and colleagues argued strongly that brain biopsy was required at the time of initiating antiviral therapy because of the high frequency of misdiagnosis. Not all practitioners agreed with that recommendation, in large measure because acyclovir is well tolerated and, perhaps, to a smaller degree, because of the evolution of MRI, which has assisted in excluding many diagnoses mistaken for HSV encephalitis. The use of CSF polymerase chain reaction and HSV-specific intrathecal antibody synthesis for the diagnosis of HSV encephalitis has rendered the controversy surrounding the issue of brain biopsy almost moot. The algorithm suggested by the authors appears quite reasonable, although brain biopsy should be incorporated into the diagnostic pathway for those patients whose CSF HSV polymerase chain reaction and specific antibody synthesis are negative and for cases in which no other diagnosis has been established.

J.R. Berger, M.D.

Sinogenic Intracranial Complications
Singh B, van Dellen J, Ramjettan S, et al (Univ of Natal, South Africa)
J Laryngol Otol 109:945–950, 1995   5–11

Background.—Although preventable, purulent sinusitis is associated with a high rate of intracranial complications with a high mortality. A series of 219 patients with intracranial sinusitis complications were described.

Study Group.—From January 1985 to December 1990, 466 patients aged 1–60 years, were seen with sinusitis. Of these, 240 had extracranial complications and 226 had intracranial complications. In this patient group, 22 had meningitis, 17 had extradural empyema, 127 had subdural empyema, 38 had brain abscess, and 15 had combined subdural empyema and brain abscess. The diagnosis of sinusitis and intracranial complications was made by CT, whereas the diagnosis of meningitis was made by culture, microscopy, and chemical investigation of cerebrospinal fluid.

Findings.—The most frequent symptoms at presentation were fever and headache. The most common localizing neurologic sign was hemiparesis. Orbital inflammation was detected in almost half of all patients in this series. Treatment consisted of immediate appropriate antibiotic therapy and surgery, performed within 12 hours of admission. In those patients with meningitis, surgery was performed only on the sinus disease. In those patients with empyema or brain abscess, the primary source of infection was evacuated by the radical frontoethmoidectomy approach after drainage of intracranial pus. The mortality rate was 16%, with the highest rate occurring in patients with meningitis.

Conclusion.—Complications from purulent sinusitis continue to have a high mortality rate. These complications can be prevented with early, appropriate treatment. Only education and recognition of this condition as potentially life-threatening can lower the mortality rate from purulent sinusitis.

▶ This large South African experience reminds us not only of the nature of the intracranial complications of sinusitis, but also of the high mortality rate associated with these conditions. These complications include meningitis, brain abscess, subdural empyema, and epidural empyema. In this series, the most common intracranial complication observed was subdural empyema, which occurred in 65% of the patients, either singly or in combination with brain abscess. However, the highest mortality rate (approaching 50%) was observed in patients with meningitis. Brain abscess, as expected, tended to involve the frontal lobes, and epidural empyemas were often associated with "Pott's puffy tumors," indicative of infection in the frontal sinus. The authors comment that malnutrition, poverty, and poor access to medical care probably contributed to the high prevalence of these disorders in their population.

J.R. Berger, M.D.

6 Epilepsy

Seizure-inducing Effects of Antiepileptic Drugs: A Review
Bauer J (Univ of Bonn, Germany)
Acta Neurol Scand 94:367–377, 1996

6–1

Background.—In patients treated with anti-epileptic drugs (AEDs), the drugs can have seizure-inducing effects. It is important to distinguish this effect from the patient's epilepsy. The various categories of AED-induced seizures were reviewed, along with the differentiation of seizures caused by AEDs vs. epilepsy.

Types of AED-induced Seizures.—Five general categories of AED-induced seizures are identified. They may represent a paradoxical reaction of the drug, such as complex focal seizures caused by carbamazepine, vigabatrin, or phenytoin. Drug-induced seizures may be related to AED-induced encephalopathy, which is common in patients taking valproate for complex focal seizures. Seizures sometimes result from AED intoxication, although this is rare. They may result from the selection of incorrect drugs to treat a given epileptic syndrome or seizure type, as when absences are provoked by carbamazepine or phenytoin. Finally, AED-induced seizures can occur in patients with mixed seizure types, especially those with West's syndrome or Lennox-Gastaut syndrome.

Identifying AED-induced Seizures.—It is essential to differentiate AED-induced seizures from those occurring in the natural course of epilepsy. This distinction can be a particular problem in patients with West's syndrome or Lennox-Gastaut syndrome, whose seizures may vary in frequency with or without AED treatment. In this group, AED-induced seizures may appear as a worsening of seizures. The possibility of AED-induced seizures must be considered when seizures increase after the start of a new therapy or an increase in dosage, or when seizures decline as the AED dosage is tapered and then increase after therapy is restarted.

Seizures may increase in patients with AED encephalopathy caused by valproate or carbamazepine. These 2 drugs are known to provoke generalized seizures in the form of absences or myoclonic seizures. In patients taking vigabatrin, seizures may be related to increased amounts of cerebral gamma-amino-butyric acid. It has been suggested that the sedative effects of AEDs may be responsible for tonic seizures in patients with Lennox-Gastaut syndrome, but this is controversial. Possible risk factors for the development of AED-induced seizures include young age, mental retardation, AED polytherapy, frequent seizures, and prominent epileptic activity in the electroencephalogram before drug treatment.

Discussion.—The problem of AED-induced seizures in patients with epilepsy is reviewed. Knowing about the potential for these effects and the risk factors for them should help to prevent or correct drug-related worsening of seizures.

▶ It is not well recognized that AEDs may induce seizures in certain circumstances. Not infrequently, I encounter this as one of the reasons for lack of seizure control or as the basis of acute loss of control. This article very nicely reviews the major drugs and mechanisms for AEDs inducing seizures.

E. Ramsay, M.D.

Risk of Accidents in Drivers With Epilepsy

Taylor J, Chadwick D, Johnson T (Walton Ctr for Neurology and Neurosurgery, Liverpool, England; Univ Forvie Site, Cambridge, England)
J Neurol Neurosurg Psychiatry 60:621–627, 1996   6–2

Background.—Driving is restricted for individuals with a history of epilepsy. However, very few studies have considered the relative risk of accident rates among such drivers. The risks of road traffic accidents for drivers with a history of single seizures or epilepsy were estimated during a 3-year period.

Methods.—A survey questionnaire eliciting driving and accident experience was completed by 16,958 drivers with a history of epilepsy. A group of 8,888 nonepileptic drivers responded to a Transport Research Laboratory survey.

Findings.—The drivers with a history of epilepsy had no overall increase in risk of accidents compared with the nonepileptic drivers after adjustment for age, sex, driving experience, and mileage. However, the drivers with epilepsy did appear to have an increased risk for more severe accidents. The risk for serious injuries was increased by about 40%. There also was a twofold increase in the risk of nondriver fatalities.

Conclusions.—The eligibility of individuals with epilepsy to drive should be based on the determination of an acceptable risk of accidents resulting in injury or serious injury rather than overall accident rates. Further study is needed to determine the acceptability of relaxing driving restrictions among individuals with a history of epilepsy.

▶ Physicians have to discuss with their patients with epilepsy the basis for driving restrictions. This article reviewed outome in a large group of patients with epilepsy and compared the outcome in the general population. Although the accident rate was not increased, the seriousness of the accident and fatality rate was worse when an accident was caused by a seizure. The laws restricting driving have a reasonable basis, and this article provides a good basis to discuss the issue with patients.

E. Ramsay, M.D.

The Prognostic Value of the Electroencephalogram in Antiepileptic Drug Withdrawal in Partial Epilepsies

Tinuper P, Avoni P, Riva R, et al (Univ of Bologna, Italy)
Neurology 47:76–78, 1996   6–3

Introduction.—There is ongoing controversy as to the prognostic value of the electroencephalogram (EEG) in seizure free patients undergoing withdrawal of antiepileptic drug therapy. Previous studies of this issue have used varying inclusion criteria, length of follow-up, and research methods. The prognostic value of EEG during antiepilephic drug withdrawal in patients with partial epilepsies was evaluated.

Methods.—The study included 120 patients with a history of epileptic partial seizures who had been seizure free for 2 to 6 years and received constant antiepileptic drug therapy. Forty-nine had complex partial seizures with or without episodic secondarily generalized attacks (CPS), 20 had simple partial seizures with or without episodic secondarily generalized attacks, and 51 had only partial secondarily generalized seizures (PSG). All patients underwent repeated EEG examinations before, during, and 3 to 36 months after withdrawal of antiepileptic drug therapy. The relation between the EEG findings and the results of antiepileptic drug withdrawal was evaluated.

Results.—Relapse occurred in 45% of patients with CPS, 100% of those with simple partial seizures, and 65% of those with PSG. The relapse rate was 69% in the 36 patients who had epileptiform EEG findings before the start of drug withdrawal and 60% in those with normal EEG findings. This difference was not significant. However, relapses occurred in 83% of 36 patients in whom the EEG got worse during drug withdrawal, compared with 54% of those whose EEG was unchanged. Further analysis showed that the predictive value of new epileptiform abnormalities occurred mainly in the PSG group.

Conclusions.—In patients who were seizure free with partial epilepsies, EEGs recorded before antiepileptic drug withdrawal cannot predict the response to drug withdrawal. However, a worsening EEG during the drug withdrawal period may predict relapse, particularly in patients with PSG. The finding of previously absent epileptic abnormalities during follow-up signals relapse in most patients with CPS and all patients with PSG.

▶ It is important to identify patients at risk for seizure recurrence when discontinuing therapy. This article found that changes in the EEG after stopping a patient's anticonvulsant drugs and, specifically, the return of epileptiform activity is predictive of return of clinical symptoms. This has been my experience and suggests that recording EEGs before and after discontinuing antiepileptic drugs will help in identifying patients that should resume therapy.

E. Ramsay, M.D.

An Assessment of Nonconvulsive Seizures in the Intensive Care Unit Using Continuous EEG Monitoring: An Investigation of Variables Associated With Mortality

Young GB, Jordan KG, Doig GS (Victoria Hosp, London, Ont, Canada; St Bernardine Med Ctr, San Bernardino, Calif)
Neurology 47:83–89, 1996   6–4

Background.—Continuous EEG (CEEG) may be an excellent method for supplementing single or serial recordings in the detection and management of nonconvulsive seizures, which are common in patients in the neurologic ICU. The factors associated with mortality and morbidity in patients in the neurologic ICU with nonconvulsive seizures and the role of CEEG in patient management were investigated.

Methods and Findings.—Forty-nine patients with nonconvulsive seizures were monitored with CEEG. The overall mortality was 33%. Fifty-nine percent of the 23 patients with nonconvulsive status epilepticus (NCSE) died. Mortality was significantly associated with age, presence of NCSE, seizure duration, hospital and neurologic ICU length of stay, and

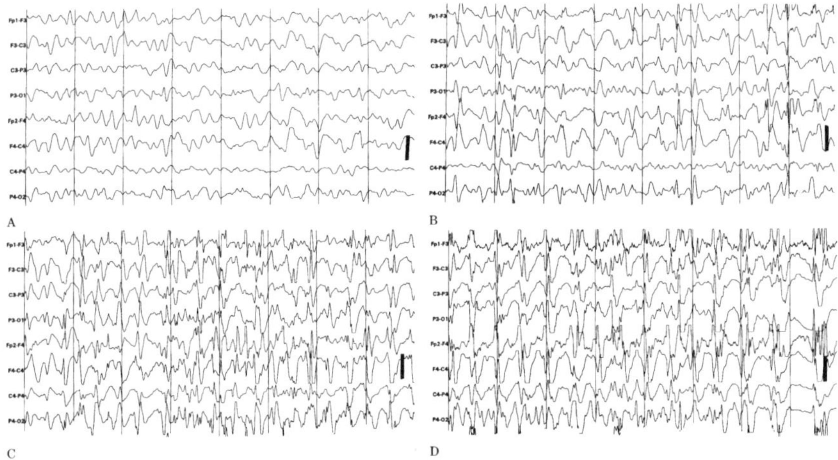

FIGURE 1.—Generalized nonconvulsive status epilepticus in a woman aged 54 years with multi-organ failure. The patient died without recovering consciousness. Between seizures, low-medium voltage posterior rhythms of medium voltage at 5–6 Hz predominated, but slower frequencies were seen in the anterior head, including intermittent delta (**A**). In the seizures (**B through D**), an incrementing pattern of irregular generalized spike-and-wave and sharp-and-slow-wave complexes occurred with poor stereotypy. These could be blocked by diazepam injection. The *thick vertical calibration bar* is 50 µV, and the time interval between the *long, thin vertical lines* is 1 sec. (Courtesy of Young GB, Jordan KG, Doig GS: An assessment of nonconvulsive seizures in the intensive care unit using continuous EEG monitoring: An investigation of variables associated with mortality. Reprinted from *Neurology* Vol. 47, pp. 83–89, 1996 by permission of Little, Brown and Company Inc.)

delay to diagnosis and etiology. In a multivariate logistic regression analysis, the only factors associated with increased mortality were seizure duration and delay to diagnosis. When consciousness impairment arose from the initial illness, the classification system of absence, simple, or complex partial status epilepticus was not adequate for acute symptomatic cases (Fig 1).

Conclusions.—Duration of NCSE and delayed diagnosis are strongly associated with mortality. Mortality also is highly correlated with etiology and seizure duration. Seizures can be detected more readily and their spread examined with CEEG.

▶ Nonconvulsive status epilepticus also has been called subtle status because the usual obvious motor manifestations are absent. This article reports the outcome in patients found in an ICU to have nonconvulsive seizures, half of which were in status epilepticus. Many patients are seen with an identified epileptic seizure and a persisting impairment of consciousness. Persisting coma secondary to continued cortical seizure activity may be underappreciated by the treating physician.

This article found that morbidity and mortality increased with seizure duration regardless of underlying etiology. The results of this article strongly support the early use of electroencephalograms in the evaluation of patients in the ICU with impaired consciousness.

E. Ramsay, M.D.

Serum Prolactin Concentrations Are Elevated After Syncope
Oribe E, Amini R, Nissenbaum E, et al (Catholic Med Ctr of Brooklyn and Queens, Jamaica, NY)
Neurology 47:60–62, 1996   6–5

Background.—It can be difficult to distinguish between syncope and epileptic seizures. Ancillary tests are sometimes needed. Previous reports suggest that serum prolactin (PRL) concentration is elevated after generalized and complex partial seizures. Reports of serum PRL after syncope have given variable results. The effects of syncope on serum PRL were prospectively evaluated.

Methods.—The study included 21 patients with a history of near fainting or syncope. All were referred for passive 60–degree head-up tilt testing. The test lasted for 45 minutes or until syncope occurred, defined as a decrease in blood pressure accompanied by symptoms and signs of reduced cerebral perfusion with transient or near loss of consciousness. Blood samples were obtained for measurement of serum PRL concentration.

Results.—Eleven patients had syncope and hypotension (mean arterial pressure, 51 mm Hg) during head-up tilt testing. Nine patients had PRL concentrations elevated above 19 ng/mL, peaking within the first 30 minutes after the onset of syncope. The mean PRL value in this group was 11 ng/mL in the supine position, increasing to 52 ng/mL after syncope. The 10

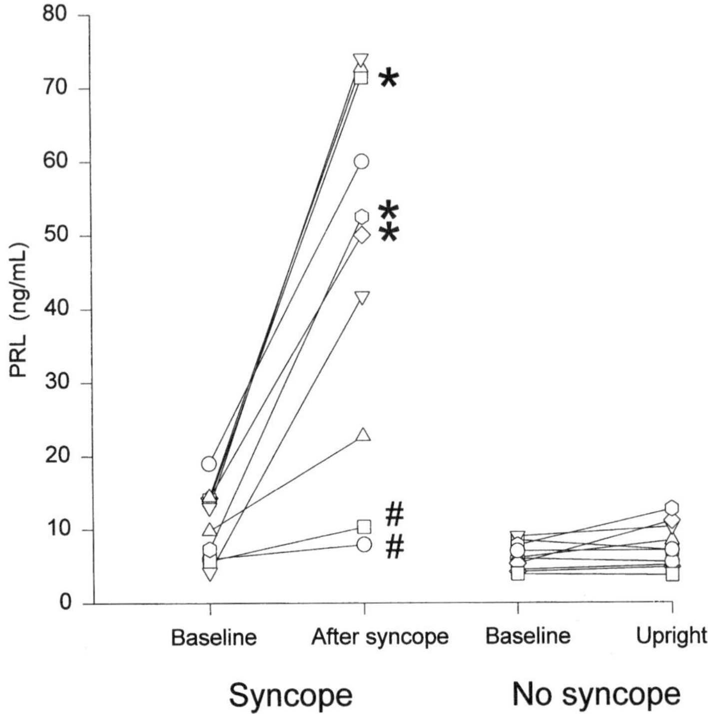

FIGURE 2.—Serum prolactin (*PRL*) concentrations before (baseline) and after syncope in patients with tilt-induced syncope (*Syncope*) and during baseline and upright tilt in patients with a normal response (*No syncope*) to upright tilt.* Patients who had "anoxic seizures" during syncope; # patients with hypotension lasting less than 1 minute. (Courtesy of Oribe E, Amini R, Nissenbaum E, et al: Serum prolactin concentrations are elevated after syncope. (Reprinted from *Neurology*, Vol. 47, pp. 60–62, 1996 by permission of Little, Brown and Company Inc.)

patients with a normal head-up tilt test had no significant change in PRL (Fig 2). Serum PRL measurement had a sensitivity of 82% and a specificity of 100%.

Conclusions.—Patients with hypotensive syncope show an increase in serum PRL concentration. The increase is similar to that observed after epileptic seizures, suggesting that serum PRL measurement will not be useful in differentiating seizures from nonepileptic attacks. It still can be a useful test to differentiate epileptic seizures and syncope from pseudoseizures, which are not associated with any change in serum PRL.

▶ After an epileptic seizure, serum PRL levels have been shown to rise dramatically and return back to baseline within 1 to 2 hours. The transient rise in prolactin levels has been used as a diagnostic tool to differentiate epileptic from non-epileptic attacks. This article very nicely establishes that PRL elevations can be produced by transient cerebral hypoperfusion and are not specific for seizures. This raised the question whether other neurologic disorders such as migraines could trigger the same transient change in PRL levels.

E. Ramsay, M.D.

The Risk of Seizure Recurrence After a First Unprovoked Afebrile Seizure in Childhood: An Extended Follow-Up
Shinnar S, Berg AT, Moshe SL, et al (Albert Einstein College of Medicine, Bronx, NY; Northern Illinois Univ, DeKalb; Columbia College of Physicians and Surgeons, New York)
Pediatrics 98:216–225, 1996   6–6

Background.—The long-term recurrence risks and prognosis in children experiencing a first unprovoked seizure have not been well documented. The authors previously reported the short-term outcomes of a cohort of children followed prospectively for a mean of 2.5 years after first seizures. A larger cohort monitored for a mean 6.3 years was reported.

Methods and Findings.—Four hundred seven children were included. Forty-two percent had subsequent seizures. The cumulative risk of seizure recurrence was 29% at 1 year, 37% at 2 years, 42% at 5 years, and 44% at 8 years (Fig 1). The median time to recurrence was 5.7 months. Fifty-three percent of recurrences occurred within 6 months, 69% within 1 year, and 88% within 2 years. Only 3% of the recurrences happened after 5 years. Multivariate analysis indicated that remote symptomatic etiology, abnormal electroencephalogram (EEG), seizure occurring during sleep, history of febrile seizures, and Todd's paresis were risk factors for seizure

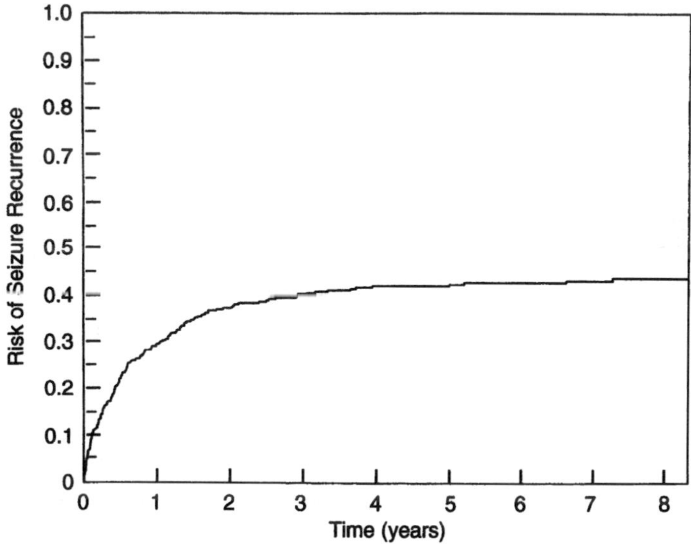

FIGURE 1.—Probability of seizure recurrence after a first unprovoked seizure (*n* = 407): Kaplan-Meier curve. (Reproduced by permission of *Pediatrics*, Vol 98, Pages 216–225, Copyright 1996.)

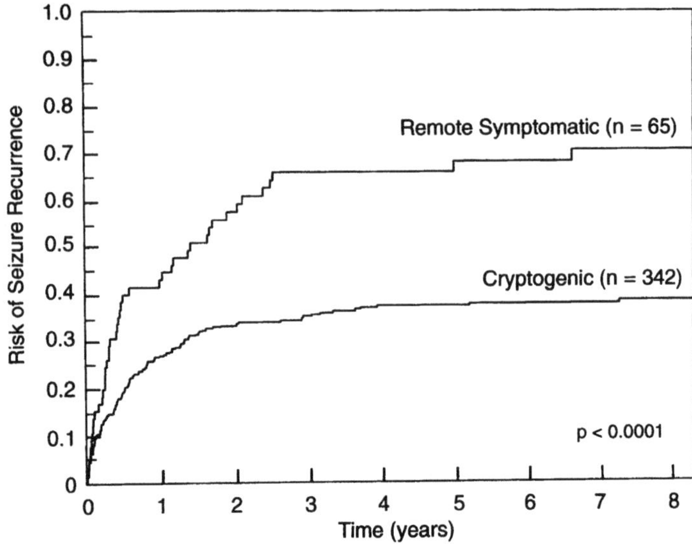

FIGURE 2.—Probability of seizure recurrence after cryptogenic and remote symptomatic first seizures (*n* = 407): Kaplan-Meier curve. (Reproduced by permission of *Pediatrics*, Vol 98, Pages 216–225, Copyright 1996.)

recurrence. In patients with cryptogenic seizures, abnormal EEG and initial seizure during sleep were the risk factors for recurrence. In patients with remote symptomatic seizures, the risk factors for recurrence were a history of febrile seizures and age of onset younger than 3 years. Etiology,

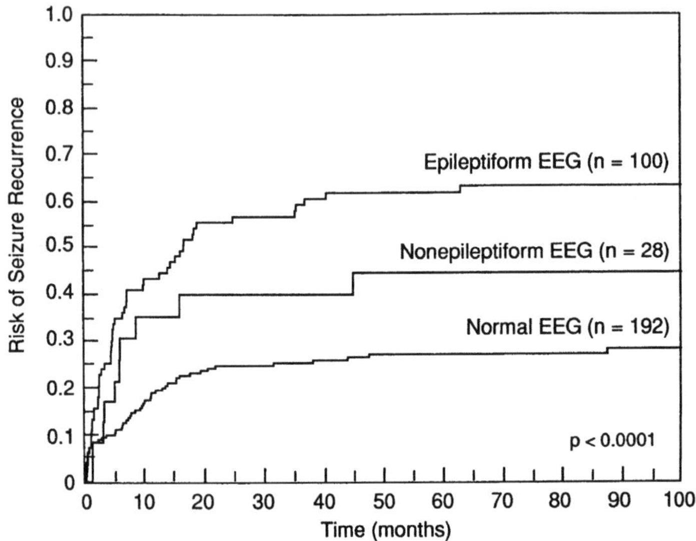

FIGURE 3.—Probability of seizure recurrence after a cryptogenic first seizure as a function of the electroencephalogram (*n* = 320): Kaplan-Meier curve. *Abbreviation: EEG*, electroencephalogram. (Reproduced by permission of *Pediatrics*, Vol 98, Pages 216–225, Copyright 1996.)

an abnormal EEG, previous febrile seizures in the overall group, and an abnormal EEG in the cryptogenic group were the risk factors for recurrences after 2 years. These risk factors are similar to those for early recurrence (Figs 2 and 3).

Conclusions.—More than half of the children with an initial unprovoked seizure do not have recurrences. Prognosis is particularly good for children with cryptogenic first seizures and a normal EEG whose initial seizure occurs while awake. The 5-year recurrence risk in this subgroup is only 21%. Late recurrences are uncommon.

▶ A recurring issue in child neurology has been the rational decision of whom to treat among those children who present with a first unprovoked afebrile seizure. Related to this is the question of how long these children, left untreated, are at risk for seizure recurrence. Shinnar and colleagues have performed the longest and most comprehensive follow-up of such children to date. Their findings bear on both the need to treat after the initial seizure and the duration of the "at-risk" period after this event. Furthermore, they dissect from this global picture risk factors that should influence decision making in this commonly encountered and critically important arena.

N. Schor, M.D.

Lamotrigine for the Treatment of Epilepsy in Childhood
Besag FMC, Wallace SJ, Dulac O, et al (St Piers Lingfield, England; Univ Hosp of Wales, Cardiff; Hôpital Saint Vincent de Paul, Paris; et al)
J Pediatr 127:991–997, 1995   6–7

Background.—Lamotrigine is an established adjunctive antiepileptic drug for adults. To determine its usefulness in pediatric patients, 5 multicenter, open-label, 12-month studies were performed with the study group consisting of children who had refractory epilepsy.

Methods.—Two hundred eighty-five children with refractory epilepsy were recruited from 37 medical centers in 11 countries. All studies used an open design in which lamotrigine was added to existing medication for 48 weeks, after a 3-month baseline period. The lamotrogine dose was individualized to the patient based on body weight and other therapy and then readjusted according to clinical response and adverse reactions. Data from all studies was pooled for this analysis. Seizure frequency and type were evaluated every 12 weeks.

Results.—Of the 285 patients initially recruited for this study, 249 received lamotrigine for at least 12 weeks, and 126 completed the 48-week study. The reasons for withdrawal were lack of benefit in 60 patients, adverse experience in 36, and withdrawal for reasons not related to the study medication in 21. Seizure frequency was reduced by at least 50% in one third of the patients in the study group. Lamotrigine was effective in reducing seizure frequency of all types, particularly typical and atypical

absence seizures and atonic seizures. Those children who also took valproate had to take lower doses of lamotrigine than the other children. The
most common adverse reactions were somnolence, rash, vomiting, and
seizure exacerbation. Rash was the most common adverse reaction leading
to treatment withdrawal, but all rashes resolved after discontinuation of
therapy.

Conclusion.—The results of this large, open-label, multicenter study of
lamotrigine as adjunctive treatment for children with refractive epilepsy
indicate that lamotrigine is well-tolerated and effective in the treatment of
many types of seizures.

▶ Lamotrigine has been approved in the United States as adjunctive therapy
in partial epilepsy. Clinical experience has suggested that the spectrum of
efficacy includes the primary generalized epilepsies and other childhood
syndromes. This paper, reporting outcome in 285 children, provides additional evidence for this, with improved control observed in absence, generalized tonic-clonic, myoclonic, and atonic seizures. Lamotrigine holds the
promise of becoming a very significant addition in the treatment of many
types of childhood seizures. Rash is the most important side effect. This
paper shows that the occurrence of rash is dependent on the rate of dosage
increase and can be reduced by a slow introduction and titration.

E. Ramsay, M.D.

**"Pseudo-BECRS": Intracranial Focal Lesions Suggestive of a Primary
Partial Epilepsy Syndrome**
Shevell MI, Rosenblatt B, Watters GV, et al (Montreal Children's Hosp;
McGill Univ, Montreal)
Pediatr Neurol 14:31–35, 1996   6–8

Background.—Benign epilepsy of childhood with rolandic spikes
(BECRS), an electroclinical entity, is the most common primary partial
epilepsy syndrome in children. Onset typically occurs between 3 and 13
years of age. It is characterized by an easily recognized seizure pattern in
a normal child, with electroencephalographic (EEG) findings limited to the
rolandic/centrotemporal regions. Seizures are usually easy to control, and
prognosis is thought to be good. Some authorities suggest that neuroimaging is not needed in patients whose findings are consistent with the
electroclinical parameters of this entity. The current report suggests that in
some patients, a negative neuroimaging study may be essential to accurately diagnose BECRS.

Patients and Findings.—The patients, 4 boys aged 7–13 years and 1 girl
aged 5 years, were seen during a 13-year period. The patients had peribuc-
cal seizures, normal neurologic evaluations, and EEG data initially suggesting BECRS. However, neuroimaging demonstrated focal lesions. Three
children had independent bilateral centrotemporal epileptiform abnormalities. In all children, CT and/or MRI showed a mass lesion in various

locations. On histologic assessment, low-grade astrocytoma was documented in 3 patients and a cavernous angioma in 1. Treatment and biopsy for the fifth patient were refused.

Conclusions.—These children had an electroclinical phenotype initially suggesting BECRS but atypical clinical features that raised the possibility of an underlying structural lesion. Thus in some patients, a negative neuroimaging study may be necessary to accurately diagnose BECRS.

▶ It is not cost-effective to request neuroimaging when evaluating children with typical clinical and electroencephalographic features of benign rolandic epilepsy, especially when other family members have a similar history. Five children are reported who were initially diagnosed with benign rolandic epilepsy and who were later shown to have symptomatic epilepsy: low-grade gliomas in 4 and a cavernous angioma in 1. Cranial MRI is indicated when the clinical features are not typical or the seizures are difficult to control. A delay in the diagnosis of a low-grade glioma in a child is not critical.

G.M. Fenichel, M.D.

Epilepsy and Attention Deficit Hyperactivity Disorder: Is Methylphenidate Safe and Effective?

Gross-Tsur V, Manor O, van der Meere J, et al (Hadassah-Hebrew Univ, Jerusalem; Univ of Gröningen, The Netherlands)
J Pediatr 130:40–44, 1997   6–9

Purpose.—Epilepsy and attention deficit hyperactivity disorder (ADHD) are both common among children. The rate of ADHD among children with epilepsy may be higher than 20%. The use of methylphenidate and other psychostimulants in children with this dual diagnosis is not accepted therapy. The safety and efficacy of methylphenidate for children with epilepsy and ADHD were evaluated.

Methods.—The study included 30 children with the dual diagnosis of epilepsy and ADHD. The age range was 6 to 16 years. The children received 2 months of treatment with anti-epileptic drugs (AED) only, followed by 2 more of treatment with AEDs plus a morning dose of 0.3 mg methylphenidate per kilogram. At baseline and before the start of methylphenidate treatment, the patients had neurologic assessment, brain CT, intelligence quotient testing, and evaluation on the Childhood Behavior Checklist. At baseline and after the end of methylphenidate treatment, they had an electroencephalogram (EEG), AED determinations, and testing on a continuous performance task. In addition, a 2-day, double-blind, crossover study was done to compare the effects of methylphenidate and placebo on EEG, AED levels, and continuous performance task.

Results.—Without methylphenidate, 25 children were seizure free and the other 5 had no more than 5 seizures per week. None of the children who were seizure free without methylphenidate had seizures with methylphenidate. Three of the other 5 children had increased seizures while taking methylphenidate. The parents believed that methylphenidate was beneficial in 70% of cases. Methylphenidate treatment did not alter the AED levels or EEG findings, and it improved performance on the continuous performance task. Only mild, transient side effects of methylphenidate were noted.

Conclusions.—The effects of methylphenidate treatment in children with the dual diagnosis of epilepsy and ADHD were studied. Methylphenidate is safe and effective in children who are seizure free on their AED treatment. It should be used cautiously in children who are still having seizures. In this situation, the behavioral and achievement benefits possible with methylphenidate must be weighed against the risk of further seizures.

▶ A large percentage of children with epilepsy also have ADHD. High doses of the stimulant drugs used to treat ADHD lower the seizure threshold and may produce convulsive seizures. Untreated ADHD can be more disabling than the infrequent occurrence of seizures. My experience has been that uses of recommended doses does not affect seizure control. However, the product information in the Physicians' Desk Reference lists "in the presence of seizures, the drug should be discontinued." This study addresses this major concern and found that a dose of methylphenidate effective in ADHD did not precipitate seizures.

E. Ramsay, M.D.

High-resolution Surface-coil MR of Cortical Lesions in Medically Refractory Epilepsy: A Prospective Study
Grant PE, Barkovich AJ, Wald LL, et al (Univ of California, San Francisco)
AJNR 18:291–301, 1997   6–10

Introduction.—Patients whose epilepsy does not respond to drug treatment are candidates for surgery. Magnetic resonance imaging plays a key role in identifying the apparent epileptogenic area. The MRI detection of multiple or large cortical abnormalities is a bad prognostic sign. High-resolution volumetric MRI can improve the visibility of focal cortical abnormalities. Whether adding surface coils to high-resolution MRI could improve the ability to identify the suspected epileptogenic zone in patients with medically refractory epilepsy was studied.

Methods.—The prospective study included 25 patients with neocortical partial epilepsy that had failed to respond to drug treatment. Each patient underwent 2 MRI studies: once with standard head coils and once with high-resolution phased-array surface coils designed specifically for evaluation of cortical lesions. The imaging studies were reviewed by 2 neuroradiologists to assess their ability to demonstrate cortical lesions. In combination with surface electroencephalogram (EEG), the MRI studies were evaluated for their ability to locate the suspected epileptogenic zone.

Results.—The surface-coil MRI studies showed 4 additional lesions that were not detected by the standard head-coil studies. The probable diagnosis was changed as a result of the surface-coil studies in 5 patients, and the epileptogenic zone was better defined in 4. Eleven patients had lobar abnormalities on EEG—surface-coil imaging demonstrated focal cortical abnormalities within the same or an adjacent lobe in 5 patients and multifocal abnormalities in 2. Six patients had abnormalities in 2 adjacent lobes only on EEG—surface-coil MRI showed focal cortical abnormalities in a single lobe in 5 of these patients and multifocal abnormalities in 1. Imaging revealed focal cortical abnormalities in 5 of 8 patients with nonfocal findings on EEG, and multifocal abnormalities in another. Seizure localization was enhanced by video/EEG telemetry in 2 of 13 patients. Of the other 11 patients in this group, surface-coil MRI revealed focal cortical lesions in 6 and provided useful prognostic information in 5.

Conclusions.—For most patients with medically refractory epilepsy, surface-coil imaging is more effective than standard head-coil MRI in detecting and differentiating focal cortical lesions. In the authors' experience, the combination surface-coil imaging and EEG provides better localization of the epileptogenic zone or useful additional prognostic information in 85% of patients. In the other 15% of patients, localization is improved by video/EEG telemetry. Surface-coil MRI may prove useful in the evaluation of patients with neocortical partial epilepsy.

▶ Ten percent to 20% of patients with epilepsy are considered to be medically refractory. In this group, resective surgery can be considered, with the best outcome found in those patients with well-defined cortical lesions. My experience has been the same as reported in this study: higher-resolution MRIs and new sequencing protocols have significantly improved our ability to identify focal lesions. This will allow us to offer surgery as a treatment option and also to improve the outcome. High-resolution MRI is the imaging study of preference in the evaluation of the patient with epilepsy.

E. Ramsay, M.D.

7 Pediatric Neurology

Long-term Prognosis of Typical Childhood Absence Epilepsy: Remission or Progression to Juvenile Myoclonic Epilepsy
Wirrell EC, Camfield CS, Camfield PR, et al (IWK Hosp for Children, Halifax, NS, Canada)
Neurology 47:912–918, 1996　　　　　　　　　　　　　　　　　7–1

Background.—Childhood absence epilepsy (CAE), characterized by numerous absence seizures per day, typically occurs in otherwise healthy children of school age. The peak age of onset is 6–7 years. Classic electroencephalography (EEG) findings are bilateral, synchronous, symmetric 3-Hz spike-and-wave discharges with normal background rhythms. Most children have remission of the seizures, but generalized tonic-clonic seizures develop in one third to one half of patients, usually during adolescence. An estimated 2.8% to 7.5% of children with an initial diagnosis of CAE progress to juvenile myoclonic epilepsy (JME). To date, no one has determined whether certain factors at the time of absence seizure onset or during the course of CAE can identify children at risk for progression to JME.

Methods and Findings.—Centralized EEG records for Nova Scotia were searched to identify all children with a diagnosis of typical CAE between 1977 and 1985. Seventy-two of 81 children with CAE (89%) could be contacted for follow-up. The mean age at seizure onset was 5.7 years, with a range of 1–14 years. The mean follow-up was 20.4 years. At follow-up, 65% were in remission. Another 17% were not taking anti-epileptic drugs (AEDs) but continued to have seizures. Eighteen percent were taking AEDs. Five of these 13 children had been seizure free in the past year. Overall, 15% of the children had progressed to JME. Factors that predicted no remission were cognitive problems at diagnosis, absence status before or during AED therapy, development of generalized tonic-clonic or myoclonic seizures after AED implementation, abnormal background on initial EEG, and a family history of generalized seizures in first-degree relatives.

Conclusion.—Remission occurred in only 65% of these children initially diagnosed as having CAE. Juvenile myoclonic epilepsy developed in 44% of those without remission. Accurately predicting remission at the time of diagnosis is difficult in most patients. The development of generalized tonic-clonic seizures or myoclonic seizures during AED therapy, however, is ominous, predicting lack of CAE remission and progression to JME.

▶ Childhood absence epilepsy, or petit mal epilepsy, has long been held by common wisdom to be a benign disorder, typically outgrown by adulthood. Child neurologists have been aware of a subgroup of somewhere between 30% and 50% of these patients who stop having absence seizures but who begin having generalized tonic-clonic seizures in adolescence.

This study identified all children with a diagnosis of typical CAE between 1977 and 1985 in Nova Scotia and asked how many of them were seizure free and without medication 10 years later. Given the outlook of child neurologists, it is not surprising that only 65% of these patients met criteria for remission of their epilepsy. What this paper adds that is new is the finding that 44% of those not in remission met diagnostic criteria for juvenile myoclonic epilepsy, rather than purely generalized tonic-clonic seizures, and the definition of predictors of nonremission. This latter included the development of myoclonic or tonic-clonic seizures while the patients were taking anticonvulsants, and abnormal EEG background at the time of diagnosis.

N.F. Schor, M.D., Ph.D.

Cerebral Infarction and Antiphospholipid Syndrome in Children

Baca V, Garcia-Ramirez R, Ramirez-Lacayo M, et al (Centro Medico Nacional Siglo XXI, Mexico City)
J Rheumatol 23:1428–1431, 1996   7–2

Background.—A clinical syndrome with widespread arterial and venous thrombosis associated with antibodies directed against phospholipids

TABLE 1.—Demographic Data and Results of Anticardiolipin Antibody and Protein C Determinations in Children With Cerebral Infarct

Patient	Age/Sex (yrs)	aCL Determinations*				Protein C Determinations† (%)	
		1st	2nd	3rd	4th	1st	2nd
		IgG/IgM	IgG/IgM	IgG/IgM	IgG/IgM		
1	13.00/M	Neg/mod				106	ND
2	15.75/M	Mod/neg	Neg/neg	Neg/neg		95	ND
3	1.50/M	Neg/mod	Neg/neg	Neg/high	Neg/neg	70	ND
4	8.00/M	Neg/neg	Neg/neg			ND	ND
5	15.00/F	Neg/mod	Neg/mod	Neg/neg		117	ND
6	1.50/M	Mod/high	Neg/neg	Neg/neg	Neg/mod	83	ND
7	2.08/F	Mod/neg	Neg/mod			78	ND
8	5.50/F	High/neg	Neg/neg	Neg/neg		86	ND
9	0.41/F	Neg/neg	Neg/neg	Neg/neg		50	70
10	5.33/F	Neg/neg				37	95

*The lapse between each anticardiolipin antibody (*aCL*) determination was 3–6 months. Anticardiolipin antibodies were expressed in GPL and MPL units: *neg* = negative (< 10 GPL or MPL); *mod* = moderate (20–100 GPL, 20–60 MPL); high (> 100 GPL, > 60 MPL).

†Normal protein C activity 66-129%. ND = not done.

(Courtesy of Baca V, Garcia-Ramirez R, Ramirez-Lacayo M, et al: Cerebral infarction and antiphospholipid syndrome in children. *J Rheumatol* 23:1428–1431, 1996.)

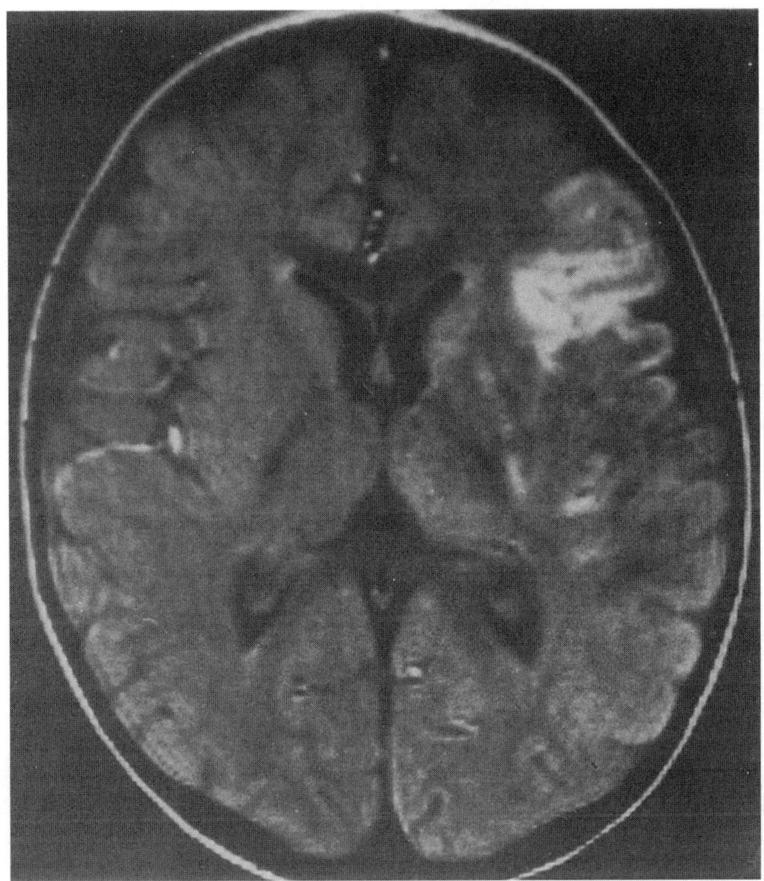

FIGURE 1.—Brain MRI shows an area of increased signal that follows the brain cortex, compatible with hemorrhagic infarct of the left temporoparietal region in a T1-weighted image. (Courtesy of Baca V, Garcia-Ramirez R, Ramirez-Lacayo M, et al: Cerebral infarction and antiphospholipid syndrome in children. *J Rheumatol* 23:1428–1431, 1996.)

(aPL) was described 15 years ago by Hughes et al. The neurologic abnormalities associated with aPL include multiple cerebral infarcts, encephalopathy, migraine-like headaches, visual abnormalities, and transverse myelitis. The most common manifestation of primary antiphospholipid syndrome is stroke. In patients with this condition, strokes are often recurrent and accompanied by transient ischemic attacks and retinal occlusive events. The prevalence of aPL in children with acute cerebral infarction was investigated.

Methods.—Ten consecutive patients, aged 0.4–15.7 years, were assessed in the first days of neurologic symptoms. The patients were 5 girls and 5 boys seen between 1992 and 1994. Prospective assessment was continued for 15.7 months.

Findings.—Seven patients had acute cerebral infarction associated with anticardiolipin antibodies (aCL). Four patients had high serum aCL levels in 2 different assessments. Temporary protein C deficiency was noted in 2 patients. Protein C and S and antithrombin III determinations were not performed in 1 patient with negative aCL, and there was no other evidence of coagulopathy in the patients. None of the patients had evidence of connective tissue disease or a family history of hypercoagulable state. After 15.7 months of follow-up, none of the children had recurrent infarction while taking aspirin (Table 1 and Fig 1B).

Conclusion.—Clinicians must identify antiphospholipid syndrome as an underlying cause of hypercoagulability in children with cerebral infarcts. Aspirin therapy may be effective in preventing recurrences.

▶ The adult neurology literature is replete with references to cerebrovascular disease in the face of lupus anticoagulants and antiphospholipid antibodies. The pediatric literature is somewhat less convincing in this regard, and most children with strokes are left without a definitive etiologic diagnosis. This study evaluates 10 children prospectively for almost 2 years from the time of their stroke. Seventy percent of these children had positive results of an aCL test at the time of their stroke. Antibody determinations fluctuated over the next 2 years in all children, although none of the children who were initially (i.e., in the acute poststroke period) negative converted to positive.

This study makes clear the need for determination of aPLs in all children with cryptogenic stroke and for studies to determine the optimum treatment modalities for aPL-associated stroke. It further emphasizes the critical nature of the timing of such determinations and the virtue of studying children for aPLs in the acute poststroke period.

N.F. Schor, M.D., Ph.D.

Treatment of Four Siblings With Progressive Myoclonus Epilepsy of the Unverricht-Lundborg Type With *N*-Acetylcysteine

Hurd RW, Wilder BJ, Helveston WR, et al (Gainesville Veterans Affairs Med Ctr, Fla; Univ of Florida, Gainesville)
Neurology 47:1264–1268, 1996   7–3

Background.—Patients with progressive myoclonus epilepsy of the Unverricht-Lundborg type (PME-UL) have spontaneous stimulus-sensitive and action myoclonus together with tonic-clonic seizures and cerebellar signs. This is an autosomal recessive condition that usually appears between 8 and 13 years of age. The patients have only mild dementia, but the rate of neurologic deterioration increases if phenytoin is given. The locus for PME-UL is on chromosome 21q22.3, and a candidate gene has been identified. The putative gene product has sodium channel proteins, as well as other homologies with sodium channels and other transmembrane proteins. The authors have found a marked increase in extracellular superoxide dismutase activity in patients with PME-UL. The activities of the sulfhydryl antioxidant *N*-acetylcysteine (NAC) include diminution of H_2O_2 production and scavenging of hydroxyl radicals. Patients with PME-UL received experimental treatment with NAC.

Methods.—The study included 4 siblings with PME-UL, aged 33–39 years. The 2 younger patients, who were more ambulatory, were first given NAC at a dose of 2 g twice a day. After 3 weeks, this was increased to 2 g three times a day. Treatment led to rapid improvement in many areas, including seizure control, mental alertness, ability to vocalize, and patient sense of well being. The subjective improvements were reflected by changes in the objective measurement of giant somatosensory evoked potentials. Treatment was then extended to the other 2 patients. The improvements persisted for up to 30 months after reaching a plateau. There were few side effects.

Discussion.—Treatment with the antioxidant NAC may bring subjective and objective improvement in patients with PME-UL. This treatment may be useful in other neurodegenerative conditions in which excessive free radical production plays a role in disease progression. Future studies are needed to tell whether early treatment with NAC can modify the course of the disease.

▶ Progressive myoclonus epilepsy is a collection of disorders characterized by nervous system degeneration accompanied by progressive polymyoclonia and dementia. The type first described by Unverricht and Lundborg is inherited in an autosomal recessive fashion and is characterized pathologically by the absence of the inclusion bodies invariably seen in other forms of this disorder. The Unverricht and Lundborg is most often seen in late childhood or early adolescence. Although recent studies have shown that the gene for PME-UL is located on chromosome 21q22.3, the specific gene and gene product responsible for this disease remain unknown.

Based on the finding of markedly increased levels of superoxide dismutase in patients with PME-UL, these authors indirectly tested the hypothesis that toxic free radicals play a role in the progression of the disease. They demonstrated in a single kindred that NAC, a free radical scavenger and glutathione precursor, slows the progression of PME-UL. The authors, therefore, speculate that the pathogenesis of PME-UL involves free radical toxicity. It is curious, in light of these findings, that patients with this disorder apparently demonstrate a decline in function from phenytoin, but not from valproate, given that both drugs have free radical–generating metabolites.

N.F. Schor, M.D., Ph.D.

Magnetoencephalographical Analysis of Focal Cortical Heterotopia

Minami T, Tasaki K, Yamamoto T, et al (Kyushu Univ, Fukuoka, Japan)
Dev Med Child Neurol 38:945–949, 1996   7–4

Background.—One of the most important causes of intractable epileptic seizures is focal cortical heterotopia. Although imaging modalities such as MRI can demonstrate the morphologic lesions of cortical heterotopia, they cannot be used for reliable functional assessment. The anatomical relationship between a lesion and epileptic foci must be determined precisely to develop an appropriate surgical strategy. The value of magnetoencephalography (MEG) for focal cortical heterotopia was illustrated.

Case Report.—Man, 20, underwent MEG recordings after receiving a diagnosis of epilepsia partialis continua. Studies were performed in a magnetically shielded room using a 37-channel first order gradiometer system. The magnetic fields of the brain were analyzed by the dipole method, in which small equivalent current dipoles are considered a source of the brain's electric currents. The estimated spike dipoles located in a limited frontocentral region corresponded to the cortical heterotopia on MRI (Fig 3).

Conclusion.—In patients with focal cortical heterotopia, the combination of MEG and MRI, in which the neuromagnetic source localizations are superimposed on MRI, clearly shows the 3-dimensional localization of epileptic foci. Thus, MEG appears to be a promising tool for routine clinical use, although further careful assessment of the technique is needed.

▶ One of the most difficult aspects of the surgical treatment of focal seizures is the determination before surgery of the precise localization of the origin of the seizures relative to the anatomical lesions presumably responsible for them. Such a determination is critical to maximization of the efficacy of the surgery and to avoiding the need for repeated operations in seizure patients. This paper describes the use of a novel technique—magnetoencephalography—which provides corollary anatomical and electrophysiologic information for the spatial identification of seizure foci and which is used here specifically in a patient with congenital focal cortical heterotopia.

N.F. Schor, M.D., Ph.D.

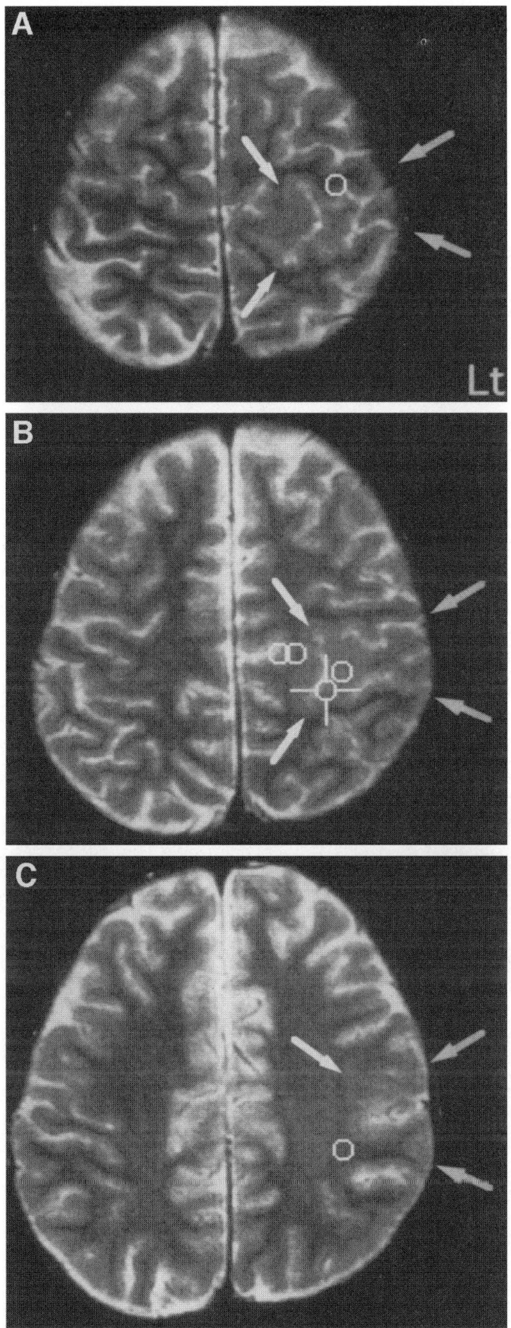

FIGURE 3.—Equivalent current dipoles of spike foci superimposed on patient's MR image. *Open circles* indicate localization of spike foci with correlation of higher than 0.99. T2–weighted MR imaging revealed focal cortical heterotopia, i.e., a focally thickened cortex exhibiting isointensity as to normal gray matter in left frontocentral white matter region (*arrows*). Spike dipoles are located only around this cortical heterotopia. (Courtesy of Minami T, Tasaki K, Yamamoto T, et al: Magnetoencephalographical analysis of focal cortical heterotopia. *Dev Med Child Neurol* 38:945–949, 1996.)

Survival at 5 Years of a Cohort of Newborn Infants With Myelomeningocele

Worley G, Schuster JM, Oakes WJ (Duke Univ, Durham, NC)
Dev Med Child Neurol 38:816–822, 1996   7–5

Background.—Comprehensive management of the medical problems seen in children with myelomeningocele has recently become accepted. Brain stem dysfunction from a Chiari type II malformation is now the most common cause of death in these patients. Between 1981 and 1990, closure of the spinal lesion was performed in all viable neonates at Duke University Medical Center. All patients received comprehensive management. Brain stem decompression was performed in all infants in whom life-threatening brain stem dysfunction developed from a Chiari type II malformation. Survival at 5 years is reported.

Methods.—Sixty-three viable neonates with myelomeningocele were referred to this medical center. A ventriculoperitoneal shunt was placed in 62 infants. Symptoms of brain stem dysfunction developed in 15 patients at a median of 3 months. Brain stem decompression was performed in 11 of the 15 patients because their symptoms appeared life-threatening. Follow-up information was collected for all 63 patients.

Results.—The probability of survival of infants with brain stem dysfunction was lower than that of infants without brain stem dysfunction (Fig 1). The distribution of levels of spinal lesions and the male/female ratio were similar for patients in whom symptoms developed and those in whom they did not. Promptness of decompression after the onset of symptoms and survival were not significantly correlated.

Discussion.—In these infants, brain stem decompression performed at a median of 8 months of age after a 3-month period of symptoms did not

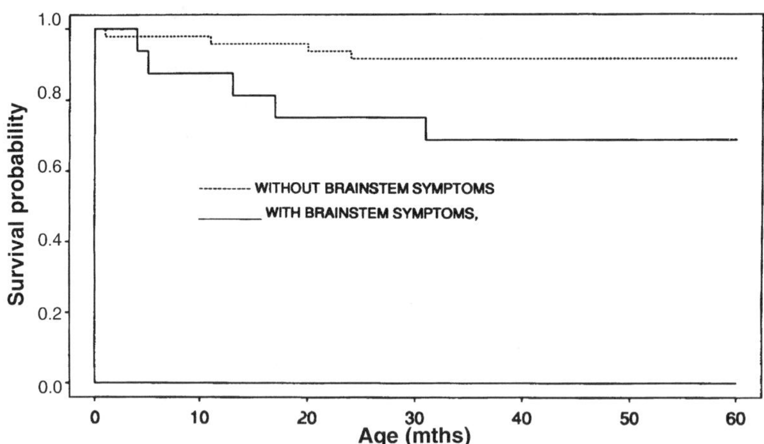

FIGURE 1.—Probability of survival of patients with (n = 15) and without (n = 48) brain stem symptoms (*P* = 0.02). (Courtesy of Worley G, Schuster JM, Oakes WJ: Survival at 5 years of a cohort of newborn infants with myelomeningocele. *Dev Med Child Neurol* 38:816–822, 1996.)

improve survival. Mortality at 5 years was 14%. The same 14% mortality was reported by McLone et al. in 2 studies of 100 infants. In the study from 1975 to 1978, the infants were monitored for 5 years. In the study from 1979 to 1984, some of the infants were monitored for 5 years. In a study by Steinbok et al. from 1971 to 1981, a mortality rate of 18% was reported for 101 infants observed for at least 8.6 years. The infants in the present study and the study by McLone et al. from 1975 to 1978 differed only in the management of brain stem dysfunction and hydrocephalus. Because the cohorts were similar in other respects, the similar mortality suggests that the management techniques did not affect mortality.

► With increasingly successful surgical closure of the primary defect and medical treatment of related infections, the survival of children with myelomeningocele has become increasingly dependent on the neurologic sequelae of this developmental anomaly. This study examines the specific determinants of survival in these children and the influence of each of several surgical procedures on survival rate. By putting the present results in the perspective of several previously performed studies and comparing the patient populations and surgical management techniques involved in each of these studies, these authors are able to begin dissecting out the influence of currently available operative treatments and underlying brain abnormalities on the survival of children with late sequelae of myelomeningocele.

N.F. Schor, M.D., Ph.D.

8 Movement Disorders

Comparison of Therapeutic Effects and Mortality Data of Levodopa and Levodopa Combined With Selegiline in Patients With Early, Mild Parkinson's Disease
Lees AJ on behalf of the Parkinson's Disease Research Group of the United Kingdom (Natl Hosp for Neurology and Neurosurgery, London)
BMJ 311:1602–1607, 1995

8–1

Background.—The Parkinson's Disease Research Group of the United Kingdom instituted a study in 1985 to compare the effects of levodopa (with a dopa decarboxylase inhibitor), levodopa combined with selegiline hydrochloride, and bromocriptine on the natural course of Parkinson's disease. Baseline disabilities improved with all 3 regimens after 1 year of continuous treatment; after 3 years, however, functional disability and physical signs had deteriorated. The mortality rate did not differ significantly among groups after 3 years. Results of an interim analysis in 1994 were reported.

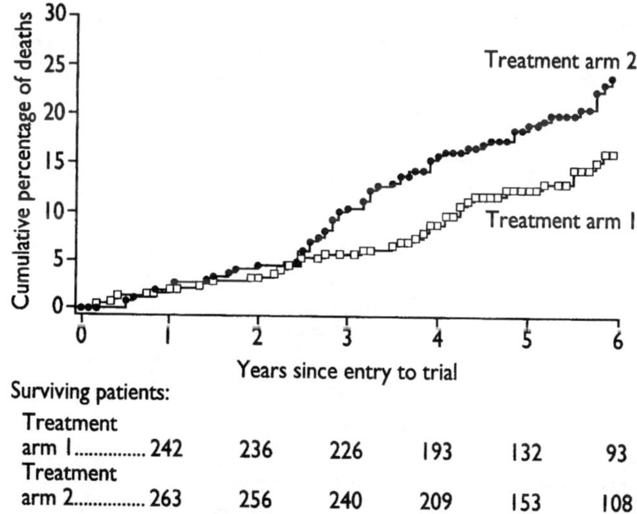

FIGURE 1.—Cumulative percentage of deaths in treatment arm 1 (levodopa alone) and arm 2 (levodopa and selegiline): Kaplan-Meier estimate. (Courtesy of Parkinson's Disease Research Group of the United Kingdom: Comparison of therapeutic effects and mortality data of levodopa and levodopa combined with selegiline in patients with early, mild Parkinson's disease. *BMJ* 311:1602–1607, 1995.)

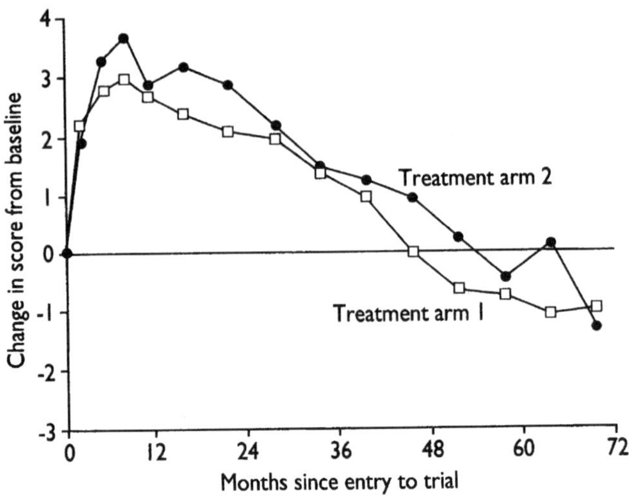

FIGURE 2.—Average change in Webster score of disability from baseline value in treatment arm 1 (levodopa alone) and arm 2 (levodopa and selegiline). (Courtesy of Parkinson's Disease Research Group of the United Kingdom: Comparison of therapeutic effects and mortality data of levodopa and levodopa combined with selegiline in patients with early, mild Parkinson's disease. *BMJ* 311:1602–1607, 1995.)

Design.—Five hundred twenty patients who had early Parkinson's disease and who were not receiving dopaminergic treatment were included in an open, long-term, prospective randomized trial. Patients in arm 1 of the study received 62.5 mg of levodopa and benserazide 3 times a day after meals. The dose was increased to 125 mg thrice daily for 3 months; further increases were left to the discretion of individual physicians. Patients in arm 2 of the study received 5 mg of selegiline once in the morning for 1 week then 5 mg twice daily for 3 more weeks. The patients continued to receive selegiline at the same dose while additional treatment with levodopa and benserazide was begun as in arm-1 patients.

Results.—Interim follow-up analysis after 5.6 years revealed that the mortality ratio among arm-2 patients compared with that of arm-1 patients was 1.57; difference in survival was significant (Fig 1). Hazard ratio was 1.49 after adjustment for age and sex but increased to 1.57 after adjustment for other baseline factors. Patients in arm 1 showed slightly, but nonsignificantly, worse disability scores than did patients in arm 2 (Fig 2). Patients in arm 2 experienced more frequent functionally disabling peak dose dyskinesias and on/off fluctuations than did patients in arm 1. Dose of levodopa required to produce optimum motor control steadily increased in arm-1, but not in arm-2, participants.

Conclusions.—Patients who have mild, previously untreated Parkinson's disease appeared to derive no clinically detectable benefit from treatment with selegiline in addition to levodopa. Mortality was significantly increased in patients who received both drugs compared with those receiving levodopa alone. Participants in arm 2 of this ongoing study were advised to discontinue use of selegiline. Follow-up of these patients and the other participants continues.

▶ In 1989, the Parkinson's Study Group of North America[1] reported that selegiline delayed progression of disability in patients who had early Parkinson's disease. The optimism generated by that report was dampened considerably, however, by the follow-up report in 1993 that the putative neuroprotective effects were confounded by mild symptomatic effects of selegiline.[2] The present report by the Parkinson's Disease Research Group of the United Kingdom casts a pall on the long-term use of selegiline. Use of this selective monoamine oxidase B inhibitor, in combination with levodopa, conferred no clinical benefit compared with levodopa alone, and the mortality rate was significantly higher with the combination treatment. The reasons for the increased mortality rate are not known, but the finding was significant enough for the investigators to inform patients of the results and to advise withdrawal from selegiline. The increased mortality rate associated with use of selegine directly conflicts with earlier data reported by Birkmayer et al.,[3] who claimed increased life expectancy when selegiline was added to a levodopa regimen. Review of mortality data by the Parkinson's Study Group of North America is eagerly awaited.

J.R. Sanchez-Ramos, Ph.D., M.D.

References

1. Parkinson's Study Group: Effect of deprenyl on the progression of disability in early Parkinson's disease. *N Engl J Med* 321:1364–1371, 1989.
2. Parkinson's Study Group: Effects of tocopherol and deprenyl on the progression of disability in early Parkinson's disease. *N Engl J Med* 328:176–183, 1993.
3. Birkmayer W, Knoll J, Riederer P, et al: Increased life expectancy resulting from addition of L-deprenyl to Madopar treatment in Parkinson's disease: A long term study. *J Neural Transm* 64:113–127, 1985.

The Effect of Deprenyl and Levodopa on the Progression of Parkinson's Disease
Olanow CW, Hauser RA, Gauger L, et al (Mount Sinai Med Ctr, New York; Univ of South Florida, Tampa; Univ of Kansas, Kansas City; et al)
Ann Neurol 38:771–777, 1995

8–2

Introduction.—If cytotoxic free radicals play a pathogenic role in Parkinson's disease (PD), then antioxidant therapy might alter the course of disease by slowing neuronal degeneration. Conversely, levodopa, through its metabolism to dopamine, might accelerate neuronal degeneration by promoting the formation of cytotoxic radicals. The monoamine oxidase type B inhibitor deprenyl—which has the potential to reduce free radical formation resulting from oxidation of dopamine—was evaluated for its effects on the progression of PD.

Methods.—One hundred one untreated patients with PD participated in the prospective, randomized, double-blind, placebo-controlled trial. The patients were 69 men and 32 women with a mean age of 66 years and an average disease duration of 3 years. They were assigned to receive either deprenyl (10 mg/day) plus levodopa/carbidopa (Sinemet 25/100), placebo-deprenyl plus Sinemet, deprenyl plus bromocriptine (5 mg), or placebo-deprenyl plus bromocriptine. The study lasted for 14 months; the final evaluations were performed 2 months after cessation of deprenyl or placebo-deprenyl and 7 days after cessation of Sinemet or bromocriptine. Disease progression was assessed on the Unified Parkinson's Disease Rating Score (UPDRS).

Results.—From the pretreatment baseline evaluation to the final visit, UPDRS declined by a mean of 5.8 points in patients receiving placebo vs. 0.4 points in those receiving deprenyl. Deprenyl had a significant effect on disease progression in the 41 patients assigned to receive Sinemet as well as in the 23 patients completing a 14-day washout of Sinemet or bromocriptine. No such difference was apparent in patients assigned to Sinemet vs. bromocriptine. The 4 groups had a similar incidence of adverse effects.

Conclusion.—Deprenyl treatment slows deterioration of the UPDRS in patients with PD. Over the same treatment period, Sinemet does not accentuate the decline in UPDRS. Although the exact mechanism is unclear, deprenyl does appear to have a neuroprotective effect. Its effects on the course of PD are not readily explained by its symptomatic effects.

▶ The designers of this study benefited from analysis of the confounded results of the Parkinson Study Group, which found that neuroprotective effects of deprenyl were masked by symptomatic effects of the drug. By assessing patients 2 months after deprenyl washout and comparing decline in disability and motor function with baseline score, the researchers were able to detect a significant slowing in deterioration after 14 months of therapy. The debate as to whether neuroprotective benefits derived from deprenyl outweigh the reported increased mortality in users of deprenyl has just begun.

J.R. Sanchez-Ramos, Ph.D., M.D.

Impact of Deprenyl and Tocopherol Treatment on Parkinson's Disease in DATATOP Subjects Not Requiring Levodopa
Shoulson I, and the Parkinson Study Group (Univ of Rochester, NY)
Ann Neurol 39:29–36, 1996
8–3

Background.—The Deprenyl and Tocopherol Antioxidant Therapy of Parkinsonism (DATATOP) trial showed that antioxidative treatment with deprenyl in patients with untreated Parkinson's disease (PD) can delay levodopa-related disability and reduce motor impairment. However, there are questions regarding whether this represents a temporary symptomatic effect or a true slowing of underlying nigral degeneration. The long-term effects of deprenyl treatment among DATATOP patients who did not require levodopa therapy were analyzed.

Methods.—Of the 800 patients entered into the DATATOP study, 310 did not reach the primary end point of requiring levodopa therapy during a mean follow-up of 21 months or require early initiation of deprenyl during a 2–month withdrawal period. One hundred eighty-nine patients were initially assigned to receive deprenyl treatment and 121 were not. All were started on an open-label trial of deprenyl, 10 mg/day. The effects were evaluated at intervals over a mean of 12 months, without knowledge of whether they had initially been assigned to the deprenyl group.

Results.—Patients initially assigned to the deprenyl group tended to reach the main end point of disability faster than patients in the non-deprenyl group (hazard ratio, 1.43). However, the patients assigned to deprenyl were more severely impaired at the start of the study. Patients in this group showed an initial benefit from active deprenyl treatment, but were subsequently more likely to require levodopa treatment.

Conclusion.—In patients with PD, antioxidative therapy with deprenyl does not significantly reduce the incidence of disability requiring levodopa therapy. Thus, the initial advantages of this treatment do not persist over the long term. Deprenyl is still a viable option for patients with early Parkinson's disease, as it does delay the need for levodopa therapy. However, there are important questions regarding its optimal dosage, the persistence of its effects, and its impact on other outcomes.

Impact of Deprenyl and Tocopherol Treatment on Parkinson's Disease in DATATOP Patients Requiring Levodopa
Penney JB Jr, and the Parkinson Study Group (Univ of Michigan, Ann Arbor)
Ann Neurol 39:37–45, 1996   8–4

Purpose.—Although levodopa provides considerable relief from the symptoms of Parkinson's disease (PD), the underlying nigral neuron loss continues, with progressive worsening of the signs and symptoms of disease. Also, years of levodopa treatment lead to motor, behavioral, and/or autonomic adverse effects. Previous reports have suggested that treatments to decrease oxidative stress in the substantia nigra neurons could slow the progression of PD, as well as slow or prevent the development of levodopa-related adverse effects. Deprenyl and tocopherol were prospectively studied for their effects on disease progression in patients with PD requiring levodopa therapy.

Methods.—The analysis was part of the Deprenyl and Tocopherol Antioxidant Therapy of Parkinsonism trial. This double-blind, placebo-controlled study examined the effects of treatment with deprenyl, 10 mg/day, and/or tocopherol, 2,000 IU/day, in 800 untreated patients with PD. Levodopa was given to patients who required symptomatic treatment, and all patients were switched to open-label deprenyl treatment after the blinded portion of the trial. This permitted an analysis of the long-term effects of deprenyl and tocopherol treatment on the subsequent development of levodopa-related side effects. The average follow-up was 35 months.

Results.—Three hundred seventy-one patients required levodopa treatment, and 352 completed the levodopa portion of the trial. Levodopa side effects were not significantly different between patients who received early vs. late treatment with deprenyl or in those who received tocopherol vs. no tocopherol. "Wearing off" was noted in approximately 50% of patients, dyskinesias in 30%, and "freezing" in 25%. By the end of the trial, all groups were comparable in their dose of levodopa and their level of disability, as measured by the Hoehn-Yahr, Schwab-England, and Unified Parkinson's Disease Rating scales. Wearing-off was more frequent in younger patients, dyskinesias were more common in women, and freezing was most likely to occur in older patients with rapidly progressive PD.

Conclusion.—Deprenyl and tocopherol antioxidant therapy does not reduce later levodopa-associated adverse effects in patients with PD. Neither does this treatment reduce the disability of PD nor the dose of levodopa required. A companion article describes the effects of deprenyl treatment in patients with PD who did not require levodopa.

▶ Before deprenyl was available in the United States, the Parkinson Study Group initiated a large, multicenter trial to test its capacity to slow progression of the illness. Deprenyl was found to delay the need for levodopa, but, unfortunately, deprenyl was also found to have a mild symptomatic effect which confounded interpretation of the results. Whether or not deprenyl slows progression of PD has been controversial since the Parkinson Study Group reported its initial findings in 1989.[1] Finally, these 2 articles (abstracts 8–3 and 8–4) published in tandem summarize the long-term follow-up of the original cohort. Patients who were originally assigned to deprenyl and who were followed for an additional 18 months tended to require levodopa earlier than those who were initially assigned placebo and then given deprenyl in open label for 18 months.

Although deprenyl at 10mg/day slowed disability and ameliorated motor impairment in early PD, this intervention did not appear to confer sustained benefits. Moreover, those patients who did reach the end point and required levodopa but who received deprenyl early or late did not differ with respect to the development of motor fluctuations and dyskinesias. Thus, deprenyl does not provide an advantage in preventing or postponing complications from levodopa therapy. If the clinician wishes to delay need for levodopa in early PD, it is rational to prescribe eldepryl, but this benefit must be weighed against the inability of deprenyl to provide sustained benefit with chronic use.

J.R. Sanchez-Ramos, Ph.D., M.D.

Reference

1. Parkinson Study Group. Effects of deprenyl on the progression of disability in early Parkinson's disease. *N Engl J Med* 321:1364–1371, 1989.

Effect of Thalamic Stimulation on Gait in Parkinson Disease

Defebvre L, Blatt J-L, Blond S, et al (Univ of Lille, France)
Arch Neurol 53:898–903, 1996

8–5

Objective.—In patients with drug-resistant parkinsonian tremor, electric stimulation of the ventral intermediate thalamic nucleus may be used as an alternative to stereotactic thalamotomy. Thalamic stimulation is as effective against tremor as thalamotomy, but with fewer adverse effects. The effects of thalamic stimulation on gait are unclear. This issue was addressed in a video motion analysis study.

Methods.—The study included 7 patients with idiopathic Parkinson's disease and large-amplitude rest tremor. The tremors were treated by long-term monopolar stimulation of the ventral intermediate thalamic nucleus. Movement analyses were done using the Vican optoelectric system (Oxford Matrics, Oxford, England) under 2 conditions: stimulation on and off. Locomotor displacement measures analyzed were cadence, walking speed, stride and step times, single and double support times, and stride and step lengths. Traces of ankle joint position were assessed for affected and unaffected lower extremities.

Results.—The patients' mean Unified Parkinson's Disease Rating Scale scores were 17 in the on condition and 26 in the off condition. Stride and step times and double support time were longer in the off condition, and step length was shorter in the off condition. However, none of the differences were significant, nor was there any significant difference in the traces of ankle joint position in the lower limbs.

Conclusions.—In patients with idiopathic Parkinson's disease, ventral intermediate thalamic stimulation for the treatment of tremor does not appear to affect gait. No clinical gait or balance disturbances are observed after thalamic stimulation, even after a bilateral procedure or previous thalamotomy. There is no difference in gait parameters in the on vs. the off position.

▶ With the resurgence of interest in surgical approaches for treatment of parkinsonism, it is important to weigh the spectrum of benefits against risks. Stereotactic thalamotomy has been shown to be effective against tremor refractory to drug treatments, but with adverse effects in 2% to 6% of patients. Electric stimulation of the ventral intermediate thalamic nucleus is just as effective as thalamotomy in control of tremor but adverse effects are less common, at least over several years. Generally, thalamic stimulation has its greatest benefit in the control of tremor with little or no effect on akinesia, and mild effects on rigidity. The research reported here shows nicely that unilateral thalamic stimulation does not improve gait and, just as important, does not induce disequilibrium or worsen gait.

J. Sanchez-Ramos, Ph.D., M.D.

Risk Factors for Peak Dose Dyskinesia in 100 Levodopa-treated Parkinsonian Patients

Blanchet PJ, Allard P, Grégoire L, et al (Hôpital de l'Enfant Jésus, Quebec; Hôpital du Saint Sacrement, Quebec)
Can J Neurol Sci 23:189–193, 1996   8–6

Introduction.—Reports vary regarding the relationship between dyskinesia and the duration and dosage of levodopa therapy. A retrospective analysis of 100 patients with Parkinson's disease was undertaken to get a clearer understanding of the risk profile of peak dose dyskinesia (PDD) in levodopa treatment.

Methods.—Records were reviewed for information regarding treatment with levodopa. Patients were evaluated clinically to confirm the diagnosis of Parkinson's disease and the presence or absence of PDD. Patients in whom PDD developed were compared with those in whom PDD did not develop regarding gender, age at disease onset, Hoehn-Yahr stage of levodopa initiation, disease duration, duration of levodopa treatment, and cumulative levodopa dose over the study period.

Results.—Patients aged 40 or younger at disease onset were significantly more likely to experience dyskinesia than older patients. Disease duration before levodopa treatment was not associated with a higher percentage of dyskinesia. Dyskinesia developed in 56% of the patients at a mean of 2.9 years after the initiation of levodopa treatment in both age groups. The daily levodopa dose was significantly higher in patients with dyskinesia than in those with no dyskinesia. No significant difference was found in dyskinesia-free survival between patients aged 60 and less and patients over 60 years of age (Fig 2). Dyskinesia-free survival was not affected by delayed initiation of levodopa by 3 years or more after disease onset (Fig 3). Patients in stages I and II at treatment onset did not differ regarding dyskinesia-free survival over time (Fig 4). No single factor was found that increased susceptibility to early dyskinesia. The cumulative levodopa doses

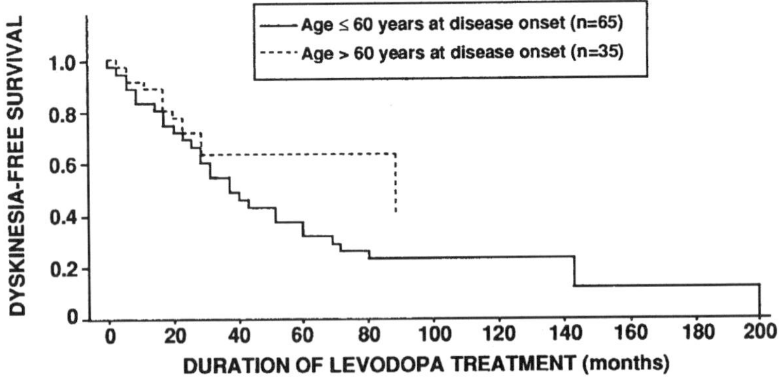

FIGURE 2.—Cumulative probability of remaining free of dyskinesia in 100 patients according to age at disease onset. (Courtesy of Blanchet PJ, Allard P, Grégoire L et al: Risk factors for peak dose dyskinesia in 100 levodopa-treated parkinsonian patients. *Can J Neurol Sci* 23:189–193, 1996.)

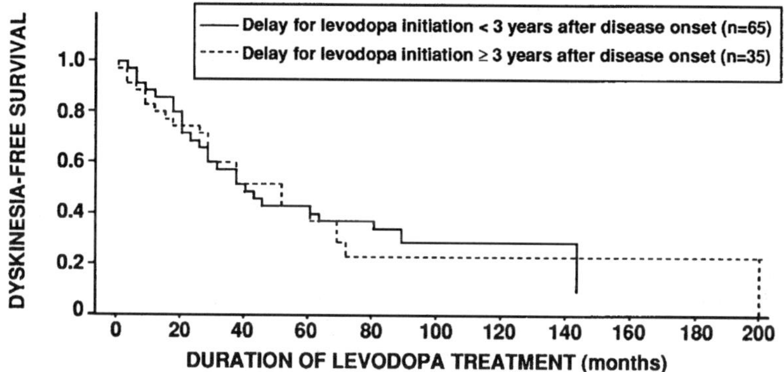

FIGURE 3.—Cumulative probability of remaining free of dyskinesia in 100 patients according to levodopa initiation delay after disease onset. (Courtesy of Blanchet PJ, Allard P, Grégoire L et al: Risk factors for peak dose dyskinesia in 100 levodopa-treated parkinsonian patients. *Can J Neurol Sci* 23:189–193, 1996.)

up to the start of dyskinesia were similar between patients with or without PDD, and the cumulative threshold dose for PDD varied greatly among patients with PDD, which suggests that dyskinesia emergence is not dose related (Fig 1).

Conclusion.—Withholding levodopa therapy did not increase the dyskinesia risk. An initial trial of dopaminomimetic agonist therapy may be continued as tolerated to postpone the emergence of dyskinesia after the onset of parkinsonian symptoms and to reduce the levodopa daily dose once it is added.

▶ This article suggests that no single factor accounts for the risk of development of dyskinesias other than a young age at onset of the disease. In this population "at risk," the appearance of dyskinesias can be expected after an average interval of 3 years following initiation of levodopa therapy, indepen-

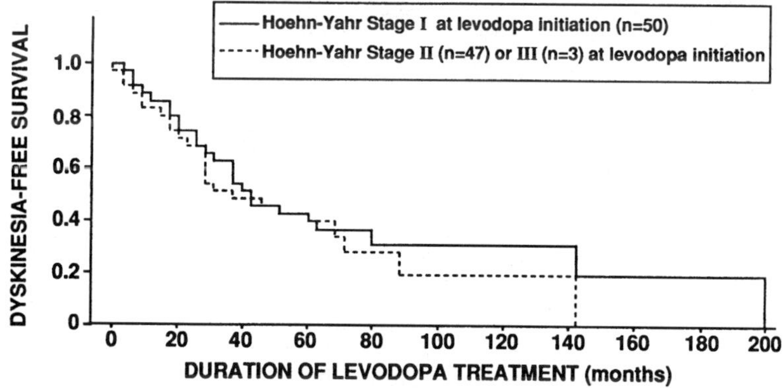

FIGURE 4.—Cumulative probability of remaining free of dyskinesia in 100 patients according to the Hoehn-Yahr stage of Parkinson's disease at levodopa initiation. (Courtesy of Blanchet PJ, Allard P, Grégoire L et al: Risk factors for peak dose dyskinesia in 100 levodopa-treated parkinsonian patients. *Can J Neurol Sci* 23:189–193, 1996.)

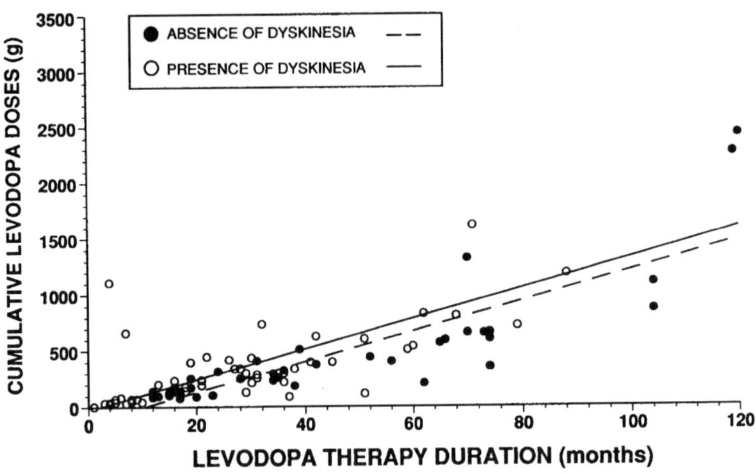

FIGURE 1.—Cumulative levodopa doses in relation to the levodopa treatment interval free of dyskinesia in patients with (*open circles*) or without (*filled circles*) dyskinesia. (Courtesy of Blanchet PJ, Allard P, Grégoire L et al: Risk factors for peak dose dyskinesia in 100 levodopa-treated parkinsonian patients. *Can J Neurol Sci* 23:189–193, 1996.)

dent of other risk factors. It follows that withholding levodopa therapy would extend the total period free of dyskinesia from disease onset. However, withholding levodopa might entail unacceptable disability. A way to avoid this problem is to initiate treatment early with a dopamine agonist such as bromocriptine or pergolide. A recent prospective, randomized, controlled study showed that initiation of treatment with bromocriptine delayed the need for levodopa an average of 2.7 years, but once levodopa therapy was initiated, motor complications, including dyskinesias, arose after a mean latency of 2.2 years.[1] This dyskinesia-free period is similar to the 1 reported in the article summarized here. Dopamine agonist monotherapy is rarely responsible for the emergence of peak-dose dyskinesias, and it is therefore reasonable to begin therapy with a trial of a dopamine agonist and to continue this as long as the patient can tolerate it in order to postpone the emergence of dyskinesia and reduce the levodopa daily dose once the latter drug is added.

J.R. Sanchez-Ramos, Ph.D., M.D.

Reference

1. Montastruc JL, Rascol O, Senard JM, et al: A randomized controlled study comparing bromocriptine to which levodopa was later added, with levodopa alone in previously untreated patients with Parkinson's disease: A five year follow up. *J Neurol Neurosurg Psychiatry* 57:1034–1038, 1994.

Post-traumatic Movement Disorders in Survivors of Severe Head Injury
Krauss JK, Tränkle R, Kopp K-H (Albert-Ludwigs-Universität, Freiburg, Germany)
Neurology 47:1488–1492, 1996

8–7

Introduction.—A variety of movement disorders, particularly tremors and dystonia, may have their origin in severe head trauma. The occurrence of posttraumatic movement disorders was analyzed in a large series of survivors of severe head injury.

Methods.—Between January 1988 and April 1992, 398 patients were consecutively admitted to the study institution with severe head trauma (defined as a Glasgow Coma Score [GCS] of 8 or less). The presence of posttraumatic movement disorders was determined by a follow-up questionnaire sent between November 1993 and January 1994 to all survivors of the early period after head injury. All patients identified as having a possible movement disorder were interviewed by telephone. Personal follow-up visits were conducted during 1994 with patients whose symptoms could not be assessed adequately over the telephone. Movement disorders were classified according to established criteria and analyzed for their possible associations with age at trauma, severity of head injury, and initial CT findings.

Results.—The severe head injury population was predominantly male (79%); the mean age at trauma was 36.2 years. Approximately one third of patients (34%) died after hospital admission. Survivors were significantly younger than nonsurvivors (mean age, 27.2 vs. 51.7). Follow-up was available for 221 of 264 survivors. In 50 of the interviewed patients (22.6%) movement disorders had developed; they were persistent in 27 cases and transient in 23. Tremor was the most common finding, reported by 42 of 50 patients. Twelve patients had disabling low-frequency kinetic tremors (2.5 to 4 Hz), dystonia, or both. These tremors developed within 2 weeks to 6 months after trauma; dystonia appeared with a latency period of from 2 months to 2 years. Patients with movement disorders had a higher proportion of lower Glasgow Coma Scores at admission than those without movement disorders. Generalized brain edema on initial CT scans was significantly associated with development of movement disorders.

Discussion.—Only 1% of all head injuries are classified as severe on the Glasgow Coma Score (a score of 8 or less). Survivors of such severe head trauma frequently experience movement disorders, but only a small percentage have disabling disorders such as kinetic tremors and dystonia.

▶ The etiologic role of head trauma in movement disorders is of increasing interest. An association between head trauma and Parkinson's disease is controversial. This epidemiologic longitudinal study reveals that in 22.6% of survivors of severe head trauma movement disorders developed, primarily postural/kinetic tremors that were transient or persistent. Parkinsonism was notably rare among these patients.

J.R. Sanchez-Ramos, M.D., Ph.D.

Restless Legs Syndrome: Clinicoetiologic Correlates

Ondo W, Jankovic J (Baylor College of Medicine, Houston)
Neurology 47:1435–1441, 1996

8–8

Introduction.—Restless legs syndrome (RLS) is a poorly understood neurologic disorder. Previous studies have emphasized broad heterogeneous inclusion criteria rather than attempting to define familial vs. sporadic or idiopathic vs. neuropathic RLS. A study of 54 patients with RLS compared their clinical and pharmacologic correlates with respect to these etiologic classifications.

Methods.—Patients were 29 women and 25 men with a mean age of 62.69 years at the time of evaluation; 53 were white and 1 was Asian. All satisfied diagnostic criteria for RLS and none had a history of exposure to dopamine-blocking agents. Most had been referred for RLS (32) or parkinsonism (10); other reasons for referral were tremor, myoclonus, tardive dyskinesia, blepharospasm, hemifacial spasm, and low back pain. All patients were interviewed and 52 completed a questionnaire. Electromyography (EMG) and nerve conduction velocities (NCVs) were obtained in 41 cases. Patients were also rated for response to medications.

Results.—The mean age at initial symptom onset was 34.13 years; symptoms were reported to occur "nearly every night" at a mean age of 46.36 years. A family history of RLS was present in 23 of 25 idiopathic cases (92.0%) vs. 2 of 15 neuropathic cases (13.3%). Symptoms consistent with RLS were reported in 58 of 246 possible first-degree relatives (23.6%) of patients with a positive family history. Compared with the familial/idiopathic patients, the sporadic/neuropathic patients were older at symptom onset and tended to have a more rapid progression. Sleep was subjectively impaired in all but 2 patients, and sleep characteristics did not differ between sporadic and familial cases or between neuropathic and idiopathic cases (Table 1). Fifteen of 41 tested patients had abnormal EMG/NCV findings. Although leg involvement is predominant in RLS, arms were often affected as well, particularly with longer duration of symptoms. All patients gained relief by walking or other volitional movement. The most effective medications were levodopa and dopamine agonists.

TABLE 1.—Subjective Sleep Characteristics

	Neuropathic (n = 15)	Idiopathic (n = 26)	Sporadic (n = 18)	Familial (n = 35)	Total (n = 54)
Sleep latency (h)	0.80 ± 0.68	0.96 ± 0.75	0.86 ± 0.85	0.97 ± 0.76	0.92 ± 0.76
Number of awakenings per night	2.27 ± 1.06	2.35 ± 1.89	2.58 ± 1.80	2.31 ± 1.58	2.45 ± 1.68
Sleep efficiency (%)	61.67 ± 14.0	70.0 ± 13.3	63.6 ± 14.4	67.2 ± 15.4	65.9 ± 15.0
Patients with witnessed leg movements (%)	13 (86.7)	19 (73.1)	13 (72.2)	27 (77.1)	41 (75.9)

(Reprinted from *Neurology*, courtesy of Ondo W, Jankovic J: Restless legs syndrome: Clinicoetiologic correlates. *Neurology* 47:1435–1441, 1996, by permission of Little, Brown and Company, Inc.)

Discussion.—Overall clinical characteristics were similar across all RLS cases: neuropathic, idiopathic, sporadic, and familial. The shared clinical characteristics of familial and neuropathic cases suggest a similar underlying pathophysiology, possibly involving the descending dopaminergic system.

▶ Restless legs syndrome, akathisia, and periodic limb movements of sleep are fascinating movement disorders that are confusing to the average practicing neurologist. All 3 involve appendicular motor restlessness but differ with respect to subjective sensations of restlessness and degree of volitional control and supressability of the leg movements. They all, most likely, involve a problem in central sensory-motor integration. This paper provides an excellent overview of clinical and etiological aspects of RLS and a practical framework for diagnosing and managing this disorder.

J.R. Sanchez-Ramos, M.D., Ph.D.

9 Neuro-Imaging

Clinical Applications of Proton MR Spectroscopy
Castillo M, Kwock L, Mukherji SK (Univ of North Carolina, Chapel Hill)
AJNR 17:1–15, 1996   9–1

Introduction.—Although MR spectroscopy (MRS) has received little attention from the clinical radiologic community, it can provide more information about tissue characterization than can MRI studies alone. Adequate MRS can be completed in only 10–15 minutes and can be added to routine MRI. The current status of MRS was reviewed, with emphasis on its clinical utility for evaluating neurologic disorders.

Principles.—In MRS, nuclei are exposed to a uniform magnetic field, then receive a radio frequency pulse that rotates them from the z-axis to the x-axis; the nuclei return to their original position in the z-axis when the pulse is turned off. Data regarding voltage variations and time elapsed during this return to the original position are transformed into a plot of peaks characterized by resonance frequency, height, and width at half-height. Resonance frequency depends on the chemical environment of the nucleus and is usually expressed as parts per million from the main resonance frequency (chemical shift). Relative measurements of the concentration of protons may be calculated from the height or area under a peak. Most MRS studies are obtained by using a localized single voxel or by sampling volume element (Fig 1). However, obtaining 1-or 2-dimensional data sets that show metabolites from adjacent compartments (encompassing a larger tissue volume) is also possible. With 2-dimensional chemical-shift proton MRS, metabolite concentrations can be superimposed on the image of an abnormality to show the distribution of metabolites (which can be represented with different colors) in a given area.

Clinical Applications.—The concentration of normal metabolites in the brain may vary with age or with pathologic conditions. Abnormal levels of N-acetyl aspartate, choline, creatinine, lactate, myoinositol, glutamate and glutamine, alanine, or lipids may be characteristic of or suggestive of particular pathologic processes. Proton MRS readily distinguishes astrocytomas from normal brain tissue but may not distinguish histologic grade. Magnetic resonance spectroscopy may help distinguish difficult cases of meningioma and may detect radiation injury before it is evident via MRI. Metabolic alterations may be revealed by proton MRS in patients who have only mild AIDS-related dementia. Abnormal proton MRS may

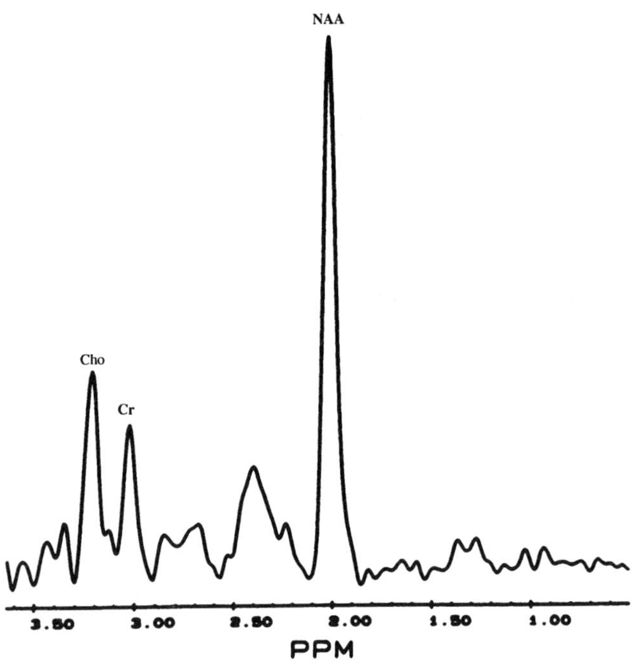

FIGURE 1.—Normal brain proton MR spectroscopy, single voxel. Proton MR spectroscopy obtained in a healthy volunteer using a single 8-cm^3 volume element in right centrum semiovale. *Abbreviations: Cho*, choline; *Cr*, creatinine; *NAA*, N-acetyl aspartate. (Courtesy of Castillo M, Kwock L, Mukherji SK: Clinical applications of proton MR spectroscopy. *AJNR* 17:1–15, 1996, copyright by American Society of Neuroradiology.)

be evident in HIV-positive newborns within as few as 10 days after birth. Magnetic resonance spectroscopy is a potential tool for early detection of Alzheimer's disease and for screening for subclinical hepatic encephalopathy. Proton MRS has been used to quantify brain lithium, characterize hamartomas, diagnose giant heterotopia, and study orbital tumors.

▶ If one believes that MRS will have a significant impact on the practice of the clinical neurosciences, then the techniques of MRS need to be understood, and the normal and abnormal biochemistry of the brain reviewed. This article brings together the critical physical principles involved in MRS and summarizes the various clinical applications. The authors describe each spectral peak (whether lowered or elevated) and how they are related to a known biochemical alteration in the brain; this serves as the base for understanding spectral alterations. N-acetyl aspartate is an indicator of neuron activity and, therefore, is shown to decrease in brain tumors. Choline is an indicator of cell membrane metabolism and reflects the cellularity of the tissue under investigation. Lactate, shown as 2 peaks, increases in states of diminished oxidative metabolism. Other important brain constituents that are seen with MRS include creatinine, glutamate, alanine, and myoinositol. Understanding the biochemical role of each of these chemicals and their place on a proton spectrum is shown in this article, which then allows one to appreciate how MRS may be of value primarily in the evaluation of brain tumors, viral infections, degenerative brain diseases, and cerebral ischemia.

R.M. Quencer, M.D.

Reproducibility of Proton MR Spectroscopic Imaging Findings

Tedeschi G, Bertolino A, Campbell G, et al (NIH, Bethesda, Md; Univ of California, Los Angeles)

AJNR 17:1871–1879, 1996   9–2

Purpose.—There are few data on the reproducibility of proton MR spectroscopic imaging in healthy subjects. This information is needed to establish the reliability of using MR spectroscopy to monitor disease progression or treatment effects over time. The intraindividual, interindividual, interregional, and intraregional reproducibility of proton MR spectroscopy was studied in healthy volunteers.

Methods.—Six healthy young adults underwent long–echo-time, multisection proton MR spectroscopy on 3 different occasions. The imaging protocol permitted simultaneous acquisition of N-acetylaspartate (NAA), choline-containing compounds (Cho), and creatine plus phosphocreatine (Cr). These signal intensities were obtained from four 15-mm sections divided into 0.84-mL single-volume elements (Fig 2). The frontal, occipital, parietal, and insular cortices; the cingulate gyrus; the centrum semiovale; the thalamus; and the caudate were the regions of interest.

Results.—In most regions of interest, the coefficient of variation (CV) was lowest for the ratio of NAA/Cr, with a range of 8.9% to 26.1%. The

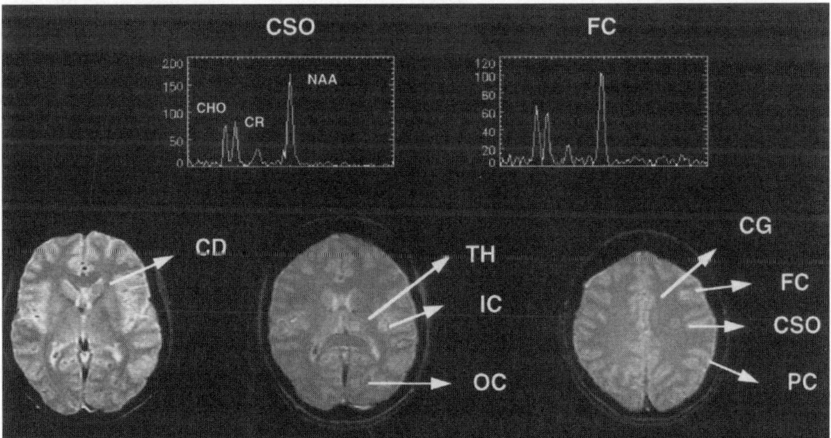

FIGURE 2.—Representative spectra from white and gray matter and location of regions of interest in 1 subject. *Abbreviations: FC,* frontal cortex; *OC,* occipital cortex; *PC,* parietal cortex; *IC,* insular cortex; *CG,* cingulate gyrus; *CSO,* centrum semiovale; *TH,* thalamus; and *CD,* caudate. (Courtesy of Tedeschi G, Bertolino A, Campbell G, et al: Reproducibility of proton MR spectroscopic imaging findings. *AJNR* 17:1871–1879. 1996, copyright by American Society of Neuroradiology.)

overall CV showed significant interregional differences. The between-subject CVs ranged from 4.2% to 8.7% for NAA/Cr, from 6.8% to 17.4% for NAA/Cho, and from 5.0% to 13.6% for Cho/Cr. Within subjects, these CVs were 2.2% to 22.2%. 12.8% to 25.8%, and 4.5% to 21.0%, respectively. The range of intraregional CVs was 12.3% to 21.2% for NAA/Cr, 13.0% to 20.4% for NAA/Cho, and 12.2 to 18.9% for Cho/Cr.

Conclusion.—Repeated proton MR spectroscopic imaging studies in normal subjects show good overall reproducibility. There are some intra-regional variations in CV, suggesting the need for caution in using proton MR spectroscopy for follow-up studies. The findings also suggest that metabolite signal intensities differ significantly among different regions of interest.

▶ With the increase in the application of MR spectroscopy to routine MRI, it becomes important to understand the normal distribution of major chemical constituents within the brain, to assure the reproducibility of obtained spectra, and to recognize that spectroscopic imaging is possible. In most centers, when proton MR spectroscopy is performed, it is in terms of single-voxel spectroscopy; spectroscopic imaging, however, is capable of vivid display of constituent metabolites.

Variations in the echo time affect the detectability of metabolites and, hence, the spectroscopic images. Magnetic resonance spectroscopic imaging can show the distribution of metabolites such as Cho, Cr, NAA, and lactate, but problems may arise when analyzing the data and the images. Brain pulsations, slight magnetic field inhomogeneities, and patient motion are among those factors which could cause variations in the display of these constituents over time and, therefore, may not be reflective of abnormalities in the brain.

If true changes, over time, are shown in spectroscopic images, a number of possibilities can be inferred, such as a diminished pool of normal neurons (decrease in NAA), an increase in Cho (cellular proliferation), and decreased oxygenation with increased glycolysis (increase in lactate). However, caution is urged during analysis of MR spectroscopic imaging because regional variations in normal metabolites exist.

R.M. Quencer, M.D.

Clinical Significance of Diffuse Dural Enhancement Detected by Magnetic Resonance Imaging

River Y, Schwartz A, Gomori JM, et al (Hadassah-Hebrew Univ, Jerusalem)
J Neurosurg 85:777–783, 1996   9–3

Background.—Diffuse dural enhancement (DDE), an uncommon finding, has been observed in patients with various types of inflammatory processes of the meninges. The clinical significance of DDE as a distinct entity apart from leptomeningeal enhancement is still not clear. The clinical significance of DDE detected on MRI was explored retrospectively.

Methods.—Clinical, imaging, and laboratory findings were assessed in 20 consecutive patients with DDE. Thirteen patients with DDE and an underlying neoplastic disease were compared with 11 consecutive patients with cytologic evidence of neoplastic leptomeningeal metastasis assessed by MRI.

Findings.—Diffuse dural enhancement was associated with an underlying malignancy in 65% of 20 patients but co-existed with leptomeningeal metastasis in only 1. Skull metastases were found in 77% of 13 patients, and cranial nerve palsies were detected in 46% of 13. The other causes of DDE were associated with CSF leak or shunting, present in 25% of 20 patients, with or without symptoms of intracranial hypotension, and with dural sinus thrombosis and pachymeningitis. In 2 patients with DDE, dural biopsy specimens were obtained, revealing a narrow rim of granulation-like tissue adhering to the dural surface facing the inner skull table. Compared with patients with DDE caused by CSF leak, patients with metastatic causes had unique findings on MR subtraction, diffusion, and perfusion studies. Diffuse dural enhancement was not found in any patients with proven leptomeningeal metastasis, but 4 initially had focal dural enhancement, and 2 had apparent leptomeningeal enhancement.

Conclusions.—Diffuse dural enhancement is not a radiographic hallmark of leptomeningeal metastasis, despite the similarities in clinical manifestations. However, DDE most often is associated with metastatic malignancies and especially with skull metastases and CSF leak. Using special MR methods, the underlying cause can be established, and the disparity in the pathophysiologic mechanisms resulting in DDE elucidated.

▶ A key point in assessing meningeal enhancement is to recognize that dural enhancement is not necessarily abnormal. Normal dura will show thin, uniform, short segment enhancement. This occurs because vessels in the dura lack tight junctions and in this respect differ from the vessels in the leptomeninges. Once it has been determined that the dural enhancement is pathologic (thick, continuous, and diffuse), it is relatively easy to differentiate between leptomeningeal enhancement and dural enhancement. The former follows the gyral and sulcal patterns of the brain, whereas the latter remains closely related to the skull vault.

This article stresses that abnormal dural enhancement may be seen in the presence of a neoplastic process (predominantly skull metastasis) or in the absence of a neoplastic process. When leptomeningeal enhancement is present, neoplasia is the common cause, and in these cases one should not expect to see an associated diffuse dural enhancement. It is therefore important to clearly differentiate the pattern of leptomeningeal enhancement from diffuse dural enhancement.

R.M. Quencer, M.D.

Tumefactive Demyelinating Lesions

Dagher AP, Smirniotopoulos J (Thomas Jefferson Univ, Philadelphia; Armed Forces Inst of Pathology, Washington, DC; Uniformed Services Univ, Bethesda, Md)
Neuroradiology 38:560–565, 1996   9–4

Background.—Some primary demyelinating diseases can manifest themselves as tumefactive lesions, such as myelinoclastic diffuse sclerosis, or Schilder's disease; acute disseminated encephalomyelitis, which is a monophasic immune reaction triggered by viral infection or vaccination; and Balo's concentric sclerosis. Twenty-one pathologically confirmed cases of large demyelinating lesions were reviewed.

Findings.—The cases were collected by a 15-year review of pathology files. The patients were 12 females and 8 males (average age, 37 years).

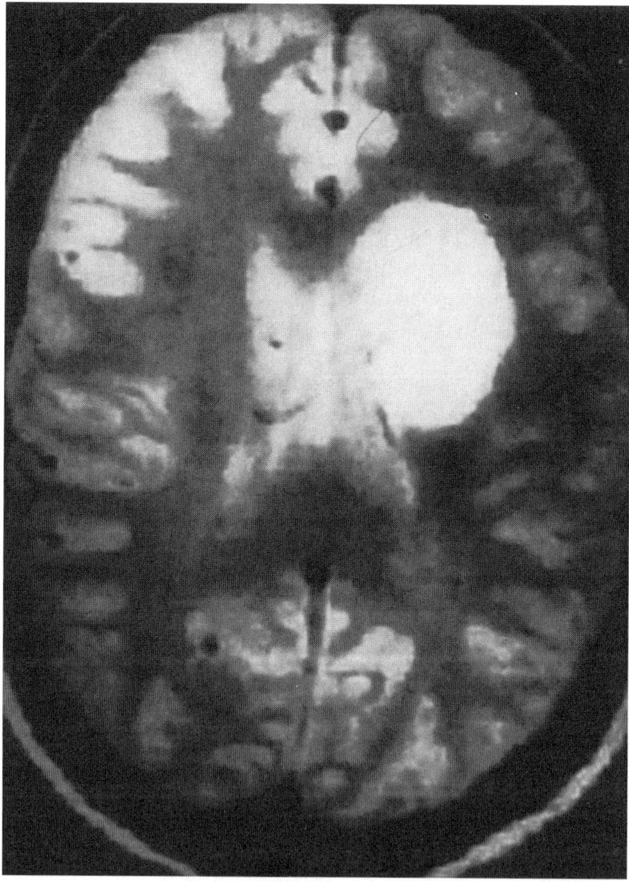

FIGURE 1.—Case of a woman, 45 years. Protein density-weighted MRI showing a single large demyelinating plaque adjacent to the lateral ventricle. (Courtesy of Dagher P, Smirniotopolous J: Tumefactive demyelinating lesions. *Neuroradiology* 38:560–565, 1996, fig 1. Copyright 1996, Springer-Verlag.)

Most patients had clinical and radiologic findings consistent with multiple sclerosis. In general, the tumefactive lesions showed relatively low density on CT scan, high signal intensity on proton-density or T2-weighted MRI scan, and relatively low signal intensity on T1-weighted MRI scan (Fig 1). The largest lesion was always found purely in white matter, not in the periventricular or infratentorial area. The average large lesion diameter was 4.6 cm, and about half of the lesions enhanced. Edema or a mass effect was present. There were no apparent cases of Schilder's disease or Balo's concentric sclerosis, although 1 patient had features of acute disseminated encephalomyelitis.

Discussion.—Patients with tumefactive demyelinating lesions have clinical, radiologic, and histologic findings similar to those of multiple sclerosis. This subgroup of patients remains ill defined, but they may have atypical symptoms, only 1 or a few lesions, prominent edema or mass effect, and an unusual lesion location. It is important to recognize the imaging features of tumefactive demyelination so as to avoid biopsy and potentially dangerous treatments.

▶ This article emphasizes the need to consider the diagnosis of a demyelinating disease even when a large mass producing enhancing lesion is seen within the brain. Clearly, additional abnormal MR signals within the white matter can help in establishing the proper diagnosis, but occasionally a single lesion is all that is seen (refer to Fig 1). The location of the lesion exclusively in the white matter along with indistinct margins of enhancement are additional clues that a tumefactive demyelinating process may be present. To avoid unnecessary biopsy, the strategy of a follow-up MR whenever these features are present is a reasonable approach. Often one will see relatively rapid change in the appearance of the mass, including decreased mass and enhancement, which would give strength to the belief that one is not dealing with a neoplastic or infectious process.

R.M. Quencer, M.D.

Acute Infectious Disorders of the Spinal Cord and Its Roots With Gadolinium-DTPA Enhancement in Magnetic Resonance Imaging

Engelter S, Lyrer P, Radü EW, et al (Univ Hosp, Basle, Switzerland)
J Neurol 243:191–195, 1996   9–5

Background.—When neurotropic infectious agents such as *Borrelia burgdorferi*, herpes zoster virus, or cytomegalovirus (CMV) affect the spinal cord, they cause acute, rapidly progressive neurologic deficits. Because the findings of serologic tests are not available in the early stages of disease, diagnostic uncertainty can result. Three patients were reported.

Case Reports.—The patients were 1 woman and 2 men, 74, 41, and 59 years of age, respectively. All had myelomeningoradiculitis caused by *Borrelia burgdorferi*, herpes zoster virus, or CMV infection. Magnetic resonance imaging of the spinal cord was performed with gadolinium diethylenetriamine pentacetic acid (Gd-DTPA). Enhancing lesions of the spinal cord or nerve roots that correlated with clinical signs were demonstrated.

Patient 3, in whom AIDS was diagnosed 11 months earlier, was seen with a 2-week history of progressive weakness of both legs and bladder and bowel dysfunction. Cytomegalovirus retinitis and proctitis had been diagnosed 1 week earlier. Cerebrospinal fluid (CSF) revealed polymorphonuclear pleocytosis, $1300/mm^3$, with no cytologic malignancy; increased protein; and an increased ratio of albumin CSF to serum without oligoclonal bands. Polymerase chain reaction identified CMV in CSF and serum. Although no abnormalities were seen on spinal MR T1-weighted, T2-weighted, or fast spin echo images, cauda equina enhancement was demonstrated in sagittal and axial images after IV Gd-DTPA. Based on clinical manifestations, early CSF findings, and enhanced spinal MRI, CMV lumbosacral polyradiculitis was diagnosed. Intravenous ganciclovir therapy was unsuccessful.

Conclusions.—In these patients, spinal MRI with Gd-DTPA demonstrated enhancing lesions of the spinal cord or nerve roots. A Gd-DTPA enhancement may reveal lesions that indicate possible inflammation associated with blood-brain-barrier changes, which could enable the diagnosis to be established before serologic findings are available.

Mitochondrial Myopathy-Encephalopathy–Lactic Acidosis–and Strokelike Episodes (MELAS) Syndrome: CT and MR Findings in Seven Children
Kim I-O, Kim JH, Kim WS, et al (Seoul Natl Univ, Korea)
AJR 166:641–645, 1996   9–6

Background.—Patients with mitochondrial myopathy-encephalopathy–lactic acidosis–and strokelike episodes (MELAS) syndrome are usually normal at birth and in early infancy, then have delayed growth, episodic vomiting, seizures, and recurrent cerebral injuries causing hemiparesis, hemianopsia, hearing loss, or cortical blindness. The imaging characteristics of patients with MELAS syndrome were described.

Methods.—Seven patients with proved MELAS syndrome were included in a restrospective study. Twelve CT scans and 15 MR images were reviewed. Patients were followed for from 3 to 39 months. Lesion distribution, enhancement pattern, presence of mass effect or atrophy, calcification, and changes on follow-up images were analyzed.

Findings.—Computed tomographic and MR images showed multiple cortical and subcortical infarctlike lesions that crossed vascular boundaries, as well as various degrees of generalized cerebral and cerebellar atrophy. In 6 patients lesions were distributed in the posterior, parietal, and occipital areas; in 5, the putamen; in 2, the caudate nucleus; in 2, the thalamus; in 2, the frontal lobe; in 1, the globus pallidus; and in 1, the brainstem. Contrast enhancement was observed in 2 of 7 MR images and in 3 of 5 CT scans. Infarctlike lesions in the early stage of the syndrome were characterized by swelling and mass effect. In 5 patients, lesions resolved with or without local tissue loss. New lesions appeared in another part of the brain in 5 patients. In 6 patients, generalized atrophy pro-

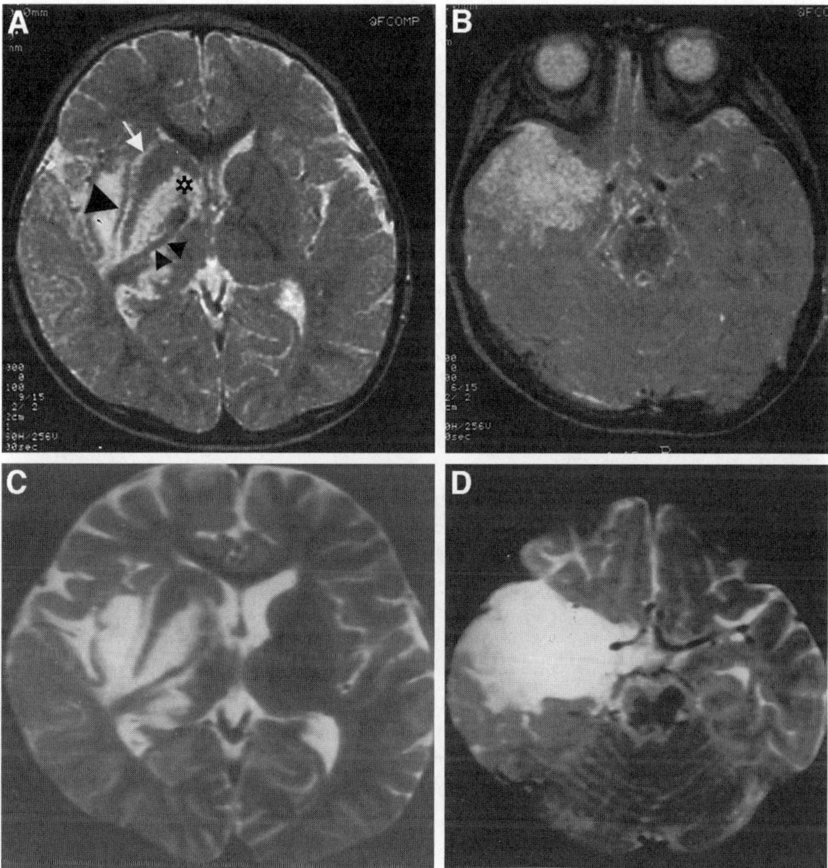

FIGURE 1.—Infarctlike lesions involving nonvascular territory in 17-month-old girl with weakness of left upper extremity (onset, 6 days before). **A** and **B**, T2-weighted MR images (2,500-3,000/100) show infarctlike areas of high signal intensity in right temporal lobe, thalamus, part of caudate nucleus (*asterisk*), globus pallidus, medial part of putamen, external (*arrow*) and extreme capsule, and insular cortex, sparing posterior limb of internal capsule (*small arrowheads*), outer part of putamen, and claustrum (*large arrowhead*). Distribution of involved area cannot be explained as specific vascular territory. Compression of frontal horn suggests acute or subacute chronology. **C** and **D**, images obtained after 8 months show persistent infarctlike lesion in right temporal lobe, basal ganglia, and thalamus and progression of generalized cortical atrophy. (Courtesy of Kim I-O, Kim JH, Kim WS, et al: Mitochondrial myopathy-encephalopathy–lactic acidosis–and strokelike episodes (MELAS) syndrome: CT and MR findings in seven children. *AJR* 166:641–645, 1996.)

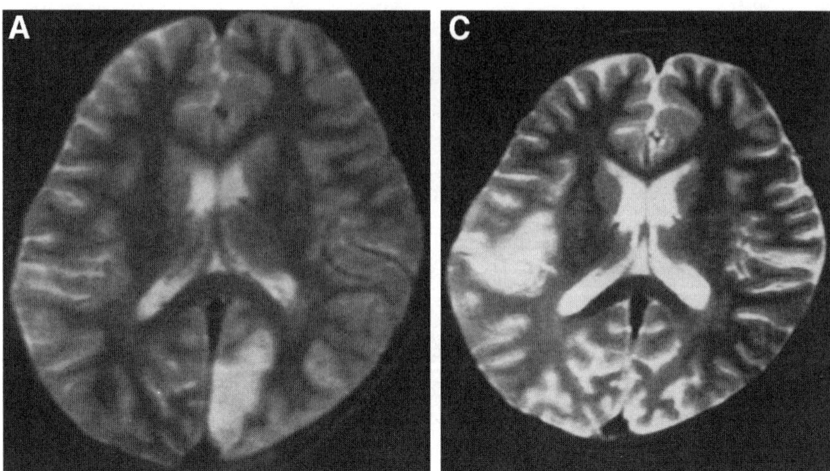

FIGURE 3.—Migrating lesions on follow-up study in 9-year-old girl with intermittent seizure and vision loss. A, T2-weighted MR image obtained 4 months after onset of seizure and 15 days after onset of vision loss shows high–signal intensity lesion in left occipital lobe. C, T2-weighted MR image obtained 7 months after A shows another small lesion in right temporoparietal area. Previously noted left temporoparietal lesion has evolved to atrophy. (Courtesy of Kim I-O, Kim JH, Kim WS, et al: Mitochondrial myopathy-encephalopathy–lactic acidosis–and strokelike episodes (MELAS) syndrome: CT and MR findings in seven children. *AJR* 166:641–645, 1996.)

gressed, being most severe in the posterior part of the cerebral hemispheres (Figs 1, 3, A, and 3, C).

Conclusion.—The imaging findings of multiple migrating infarctlike lesions not limited to a specific vascular territory suggest MELAS syndrome. This is especially so when the lesions are observed in the basal ganglia and posterior part of the cerebral hemisphere in children.

▶ The diagnosis of MELAS can be difficult to establish because of its varied clinical and radiographic presentations. Attesting to this difficulty is the need to often obtain a muscle biopsy specimen to solidify the diagnosis when transitory (Fig 1, A and B) nonenhancing gray matter lesions do not suggest the proper diagnosis. The wide range of ages at presentation (infants to young adults) compounds this problem and often an initial diagnosis of an inflammatory process or an infiltrating low-grade tumor is suggested. The predominance of a posteriorly located abnormality (occipital/posterior parietal) with minimal enhancement and mass effect can suggest the diagnosis in the proper clinical setting.

R.M. Quencer, M.D.

Patients With Antiphospholipid Antibodies: CT and MR Findings of the Brain

Provenzale JM, Barboriak DP, Allen NB, et al (Duke Univ, Durham, NC; VA Hosp, Durham, NC)
AJR 167:1573–1578, 1996   9–7

Introduction.—Patients with antiphospholipid antibodies (APAs) are reported to be at increased risk of stroke. There are few published series, however, regarding the neuroradiologic manifestations in patients with APA. A review of patients with APA who underwent CT or MRI was conducted to determine the spectrum of neurologic findings in such populations.

Methods.—Patients were identified through a review of files of coagulation laboratories at a tertiary care hospital. From January 1992 to August 1995, 110 patients with APA were identified who were younger than 65 years, were without other causes of a hypercoagulable state, and had a record of CT or MR studies. This group included 77 women and 33 men with an average age of 40.6 years. Twenty-two had systemic lupus erythematosus (SLE) and 88 were negative for SLE. Imaging study results were abnormal in 59 cases (54%), including 50 non-SLE patients and 9 with SLE. Abnormalities in these patients were categorized as large infarcts, cortical infarcts, lacunar infarcts, hyperintense white matter foci on

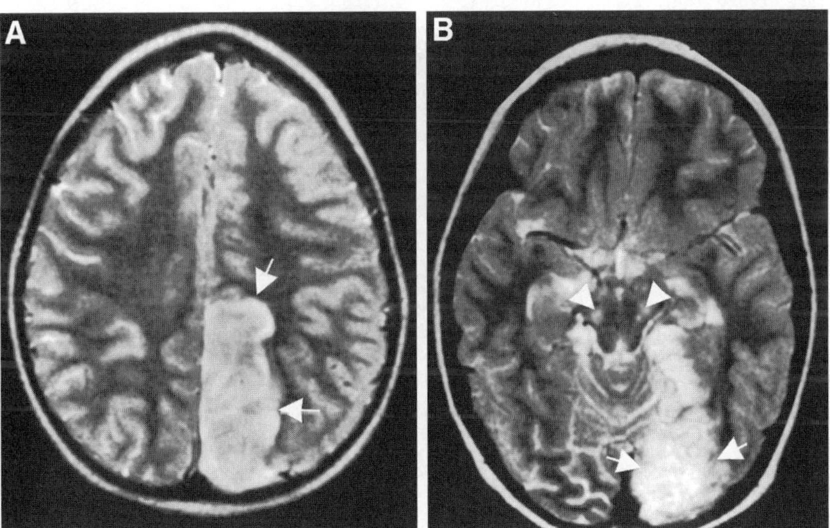

FIGURE 1.—Imaging in a 10-year-old girl with subacute onset of obtundation and hemianopsia secondary to stroke. Echocardiography (not shown) obtained for evaluation of source of embolus had normal results. Ten days after onset of stroke, deep vein thrombosis of leg, consistent with hypercoagulable state, developed. A, fast spin-echo proton-density–weighted (3400/38 [TR/TE]; excitation, 1) MR image in axial plane shows infarction (*arrows*) within left posterior cerebral artery. B, T2–weighted (3400/108) image in axial plane shows infarction extending into left medial temporal lobe (*arrows*) and at multiple sites within high mesencephalon (*arrowheads*). (Courtesy of Provenzale JM, Barboriak DP, Allen NB, et al: Patients with antiphospholipid antibodies: CT and MR findings of the brain. *AJR* 167:1573–1578, 1996.)

T2-weighted images, or dural sinus thrombosis. White matter foci were classified as small (less than 5 mm) or large (greater than 5 mm).

Results.—The most common abnormalities were large infarcts and hyperintense white matter foci, seen in 24 and 19 patients, respectively. At least 1 large lesion was present in 95% of patients with hyperintense white matter, and 76% had 5 or more small foci and/or 3 or more large foci. Less common findings were small coronal infarcts, lacunar infarcts, and dural sinus thrombosis, seen in 11, 10, and 5 patients respectively. Abnormalities were frequent in both SLE (57%) and non-SLE (41%) groups, but large infarcts were more likely to be present in the non-SLE group (26%) than in the SLE group (5%).

Discussion.—There is an increased prevalence of APA in patients with SLE and in non-SLE patients with ischemic cerebrovascular disease or other unexplained thrombosis. Compared with the general stroke population, those with APA are younger (Fig 1) and have a high rate of recurrence of thrombo-occlusive disease. Common abnormalities in patients with APA are infarcts of various sizes and hyperintense white matter foci. Detection of APA is important because many patients will require long-term anticoagulation.

▶ The importance of recognizing the role of APAs as a cause of gray or white matter infarcts, particularly in young patients, is emphasized in this paper. Based on this information, it is interesting to speculate about the possibility of APA and spinal cord dysfunction. Frequently, one is faced with a patient with an acute transverse myelopathy in whom a definitive diagnosis cannot be established. Perhaps an arterial or venous thrombosis may be the underlying cause, and such cases parallel the intracranial vascular abnormalities described by Provenzale et al.

R.M. Quencer, M.D.

10 Sleep Disorders

Sleep Apnea After 1 Year Domiciliary Nasal-Continuous Positive Airway Pressure and Attempted Weight Reduction: Potential for Weaning From Continuous Positive Airway Pressure
Noseda A, Kempenaers C, Kerkhofs M, et al (Hôpital Erasme, Brussels, Belgium; Université Libre de Bruxelles, Belgium)
Chest 109:138–143, 1996 10–1

Background.—Nasal-continuous positive airway pressure (N-CPAP) has revolutionized the treatment of sleep apnea syndrome (SAS). However, discontinued treatment results in recurrence, and few studies have assessed the long-term effects of regular continuous positive airway pressure (CPAP) treatment. Weight loss, which reduces pharyngeal collapsibility, is thought to be effective in obese patients with SAS. The effects of 1–year treatment with domiciliary N-CPAP and attempted weight loss on the severity of SAS and on the potential for weaning from CPAP were studied.

Methods.—Ninety-five patients with a baseline apnea hypopnea index of more than 10/h were treated with N-CPAP at home. All patients underwent dietary counseling, and those with a body mass index that exceeded 40 kg/m² underwent single ring vertical gastroplasty. At 1 year, a full-night polysomnography without CPAP was performed, and the results compared with baseline polysomnography.

Findings.—Thirty-nine patients compliant with CPAP were included in the final analysis. Mean weight had declined from 108.3 to 99.7 kg as a result of dietary counseling (in 36 patients) and gastroplasty (in 3). Apnea hypopnea index, maximal duration of apnea or hypopnea, minimal oxy-hemoglobin saturation, and stage shift index were significantly improved. The decline in apnea hypopnea index was associated with the decrease in body mass index and in stage shift index. Weaning from CPAP was proposed to 6 patients and was successful in 4—3 with weight losses that ranged from 29 to 94 kg and 1 with unchanged normal weight (Fig 2).

Conclusions.—One-year domiciliary N-CPAP combined with weight loss led to significant improvement in breathing during sleep and in sleep

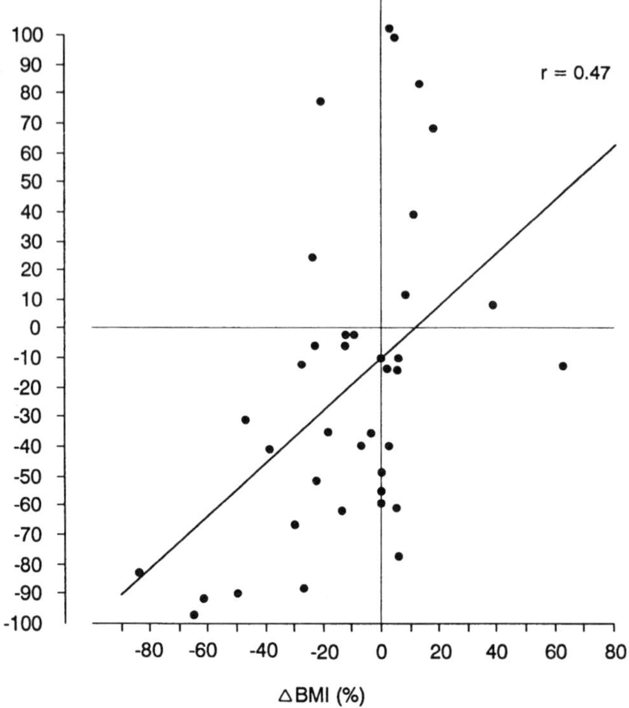

FIGURE 2.—Change in apnea hypopnea index (AHI) between baseline and 1–year measurements (*open triangle AHI*), plotted against the parallel change in body mass index (BMI) (*open triangle BMI*), in 39 patients with sleep apnea syndrome receiving domiciliary nasal-continuous positive airway pressure. The *open triangle AHI* is calculated as 1 year AHI minus baseline AHI, divided by baseline AHI and expressed as a percentage. The *open triangle BMI* is expressed as 1 year BMI minus baseline BMI, divided by baseline BMI minus ideal BMI (22 kg/m^2) and expressed as a percentage. (Courtesy of Noseda A, Kempenaers C, Kerkhofs M, et al: Sleep apnea after 1 year domiciliary nasal-continuous positive airway pressure and attempted weight reduction: Potential for weaning from continuous positive airway pressure. *Chest* 109:138–143, 1996.)

fragmentation. Weaning from CPAP was successful in 4 patients, 3 of whom had lost a substantial amount of weight.

▶ This article highlights the importance of weight reduction (and avoidance of weight gain) in the long-term management of SAS. As most of us realize, meaningful weight reduction can't be done quickly, even under the best of circumstances. Because patients without substantial weight loss quickly revert to SAS off CPAP, it is important that the clinician as well as the patient fully appreciate the implications of untreated SAS.[1] Also of note is that the occasional cure with CPAP (10% in this report), and substantial weight loss may be especially satisfying to the patient and the treating professionals. For those who are unable to accomplish the required weight loss, CPAP remains effective and well tolerated by most patients.

B. Nolan, M.D.

Reference

1. He J, Kryger MH, Zorick FJ, et al: Mortality and apnea index in obstructive sleep apnea: Experience in 385 male patients. *Chest* 94:9–14, 1988.

The Reliability of the Diagnostic Features in Patients With Narcolepsy
Folkerts M, Rosenthal L, Roehrs T, et al (Henry Ford Hosp, Detroit)
Biol Psychiatry 40:208–214, 1996   10–2

Background.—The criteria of short sleep latencies on the multiple sleep latency test (MSLT) and multiple sleep-onset rapid eye movement periods (SOREMPs) have been found to be very sensitive and specific for the diagnosis of narcolepsy. However, the reliability of polysomnographic findings in patients with this syndrome has not been established. The test-retest reliability of the sleep polysomnographic features in patients with polysomnographically diagnosed narcolepsy was determined.

Methods.—Thirty adults with narcolepsy and 30 healthy control subjects matched for age and sex were included in the study. The control subjects were divided into high- and low-MSLT groups. All subjects completed 2 polysomnographic assessments with at least 5 days between laboratory tests.

Findings.—Patients with narcolepsy had lower sleep efficiencies and high stage 1% when compared with the low-MSLT control group. When compared with both control groups, the narcoleptic patients had more awakenings and less stage 2%. The patients also had a shorter latency to stage 1 than the high-MSLT group did, although it was similar to that of the low-MSLT group. Narcoleptic patients had a greater number of SOREMPs than did the 2 control groups. The MSLT scores were stable across the 2 assessments and showed a significant association. Twenty-eight narcoleptic patients had 2 or more SOREMPs on reassessment as compared with 0 in the control groups.

Conclusions.—Polysomnographic findings are reliable in patients with narcolepsy. Multiple SOREMPs differentiated narcoleptic from normal subjects.

▶ Interviewing subjects for symptoms of cataplexy is clearly subjective even when performed by persons who have considerable experience with sleep disorders. Human leukocyte antigen testing has thus far provided only a high degree of probability that a subject *does not* have narcolepsy if lacking characteristic markers. In our sleep disorders center we also use urine testing between the overnight sleep recording and the MSLT to check for potential agents that may influence the recording. Unfortunately, neither short mean sleep latency nor multiple SOREMPs are limited to narcolepsy. Sleep apnea or other primary sleep disorders can usually be excluded in most instances by the overnight sleep recording. In addition, SOREMPs have been found in other nonnarcoleptics. Thus, the authors highlight the importance of reviewing not only the history but also the test results with an accomplished clinical sleep specialist. The utility of the MSLT is that it provides reasonably objective measures for sleepiness and SOREMPs.

B. Nolan, M.D.

Effects of Sleep and Sleep Stage on Epileptic and Nonepileptic Seizures

Bazil CW, Walczak TS (Mount Sinai School of Medicine, New York; Columbia Presbyterian Med Ctr, New York)
Epilepsia 38:56–62, 1997

10–3

Objective.—The effects of sleep on epilepsy are not clear, although the available evidence suggests that sleep promotes seizures in patients with epilepsy. Gaining insight into the relationship between epilepsy and sleep could provide clues to the ways in which seizures commence and spread. Continuous video-electroencephalographic (EEG) monitoring was used to compare seizures occurring during sleep vs. wakefulness.

Methods.—The retrospective analysis included video-EEG monitoring data on 1,116 seizures in 188 patients. For each incidence, information on the type of seizure, site of onset of partial seizures, sleep state at onset, and occurrence of secondary partial seizures was recorded. Twenty percent of the seizures occurred during sleep; these were further analyzed to determine the sleep state in which they occurred.

Findings.—Sixty percent of subclinical seizures occurred during sleep, as did 45% of primary generalized tonic-clonic seizures and 31% of complex partial seizures (CPSs). The rate of secondary generalization was 35% for CPSs occurring during sleep vs. 18% for those occurring during wakefulness. There was no difference in the rate of secondary generalization of frontal lobe CPSs during sleep and wakefulness—about 20% each. However, 45% of temporal lobe CPSs occurring during sleep generalized, compared with 19% of those occurring during wakefulness. Thirty-seven percent of frontal lobe seizures occurred during sleep, compared with 26% of temporal lobe seizures. Complex partial seizures tended to occur during stage 1 and 2 sleep and not during rapid eye movement sleep. Seizure duration was longer for those starting during slow-wave sleep, compared with seizures starting during wakefulness or stage 2 sleep. There were few psychogenic nonepileptic seizures between 12 AM and 6 AM, and none during sleep.

Conclusion.—Seizure patterns are different for seizures occurring during sleep vs. wakefulness. Temporal lobe CPSs are more likely to generalize if they occur during sleep. Frontal lobe seizures are more likely to occur during sleep than temporal lobe seizures. Psychogenic nonepileptic seizures do not occur during sleep, whereas CPSs often do. The mechanisms by which sleep influences seizures are unclear.

▶ This study provides additional evidence that continuously monitored patients experience observable differences in the pattern of their seizures during sleep states as compared with wakefulness. Differences are also observed for different sleep stages. These results highlight the importance of taking into consideration sleep differences when assessing clinical, as well as electrographic, descriptions and estimates of seizure frequency. Advances in continuous monitoring and identification of such state-specific differences, as well as development of treatment strategies to deal with them, should bring greater benefit to current and future seizure patients.

B. Nolan, M.D.

Sleep Apnea in Patients With Transient Ischemic Attack and Stroke: A Prospective Study of 59 Patients
Bassetti C, Aldrich MS, Chervin RD, et al (Univ of Michigan, Ann Arbor)
Neurology 47:1167–1173, 1996   10–4

Objective.—There is evidence suggesting that habitual snoring and sleep apnea (SA) are related not only to cardiovascular disease but also to stroke. However, there is little information about the frequency of SA in patients with acute cerebrovascular disease. The frequency of habitual snoring and SA in patients with transient ischemic attack (TIA) and stroke were prospectively determined.

Methods.—The analysis included 59 patients, 36 with stroke and 23 with TIA. There were 33 men and 26 women (mean age, 62 years). All patients were studied on a standard protocol, including the Epworth Sleepiness Score (ESS) to assess snoring and daytime sleepiness; the Sleep Disorders Questionnaire (SDQ-SA), a validated SA score; and the Scandinavian Stroke Scale (SSS). Patients with habitual snoring and an ESS of greater than 10 were considered to have clinically probable SA (P-SA). Women with an SDQ-SA score of 32 or greater and men with an SDQ-SA score of 36 or greater were also considered to have P-SA. Thirty-six patients underwent polysomnography (PSG) within a mean of 12 days after their stroke or TIA. Patients with an Apnea-Hypopnea Index (AHI) of 10 or greater on PSG were considered to have SA. A group of 19 age- and sex-matched controls was studied for comparison.

Results.—Of the patients who underwent PSG, 58% were habitual snorers and 58% were considered to have P-SA. Similar percentages were noted in those who did not have PSG (52% and 50%, respectively). Sixty-nine percent of patients undergoing PSG met the criterion for SA, compared with 15% of controls. There was no difference in the frequency of SA for patients with stroke vs. those with TIA. Furthermore, 55% of the patients undergoing PSG had an AHI of 20 or greater, with a minimal oxygen saturation of less than 85%. Sex and age were unrelated to the severity of SA. However, the AHI was significantly higher for habitual snorers, patients considered to have P-SA, or those with severe strokes (i.e., an SSS or less than 30). The clinical criteria for P-SA were 64% sensitive and 67% specific in predicting the diagnosis of SA.

Conclusion.—This prospective study found a high frequency of SA in patients with recent TIA or stroke. Although clinical findings cannot always predict the presence of SA, it is more frequent in patients with habitual snoring, a high SDQ-SA score, or severe stroke. The possibility of SA should be considered in patients with acute cerebral ischemia. Further study will tell whether treating SA has any impact on the course of cerebrovascular disease.

▶ On the face of it, it would seem that sleeping with frequently recurring significant hypoxemia, bradycardia, and other disturbing pathophysiologic changes would be chancy at best. Putting those risks together with the other potential risk factors for cerebrovascular disease found in many older individuals would seem to signal a particularly dangerous combination. Patients with impaired arterial flow and poor collateral circulation may be particularly vulnerable to interference with their supply of needed oxygen, which is, in turn, dependent on a patent airway. Proving these kinds of suppositions is the subject of this prospective clinical study, which offers useful data to support these lines of reasoning. Awareness of these risks should highlight the importance of suspecting, confirming, and treating SA in patients with cerebrovascular disease.

B. Nolan, M.D.

Hypersomnia Following Paramedian Thalamic Stroke: A Report of 12 Patients

Bassetti C, Mathis J, Gugger M, et al (Inselspital-Univ, Bern, Switzerland)
Ann Neurol 39:471–480, 1996   10–5

Background.—Organic hypersomnia can be caused by paramedian thalamic stroke (PTS). In the absence of systematic sleep-wake studies, organic hypersomnia has been attributed to disruption of ascending activating impulses and viewed as a "de-aroused" state. However, increased evidence has suggested that the thalamus has a role in sleep regulation, which raises the possibility that a sleep disturbance contributes to hypersomnia in PTS.

Methods and Findings.—Twelve patients with MRI-proved isolated PTS and hypersomnia were studied. The patients slept from 10 to more than 20 hours a day. The severity of hypersomnia was paralleled by nocturnal polysomnographic findings. In all patients, stage I non-rapid eye movement (NREM) sleep was increased and stage 2 NREM sleep and numbers of sleep spindles were reduced. Slow-wave NREM sleep was often decreased in patients with severe hypersomnia, but no major changes occurred in REM sleep. Daytime sleep behavior was associated primarily with stage 1 sleep by electroencephalogram. Hypersomnia was not correlated with the results of nap tests.

Conclusions.—Hypersomnia after PTS is associated with deficient arousal during the day and insufficient spindling and slow-wave sleep

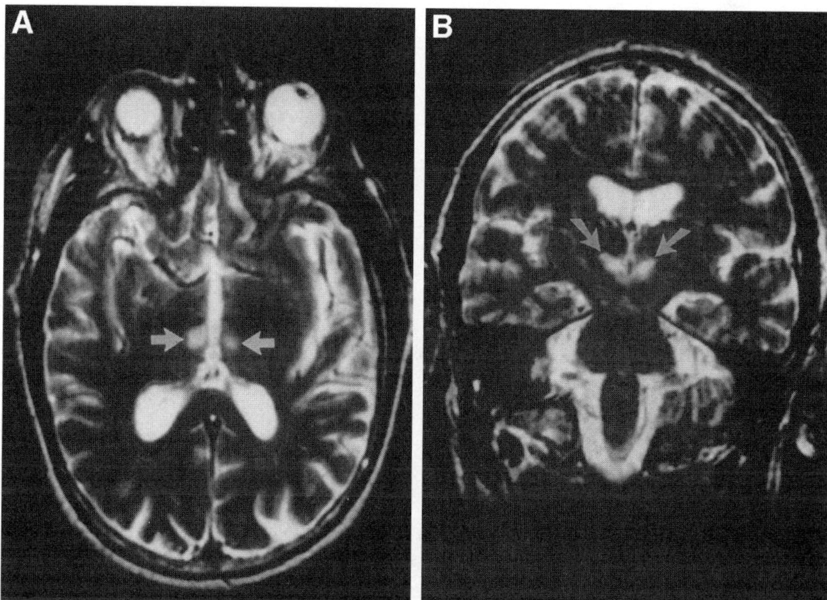

FIGURE 1.—T2–weighted axial (**A**) and coronal (**B**) brain MRI scans of Patient 1 showing a "butterfly-shaped" bilateral paramedian thalamic stroke (*arrows*). (Courtesy of Bassetti C, Mathis J, Gugger M, et al: Hypersomnia following paramedian thalamic stroke: A report of 12 patients. *Ann Neurology* 39:471–480, 1996, by permission of Little, Brown, and Company Inc.)

production at night. These data support the hypothesis that the paramedian thalamus serves a dual function as a final common pathway for both maintenance of wakefulness and promotion of NREM sleep (Figure 1).

▶ Based on their experience, the authors suggest that the sleep abnormalities identified in their patients support a potential dual role for the normally functioning thalamus. They propose that the appearance of hypersomnolence is due to interruption of the normal thalamic function to maintain wakefulness, and that an additional function of the thalamus is to promote NREM sleep. This article helps to promote further understanding of the pathophysiology of sleep and wake alteration with thalamic lesions. As the authors point out, thalamic disorder may also be associated with a clinical presentation that has been described as insomnia. The extended discussion and review also suggests that in disordered states of thalamic function, meanings for such conventional terms as hypersomnolence, insomnia, sleep, and even wakefulness itself may become less obvious.

B. Nolan, M.D.

11 Neuro-Otology

Particle Repositioning Maneuver: Effective Treatment for Benign Paroxysmal Positional Vertigo
Fung K, Hall SF (Queen's Univ, Kingston, Ont, Canada)
J Otolaryngol 25(4):243–248, 1996   11–1

Introduction.—Benign paroxysmal positional vertigo (BPPV) is a common labyrinthine disorder that has an incidence of 64 per 100,000 per year. Patients typically experience brief, intermittent, severe attacks of whirling vertigo on sudden posture change. The Dix-Hallpike position test is used to confirm the diagnosis. With the patient sitting in the head-hanging position, the head is rotated so that the affected side is down. Characteristic findings include a brief latent period followed by rotary nystagmus and intense vertigo that lasts several minutes, reversal on assuming the upright position, and fatigability on repetition. The particle repositioning maneuver (PRM) is a mechanical procedure. It displaces canaliths from the posterior semicircular canal (PSC) from the ampulla through the common crus into the utricular sac where they can no longer cause nystagmus and vertigo. The short-term and long-term efficacy of the PRM in treating BPPV was evaluated.

Methods.—Sixty-five consecutive patients with BPPV were placed into 1 of 3 categories: (1) self-limited BPPV, (2) "episodic" BPPV, or (3) "prolonged" BPPV. Patients underwent PRM. They were asked to call in 1 week to report the status of their condition. If they did not respond within 2 weeks, they were contacted. The 3 patients with bilateral disease were counted as 2 people each, so that 68 ears with BPPV were evaluated.

Results.—Fifty-seven ears (83.8%) had no evidence of residual disease immediately after PRM, 10 ears (14.7%) had partial improvement, and 1 ear (1.5%) had no improvement. Eighteen ears (26.5%) had secondary nystagmus. Factors not predictive of outcome were secondary nystagmus, gender, and duration of symptoms. Rates of disease-free outcome were 91.4%, 80.0%, and 50.0% for self-limited, episodic, and prolonged BPPV, respectively. Rates of partial improvement were 33.3%, 20.0%, and 8.6%, respectively, for self-limited, episodic, and prolonged BPPV. The patient with treatment failure had a history of head trauma and severe hearing loss and tinnitus. At a mean follow-up of 18.7 months, 43 ears (67.2%) had no history of recurrence and 22 ears (34.4%) had partial or complete recurrence. The mean latency before post-PRM recurrence was 4.6 months.

Four patients returned for 1 subsequent PRM, and 1 patient had 2 subsequent PRMs. These patients had no recurrences. The other 17 patients with recurrence did not return for subsequent PRM. The final outcome was no symptoms in 48 ears (72.6%), mild symptoms in 14 ears (22.6%), and treatment failure in 3 ears (4.8%). Four of 5 patients for whom BPPV was caused by trauma were completely cured.

Conclusion.—The PRM may be considered a simple, cost-effective, and efficacious treatment modality that can give immediate relief of BPPV symptoms. Outcomes are excellent in ears with problematic free-floating canaliths.

▶ Benign paroxysmal positional vertigo is the most common cause of spells of vertigo, with an incidence of 64 cases per 100,000 per year. It is usually caused by free-floating debris from the utricle (otoconium) in the posterior semicircular canal. The canalith repositioning maneuver (CRM), referred to as the particle repositioning maneuver in this paper, has become the standard form of treatment. Several papers have shown CRM to be effective in 80% to 90% of patients. The current paper found that CRM is most effective (91.4%) in patients with self-limited positional vertigo (first episode within the past 12 months with no periods of remission). Patients with a prolonged course of symptoms (more than 1 year without remission) have a 50% chance of remission after treatment, and patients with episodic BPPV (positional vertigo with periods of remission and relapse for an undefined time) have a success rate of 80% with CRM treatment. The authors also looked at the chance of recurrence of BPPV after CRM treatment over the course of 2–39 months (mean, 18.7 months). Thirty-four percent had recurrence with a mean latency of 4.6 months after treatment. The number of patients with recurrence was too small to determine whether this varied depending on the history of BPPV before treatment (self-limited, episodic, and prolonged). The conclusion that CRM is a simple and efficacious treatment that provides immediate and long-term relief is valid. The paper has 1 minor misconception. The type of nystagmus that occurs in patients with BPPV should not have been described as rotary nystagmus. The majority of patients have upbeat and torsional nystagmus.

R.J. Tusa, M.D., Ph.D.

Evaluation of Investigations to Diagnose the Cause of Dizziness in Elderly People: A Community-based Controlled Study

Colledge NR, Barr-Hamilton RM, Lewis SJ, et al (Univ of Edinburgh, Scotland; Royal Infirmary of Edinburgh NHS Trust, Scotland; Western Gen Hosp, Edinburgh, Scotland; et al)
BMJ 313:788–792, 1996   11–2

Introduction.—About 30% of people age 65 and over report problems with dizziness. Dizziness is the most common complaint in office visits for patients over age 75. It is a difficult diagnostic problem in elderly patients because it has many potential causes and patients have difficulty describing the complaint. Findings in 149 research subjects age 65 years and over experiencing dizziness were compared with those of 97 nondizzy elderly controls. An investigational algorithm was designed.

Methods.—All research subjects were assessed by physical examination, blood testing, electrocardiography (at rest and over 24 hours), electronystagmography, posturography, MRI of the head and neck (84% and 89% of dizzy and control research subjects, respectively), hospital anxiety and depression scores, hyperventilation, carotid massage, and the Hallpike maneuver.

Results.—No significant between-group differences were observed for blood profile, electrocardiography, electronystagmography, or MRI. There were significant between-group differences in posturography, physical examination, dizziness provocation, and psychological assessment. Of 149 research subjects for whom a cause of dizziness could be determined, 126 had more than 1 cause of dizziness. The causes of dizziness were central vascular disease (105 patients), cervical spondylosis (98), anxiety or hyperventilation (48), poor vision (23), postural hypotension (14), benign positional vertigo (6), and other (38). There were only 3 patients with a single diagnosis of anxiety or hyperventilation and no patients with a diagnosis of poor vision only.

Conclusion.—Findings indicate 5 key messages regarding evaluation of elderly persons with the complaint of dizziness: (1) dizziness may be diagnosed in most elderly persons by examination of the neurologic and locomotor systems and augmented by simple dizziness provocation testing; (2) expensive diagnostic testing is rarely helpful; (3) the most common causes of dizziness are central vascular disease and cervical spondylosis; (4) poor vision and anxiety often accompany, but rarely are the cause of, dizziness; and (5) there is a definitive role for the general practitioner in the assessment of dizziness in the elderly.

Clinical Significance.—General practitioners may be confident that clinical assessment with provocation of dizziness will identify the cause of dizziness in most elderly people. Poor vision, anxiety, and smoking should be explored and actively managed. Patients with blackouts and those whose symptoms and signs do not fit clearly defined diagnostic criteria should be referred. Otolaryngologic assessment will rarely be of use in the elderly because vestibular disease is infrequent. Geriatricians may be the most appropriate specialists for further assessment because of their experience with multisystem disease.

▶ Most population studies on the etiology of dizziness concern patients seen in neurology and otolaryngology specialty clinics. This paper examines the cause of dizziness in a community-based sample of subjects 65 years of age and older (149 patients with dizziness, 97 age-matched controls without dizziness). Some interesting points result from the study because it is a population-based study:

1. Of all forms of dizziness, vertigo is uncommon; 116 patients were unsteady, 89 were lightheaded, and 37 had vertigo (some patients had more than 1 symptom).

2. Testing is generally unhelpful; there were no significant differences on MRI or electronystagmography between the patient and control groups. Posturography was frequently abnormal in the patient group, reflecting their complaint of unsteadiness.

I agree with the distribution of presenting symptoms and the results of electronystagmography and MRI in this paper. More work will have to be done to validate the etiology of dizziness in this population. This paper suggests that central vascular disease and cervical spondylosis accounted for the majority of the problems, but this was based only on physical examination. It is not clear to what extent these disease processes are concomitant problems or true causes of dizziness.

R.J. Tusa, M.D., Ph.D.

Isolated Vertigo as a Manifestation of Vertebrobasilar Ischemia
Gomez CR, Cruz-Flores S, Malkoff MD, et al (Saint Louis Univ, St Louis)
Neurology 47:94–97, 1996   11–3

Background.—When associated with other neurologic symptoms, vertigo is a common symptom of vertebrobasilar ischemia. However, vertigo by itself is usually attributed to more benign causes, especially peripheral vestibular disorders. The current paper demonstrates that isolated episodes of vertigo are sometimes the only manifestation of vertebrobasilar ischemia.

Methods and Findings.—All records of the Saint Louis University Stroke Registry between January 1992 and September 1993 were analyzed retrospectively. Of 600 patients admitted, 30 had transient ischemic attacks (TIAs) in the vertebrobasilar circulation. Six of these patients had episodic vertigo of at least 4 weeks' duration as the only initial symptom. All 6 patients had 1 of 2 patterns of vascular abnormalities: focal basilar stenosis (present in 2 patients) and reduced flow in the entire vertebrobasilar system (in 4). Treatment consisted of warfarin in 5 patients and aspirin in 1. Brain stem infarctions developed in 2 patients, 1 of whom died.

Conclusions.—Isolated vertigo may be the only indication of vertebrobasilar ischemia. Vertebrobasilar insufficiency should be suspected in patients with significant risk factors for cerebrovascular disease; patients who have frequent episodes of vertigo that begin suddenly, last for minutes, and recur during days or weeks; and patients who have no hearing loss or tinnitus. It is important to note that 2 patients in the current series had brain stem infarctions, 1 of which was fatal.

▶ Spells of vertigo lasting less than a minute are usually the result of benign paroxysmal positional vertigo, which is a mechanical problem in the inner ear. Occasionally, transient ischemia in the distribution of the vestibular artery can result in vertigo without other cranial nerve or long-tract signs. This artery is a branch of the anterior inferior cerebellar artery and receives virtually no collateral flow. In this retrospective study from a university stroke registry, isolated vertigo was the initial symptom in 6 of 129 patients discharged from the hospital with a diagnosis of TIA. All 6 had either focal basilar artery stenosis or diffuse low flow in the vertebral basilar circulation. Brain stem stroke later developed in 2 patients. This diagnosis should be considered in any patient with significant risk factors for cerebrovascular disease who has spells of non–positional-induced vertigo that last for minutes. In the few studies published it appears that brain stem stroke can be prevented with adequate anticoagulation.

R.J. Tusa, M.D., Ph.D.

Arterial Dissection of the Vertebrobasilar Systems: A Possible Cause of Acute Sensorineural Hearing Loss

Nagahata M, Hosoya T, Fuse T, et al (Yamagata Univ, Japan)
Am J Otol 18:32–38, 1997

11–4

Background.—Acute sensorineural hearing loss (ASNHL) develops rapidly, within hours or a few days, and can range from mild to total in severity. Conditions known to cause ASNHL include viral infection, vascular disorders, and acoustic neurinoma. Vertebrobasilar dissection, now reported with greater frequency because of advances in neuroimaging methods, may also be a cause of ASNHL. The 3 patients reported here all had confirmed vertebrobasilar dissection and ASNHL.

Methods.—Patients were identified through a review of MR scans of 37 patients with ASNHL who were treated at the study institution between September 1993 and March 1995. All patients had proton density and T2–weighted axial images and 3–dimensional spoiled gradient-recalled acquisition in steady state imaging with gadopentetate dimeglumine, obtained with a 1.5 T MR system. Twenty-three patients also had T1–weighted images for review and 4 underwent vertebral angiography.

Results.—The presence of vertebrobasilar dissection was confirmed in 3 of 37 patients by vertebral angiography and/or 3–dimensional MR images. These patients, all women, were aged 63, 69, and 73 years. All 3 had a history of hypertension and 2 had diabetes mellitus. Initial symptoms, in addition to hearing loss, included a sensation of fullness in an ear, nausea, vertigo, and tinnitus. Hearing loss and symptoms appeared suddenly and patients were admitted to hospital within a few days. Treatment in 2 cases consisted of hydroxyethylated starch (1,000 mL/day) for reduction of viscosity of the blood and high-dose steroids (prednisolone, 200 mg/day) for 3 days. Audiograms showed flat loss in 1 patient and high-tone loss in the other 2 patients. All 3 experienced improvement.

Discussion.—Although circulatory disorders are considered to be an important cause of ASNHL, no studies have examined the potential role of vertebrobasilar dissection. Two possible mechanisms of acute hearing loss resulting from vertebrobasilar dissection are proposed: first, an extension of an intramural hematoma leading to occlusion or stenosis of branching vessels, or second, a distal artery-to-artery embolism arising from local thrombosis at the stenotic segment of the dissected artery. Early anticoagulant therapy may resolve the hearing loss and prevent the occurrence of more severe ischemic attacks.

▶ Acute sensorineural hearing loss is a medical emergency. Timely medical intervention may partially reverse the problem. Viral labyrinthitis, and occasionally, acoustic neuromas have been thought to be the most common cause, but there is increasing awareness that ischemia from embolism or thrombosis to the labyrinthine artery (usually a branch from the anterior inferior cerebellar artery) is also a common cause. For that reason, neurologists and neurosurgeons can be called upon to help with the diagnosis and management.

This article describes ASNHL after arterial dissection of the vertebral artery near the junction of the basilar artery. Of 37 consecutive patients with ASNHL, 3 had a dissection diagnosed on MRA and/or angiography. Magnetic resonance imaging with eighth nerve cuts and MRA should be ordered for all patients with ASNHL to rule out acoustic neuroma and vertebral basilar disease. The article does not discuss management of dissection, but one should treat the patient with coumadin, as with other dissection syndromes, to prevent embolism or propagation of clot.

R.J. Tusa, M.D., Ph.D.

Auditory and Vestibular System Findings in Patients with Vertebrobasilar Dolichoectasia

Passero S, Nuti D (Universitá di Siena, Italy)
Acta Neurol Scand 93:50–55, 1996   11–5

Objective.—In patients with vertebrobasilar dolichoectasia (VBD), cranial nerve deficits can develop, most commonly involving the nerves crossing the cerebellopontine cistern. The facial nerve is the most frequently affected, followed by the trigeminal nerve. Relatively little is known regarding the findings related to impairment of the vestibulocochlear nerve. The auditory and vestibular changes occurring in patients with VBD were presented.

Methods.—The study included 23 patients with VBD, all with auditory-vestibular symptoms and/or isolated or multiple cranial nerve deficits. As depicted on imaging studies, the basilar artery was judged to be elongated if it lay lateral to the margin of the clivus or dorsum sellae at any point, or if its bifurcation lay above the plane of the suprasellar cistern. If the artery measured greater than 4.5 mm in diameter, it was considered ectatic. The patients' results on auditory and vestibular testing were analyzed.

TABLE 2.—Abnormal Neuro-Otologic Findings in 23 Patients With Vertebrobasilar Dolichoectasia in Relation to Clinical Presentation

Neuro-otological findings	Group I ($n=10$)	Group II ($n=13$)	Total ($n=23$)
Nystagmus			
central origin	3	4	7
peripheral origin	3	3	6
Abnormal saccades	1	5	6
Abnormal smooth pursuit	3	7	10
Canal paresis/paralysis			
unilateral	4	3	7
bilateral	1	4	5
Unilateral SNHL	2	5	7
Abnormal ABR			
absent	1	2	3
abnormal I–III, I–V		2	2
abnormal I–V, III–V	1	2	3
Absent SR			
VII	3		3
VIII	1	2	3

Abbreviations: SNHL, sensorineural hearing loss; *ABR,* auditory brain stem response; *SR,* stapedius reflex.

(Courtesy of Passero S, Nuti D: Auditory and vestibular system findings in patients with vertebrobasilar dolichoectasia. *Acta Neurol Scand* 93:50–55, copyright 1996, Munksgaard International Publishers Ltd., Copenhagen, Denmark.)

Findings.—The results showed specific evidence of auditory and/or vestibular impairment in 83% of patients. Forty-seven percent of the abnormal results were consistent with peripheral impairment, 16% with central dysfunction, and 37% with both peripheral and central dysfunction. Nystagmus was the most common abnormality, followed by abnormalities of visual ocular control and significant sensorineural hearing loss (Table 2). Most patients' test results were consistent with their symptoms, but sometimes the tests disclosed clinically inapparent auditory-vestibular abnormalities.

Conclusion.—Patients with VBD may have auditory-vestibular dysfunction. These abnormalities are largely related to compression of the vestibulocochlear nerve, although brain stem–cerebellar ischemia and impaired blood supply of the vestibular labyrinth may be present as well. Patients with VBD should have a neuro-otologic examination to detect clinical and subclinical dysfunction of the auditory-vestibular systems and to gain clues as to the site of the lesion.

▶ There have only been a handful of case reports on vestibular and hearing disorders caused by dolichoectasia. This study includes 23 new cases and is the largest series to date. This entity is more common then previously believed. The cases are seen either with peripheral (eighth nerve) or central (vestibular nucleus and cerebellar flocculus) deficits. Dolichoectasia should be distinguished from compression of the eighth nerve from the anterior inferior cerebellar artery or one of its branches (vascular loops). There is no discussion of management, but the article does emphasize the need for neuro-otologic evaluation of patients with VBD to identify subclinical dysfunction, as the cerebellopontine angle cistern is the most frequently involved area.

R.J. Tusa, M.D.

Idiopathic Dandy's Syndrome
Syms CA III, House JW (Wilford Hall Med Ctr, San Antonio, Tex; House Ear Inst, Los Angeles)
Otolaryngol Head Neck Surg 116:75–78, 1997   11–6

Background.—Dandy's syndrome was first described in patients who had undergone bilateral vestibular nerve section for Meniere's disease. After surgery, they experienced "jumbling" of objects in their visual fields while in motion and difficulty in walking in the dark. Surgery is now an infrequent cause of Dandy's syndrome, but it can result as well from ototoxicity, tumors, and infections. Patients with idiopathic Dandy's syndrome were examined to determine whether they differed from those with a known cause.

Methods.—From January 1984 through June 1994, 110 patients seen at the study institution received a diagnosis of Dandy's syndrome. Medical records were available for 105 cases. Charts were retrospectively reviewed and data collected on demographic variables, clinical history, physical examination, laboratory test results, cause, and follow-up.

Results.—Approximately one third of patients (34) had no known cause of Dandy's syndrome. The most common clinical diagnoses (Table 1) in the remaining 71 patients were ototoxicity, Meniere's disease, infection, and vascular disease. Except for a higher proportion of women in the idiopathic group, the baseline characteristics of those with known and unknown causes were similar. In addition, the 2 groups did not differ significantly in symptoms of vertigo, imbalance, motion sickness, dizziness, problems in walking in the dark, tinnitus, or visual disturbance. Ear examinations, gait, and the Rhomberg and sharpened Rhomberg tests

TABLE 1.—Clinical Diagnosis in Patients With Dandy's Syndrome

Clinical diagnosis	No. of patients
Ototoxic	16
Meniere's disease	16
Infection	11
Vascular	12
Autoimmune	6
Trauma	6
Hereditary	2
Tumor	2
Unknown	34
Total	105

(Courtesy of Syms CA III, House JW: Idiopathic Dandy's syndrome. *Otolaryngol Head Neck Surg* 116:75–78, 1997.)

yielded similar results in the 2 groups. Abnormal audiographic findings were more common in the known-cause group (81%) than in the idiopathic group (47%). Symptoms were unchanged in most patients after a mean follow-up of 6.5 years. Some improvement was reported by 28% of the known-cause group and 40% of the idiopathic group. None of the clinical variables were predictive of subjective outcome.

Discussion.—The diagnosis of Dandy's syndrome can be difficult; a specific cause is often not found and the outcome cannot be predicted. Patients with balance problems without a known cause should be questioned regarding symptoms of oscillopsia and worsening of balance in the darkness.

▶ Dysequilibrium caused by bilateral vestibular hypofunction is frequently missed on examination. This is unfortunate because this cause for dysequilibrium responds well to vestibular rehabilitation. One of the reasons why bilateral vestibular hypofunction is missed is that it is usually not associated with vertigo or hearing loss. In this review of 105 patients, the authors could not come up with the cause in 34 cases (32%). More than half of these patients had normal results on audiography. The authors do not discuss the prevalence of bilateral vestibular defects among patients seen with dysequilibrium, but in our own database of 450 patients, 18% were found to have bilateral vestibular hypofunction. We need to keep this entity in mind when faced with patients complaining of dysequilibrium.

R.J. Tusa, M.D., Ph.D.

Pulsatile Tinnitus Associated With Congenital Central Nervous System Malformations

Wiggs WJ Jr, Sismanis A, Laine FJ (Med College of Virginia, Richmond)
Am J Otol 17:241–244, 1996   11–7

Background.—Pulsatile tinnitus (PT) is a rare otologic symptom. This report describes 3 patients with PT associated with congenital CNS malformations: 2 patients with type I Arnold-Chiari malformations and 1 patient with congenital stenosis of the sylvan aqueduct.

Case 1.—Woman, 44, had a 2–month history of PT, with fluctuating hearing loss and episodic vertigo. She had a history of headache and blurred vision. Results of otoscopic head and neck examination, auditory evoked brain stem response (ABR), and electronystagmography were all normal. Neuro-ophthalmologic consultation revealed bilateral mild disc edema/hyperemia. Magnetic resonance imaging showed cerebellar tonsils herniating through the foramen magnum, suggesting a type I Arnold-Chiari malformation. Lumbar puncture showed increased CSF opening pressure. Posterior fossa decompression resolved the PT and headaches and normalized hearing. The patient remains asymptomatic.

Case 3.—Woman, 23, was seen for right PT of 4 months duration and headache. Results of otoscopic head and neck examination, neuro-ophthalmologic consultation, and ABR were normal. Auscultation demonstrated PT. Magnetic resonance imaging revealed dilated lateral and third ventricles, hydrocephalus, empty sella with displaced pituitary, and stenosis of the aqueduct of Sylvius. The patient declined a ventriculoperitoneal shunt and the PT persists.

Conclusion.—Pulsatile tinnitus can be caused by congenital CNS malformations in some patients. The occurrence of PT in these patients is secondary to turbulent blood flow in the dural venous sinuses caused by elevated intracranial pressure. Any hearing loss is the result of a masking effect of the PT. The treatment of PT in these patients should normalize the intracranial pressure, which will eliminate PT and restore normal hearing.

▶ Pulsatile tinnitus can occur from a number of disorders but is most frequently seen in patients with increased intracranial pressure. Thirty percent of all individuals with pseudotumor cerebri may experience this annoying symptom. The evaluation of patients with PT is well described in the otology literature but has received very little discussion in the neurology and neurosurgery literature. The senior author of this paper (Dr. Sismanis) has published a number of important papers about this disorder. This paper discusses PT in patients with increased intracranial pressure (2 patients with fairly mild Arnold-Chiari I malformations and 1 patient with cerebral aqueduct stenosis). The approach to patients with PT is nicely described in this paper.

R.J. Tusa, M.D.

12 Headaches

Long-term Outcome of Patients With Headache and Drug Abuse After Inpatient Withdrawal: Five-year Follow-up
Schnider P, Aull S, Baumgartner C, et al (Univ Clinic for Neurology, Vienna)
Cephalalgia 16:481–485, 1996   12–1

Background.—Patients with frequent migraine attacks or tension-type headaches often start overusing ergotamine and/or analgesics. This leads to chronic, daily, drug-induced headaches. In treating these patients, the drug abuse must be dealt with before the headaches can be managed. Most previous studies of these patients have not included a lengthy follow-up, nor have they defined drug abuse according to the International Headache Society (IHS) criteria. Results of a 5-year follow-up study of the effects of inpatient withdrawal therapy in patients with headache and drug abuse were reported.

Methods.—The study included 54 patients with chronic daily headache and ergotamine and/or analgesic abuse, as defined by the IHS criteria. All patients underwent inpatient withdrawal therapy, with abrupt discontinuation of all drugs. The patients received metoclopramide, diazepam, prothipendyl, and sometimes other drugs during the 10-to 11-day withdrawal therapy. Thirty-eight patients were re-examined after a 5-year observation period.

Results.—At follow-up, 50% of the patients reported having headaches on only 8 days per month or less. Forty-seven percent had no or only mild headaches. The frequency of headaches was closely related to the length of time the patient had abused drugs, whereas the intensity of headaches was related to the number of tablets taken per month. Changes in the frequency and intensity of headache were noted from the end of treatment to 2 years afterward, with no change thereafter. Drug abuse recurred in 40% of patients. Outcomes were somewhat better for patients with migraine than for those with tension-type headache or a combination of the 2.

Conclusion.—For patients with chronic daily headache and ergotamine and/or analgesic abuse, inpatient drug withdrawal is a treatment with long-term efficacy. Half of patients still have a substantial improvement in the frequency and intensity of headaches after 5 years. Sixty percent remain free of drug relapse. The results encourage the use of inpatient drug

"

withdrawal therapy for patients with chronic headaches related to drug abuse.

► Patients with chronic daily headaches constitute a major and challenging therapeutic problem. We now know that this type of headache is frequently a consequence of, or is maintained by, immoderate use of analgesic/ergotamine medication. All too many of these patients are in a vicious cycle of headache and medication misuse. All physicians who treat large numbers of patients with headaches know that acute treatment of these patients by exclusion of all analgesics and ergots is effective in a large proportion of them. The great value of the investigation abstracted here lies in the finding that after 5 years of follow-up, many of these patients are doing very well. That is welcome news, indeed, and should indicate that although eliminating the medication abuse is often difficult and time-consuming, the potential for both acute and long-term benefits are enormous.

R.A. Davidoff, M.D.

Headache of Recent Onset in Adults: A Prospective Population-based Study
Duarte J, Sempere AP, Delgado JA, et al (Gen Hosp of Segovia, Spain)
Acta Neurol Scand 94:67–70, 1996   12–2

Introduction.—Headache is a common symptom that prompts 1,600 patients per 100,000 to consult their family physician each year. This complaint may lead many physicians to order CT or MRI to rule out organic causes of headache. Headaches of recent onset, particularly in middle-aged or elderly patients, are of particular concern. Not many prospective investigations have been conducted on headaches of recent onset.

Methods.—One hundred consecutive patients with headache of recent origin were evaluated to determine the diagnostic role of neuroimaging in patients with normal neurologic examination. All patients underwent cranial CT with and without IV contrast when possible, cranial MRI, erythrocyte sedimentation rate determinations in all patients over the age of 60, lumbar puncture, blood tests, MR angiography, and temporal artery biopsy. Headaches were classified according to criteria of the International Headache Society.

Results.—The mean patient age was 46.2 years. Eighty of 100 patients had normal neurologic examinations. Thirty-nine percent of the patients had organic headaches. Of these, 26% had normal neurologic examinations. Of the patients with normal neurologic examinations who underwent CT, 22.5% had pathology consisting of intracranial tumors in 13, hydrocephalus in 2, arachnoid cyst in 1, toxoplasmic abscess in 1, and parenchymal hemorrhage in 1. An intracranial tumor was diagnosed in 16% of 80 patients with normal neurologic examinations.

Conclusion.—Headaches of recent onset may not necessarily be benign. Tumors were diagnosed in 21% of the patients with headache of recent onset. All adult patients with nonvascular headache of recent onset and no previous history should undergo neuroimaging evaluation regardless of the characteristics of the headache or findings of the neurologic examination. Temporal arteritis should be considered in elderly patients.

▶ Far too many CT and MRI examinations are ordered in patients with all types of headaches merely because the tests are available, patients assume that they need them, and physicians believe that they are required as a precaution against charges of malpractice. In this regard, the results of this prospective study are worthy of thought. The results indicate that imaging procedures are needed in adult patients with headaches of recent onset who do not fulfill the criteria for migraine or cluster headache. They also demonstrate that a normal neurologic examination is not sufficient to rule out intracranial pathology. In addition, the results indicate that a large number of brain tumors call attention to themselves by headache rather than by other symptoms.

R.A. Davidoff, M.D.

History of Migraine and Risk of Cerebral Ischaemia in Young Adults

Carolei A, and the Italian National Research Council Study Group on Stroke in the Young (Univ of L'Aquila, L'Aquila-Collemaggio, Italy)
Lancet 347:1503–1506, 1996

12–3

Background.—A history of migraine has been proposed as a risk factor for stroke, especially among young women. To further investigate this relationship, the occurrence of a history of migraine with or without aura was noted in a prospective case series of young adults with transient ischemic attack (TIA) or stroke and matched controls.

Methods.—Participating were 308 patients aged 15–44 years with either TIA or stroke and 591 age- and sex-matched controls. Participants were recruited by neurologists at 7 referral university general hospitals.

Results.—The proportion of patients with a history of migraine (14.9%) was higher than that of controls (9.1%). Subgroup analyses revealed that in women and in those younger than 35 years, a history of migraine did emerge as a risk factor for cerebral ischemia. In men and in those older than 35 years, atherogenic risk factors were more significant. A history of migraine was a significant risk factor in patients with TIA but not in those with stroke. Patients with previous migraines with aura were at risk of stroke; patients with migraines without aura were at risk of TIA.

Conclusions.—The rare association of migraine with cerebral ischemia appears to be limited to women younger than 35 years. Taking measures to prevent the unlikely occurrence of stroke in all women with migraine is impractical, but comorbidity in the presence of migraine with aura deserves further clinical evaluation.

▶ This is a very large study that deals with an extremely important issue, namely, whether stroke and migraine are correlated. This publication in a leading journal (*Lancet*), is well carried out, involves a large number of patients, and shows that the association is uncommon and limited to women under age 35. All of this is clinically relevant.

M.D. Ginsberg, M.D.

A Double-blind Study of Subcutaneous Dihydroergotamine vs Subcutaneous Sumatriptan in the Treatment of Acute Migraine

Winner P, Ricalde O, Le Force B, et al (Palm Beach Headache Ctr, West Palm Beach, Fla; Keesler Med Ctr, Keesler Air Force Base, Miss; Lackland Med Ctr, Lackland Air Force Base, Tex; et al)
Arch Neurol 53:180–184, 1996

12–4

Background.—Serotonin receptor binding is believed to be the main mechanism in migraine relief. Dihydroergotamine mesylate (DHE-45) and sumatriptan succinate both work in this way. However, there have been no published studies that have compared these 2 agents. The effects of subcutaneous DHE-45 and sumatriptan on initial and persistent pain relief in patients with migraine were compared in a multicenter, double-blind trial.

Methods.—By random assignment, patients with moderate or severe head pain received 1 mg of subcutaneous DHE-45 or 6 mg of subcutaneous sumatriptan. The patients rated head pain, functional ability, nausea, and vomiting at baseline and at 0.5, 1, 2, 4, and 24 hours after administration. A second injection of the same medication was administered if pain persisted after 2 hours, and self-ratings were obtained 0.5 and 1 hour later.

Findings.—Two hundred ninety-five patients were evaluable. Pain relief at 2 hours was documented in 73.1% of the patients given DHE-45 and in 85.3% of those given sumatripten. Headache relief at 3 and 4 hours did not differ significantly between groups. At 24 hours, 89.7% of those given DHE-45 and 76.7% of those given sumatripten had relief. Headache recurred within 24 hours after treatment in 45% of the sumatripten group and in 17.7% of the DHE-45 group. No serious adverse effects occurred with either drug.

Conclusions.—Both DHE-45 and sumatripten effectively alleviate the initial pain of migraine headache. Sumatriptan had a faster onset of relief, but by 3 hours the 2 agents were equally effective. The relief attained with DHE-45 was more sustained, with significantly less headache recurrence. With both agents, efficacy did not require concomitant antiemetic administration.

▶ Activation of the trigeminovascular system with antidromic release of neuropeptide transmitters has been implicated in a process of neurogenic inflammation that sensitizes nociceptive nerve fibers, innervates dural and pial vasculature, and produces the pain of migraine. Activation of 5-HT$_{1D}$ receptors located on the presynaptic terminals of trigeminovascular fibers appears to block the release of endogenous peptides from these fibers. Both ergots and sumatriptan possess high affinity for the presynaptic serotonin receptors, and this appears to be their main mechanism of action to abort acute attacks. Sumatriptan is very selective in its action, but dihydroergotamine is known to bind at a number of biogenic amine receptor sites. It may be that binding to these latter additional sites is responsible for the sustained actions of dihydroergotamine. Alternatively, differences in pharmocokinetics may be responsible for the differences in duration. In any event, it is valuable to have a study that convincingly demonstrates that dihydroergotamine is superior to sumatriptan for recurrence of headaches. Physicians will have to weight the advantages of an automatic sumatriptan injector that allows self-administration vs. the difficulties many patients experience in giving themselves injections of dihydroergotamine.

R.A. Davidoff, M.D.

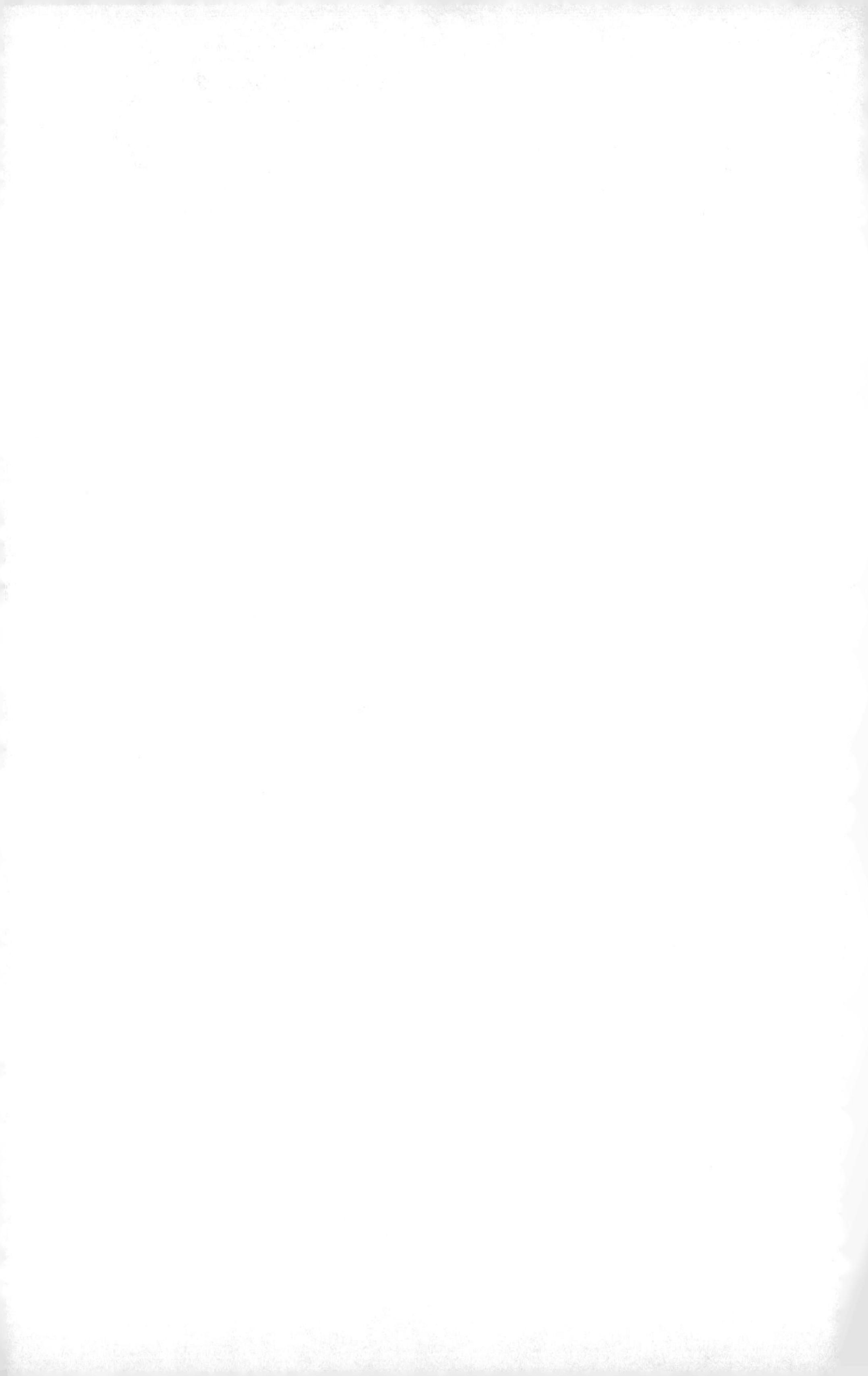

13 Behavioral Neurology

Word Comprehension: The Distinction Between Refractory and Storage Impairments
Warrington EK, Cipolotti L (Natl Hosp for Neurology and Neurosurgery, London)
Brain 119:611–625, 1996

13–1

Background.—The system that processes, stores, and retrieves information about the meanings of words, facts, objects, and concepts is called semantic memory. Impairments of semantic memory may affect only 1 domain of knowledge. The temporary unavailability of stored representations is termed an "access deficit." Word comprehension deficits in patients with cortical degenerative conditions were observed by using procedures identical to those previously used to evaluate access dysphasia.

Methods.—A series of experiments compared residual word comprehension skills between 2 patients with an access dysphasia and 4 patients with cortical degenerative conditions. Word-picture matching tests were used to assess the effects of rate of presentation, word frequency, semantic relatedness, and consistency.

Results.—Only patients with access dysphasia had word comprehension performance affected by the presentation rate (the response-stimulus interval). The performance of patients with access dysphasia was also more influenced by the semantic relatedness of the stimulus arrays. Only performance of patients with degenerative conditions, however, was strongly determined by word frequency. Response inconsistency occurred only in patients with access dysphasia.

Conclusions.—These findings differentiate word comprehension performance between these 2 types of patients, thus identifying 2 types of word comprehension impairment. A unitary account of the performance pattern of patients with access dysphasia in terms of refractoriness was previously proposed and is substantiated. Also advanced is a unitary account of patients with degenerative conditions in terms of storage deficit. Refractoriness and storage deficits may reflect 2 sources of injury to the stored representations underpinning a word rather than a dichotomy between deficits affecting the stored representations themselves and the procedures of accessing semantic representations. These findings raise implications for neurologic diagnosis and therapeutic intervention. For example, patients whose word comprehension performance is characterized by a rate-of-presentation effect might be more likely to have vascular or space-occupying lesions, whereas patients with pure cortical degenerative conditions might not show a rate effect. Therapeutically, repetition of an item may not be beneficial for patients with a refractory impairment; a wide vocabulary might be more advantageous.

▶ Disturbances of semantic memory have been documented in patients with cortical neurodegenerative conditions, with the rate of stimulus presentation presumably having little effect on performance. The latter feature is felt to reflect a fixed defect in semantic storage. A similar phenomenon occurs in some dysphasic patients, in whom, by contrast, slower stimulus presentation rates tend to result in significantly improved performance. This has been interpreted as indicating a disturbed "access" to stored representations in the latter group of patients. Warrington and Cipolotti's study addresses the empirical weaknesses in previous formulations of the concept of "storage" vs. "access" defects in semantic memory, thereby providing a stronger basis to understand the operation of this faculty from the cognitive perspective.

R. Kultis, M.D.

Neural Substrates of Facial Recognition

Andreasen NC, O'Leary DS, Arndt S, et al (Univ of Iowa, Iowa City)
J Neuropsychiatry Clin Neurosci 8:139–146, 1996   13–2

Background.—Human beings learn to identify those around them shortly after birth on the basis of complex variations in facial features. Facial recognition may involve several different systems in the human brain. The neural substrates of facial recognition in the intact human brain were examined through the use of positron emission tomography (PET).

Methods.—Cerebral blood flow was measured with PET in 17 healthy volunteers while they performed 3 facial recognition tasks: recognizing new faces, recognizing familiar faces, and recognizing sex. For testing of familiar face recognition, participants were taught to recognize 18 faces 1 week before testing, with review 1 day before testing. Recognition of new

FIGURE 1.—Three orthogonal views are shown for each of the 3 tasks. Statistical maps (*t*-maps) of the PET data showing regions significantly activated are superimposed on a composite MR image derived by averaging the MR scans from the subjects. The value of *t* is shown on the color bar at the *right*. Two types of statistical maps are provided. The "peak map" (*left panels*) shows the small areas where all contiguous voxels exceed the predefined threshold for statistical significance (3.61). The "*t*-map" (*right panels*) shows the value of *t* for all voxels in the image and provides a general overview of the landscape of increases in blood flow during the task. The planes have been chosen to illustrate the location of the relevant activity for each specific task. The categorizing-faces task (**A**) primarily activates the left frontal and inferior temporal regions. The recognizing-new-faces task (**B**) primarily activates the right frontal, anterior cingulate, right parietal, and left cerebellar regions. The recognizing-familiar-faces task (**C**) primarily activates the left lingual and fusiform gyri of the inferomedial temporoparietal visual association cortex, although
(Continued)

FIGURE 1 (cont.)

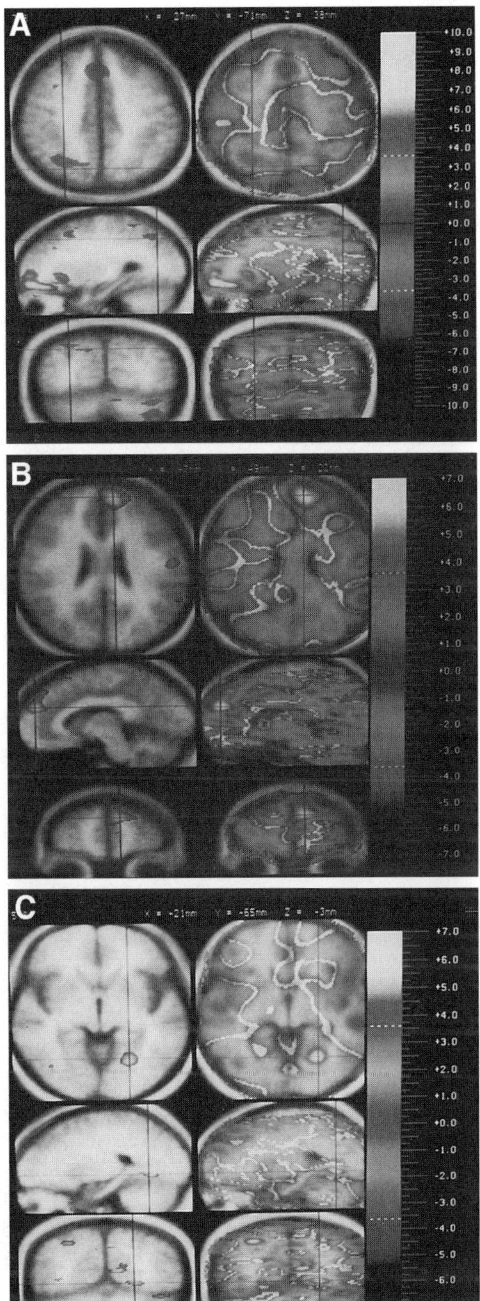

a smaller area is also seen on the right (and therefore not visualized in this figure). This suggestion of bilateral fusiform activity is consistent with human lesion literature that suggests that a bilateral injury is necessary for the production of prosopagnosia. (Courtesy of Andreasen NC, O'Leary DS, Arndt S, et al: Neural substrates of facial recognition. *J Neuropyschiatry Clin Neurosci* 8:139–146, 1996.)

faces was evaluated by exposing the participants to 18 new faces 1 minute before PET monitoring. During PET monitoring, participants were asked which faces were "learned" or "not learned" and which faces appeared male or female.

Results.—Performance of these tasks activated 3 different brain pathways (Fig 1). Categorization of sex involved the left inferior temporal lobe and left frontal cortex. Recognition of new faces involved a predominantly right frontal–right parietal–left cerebellar network, and recognition of familiar faces involved the left lingual and left and right fusiform gyri.

Conclusions.—Performance of these routine daily activities appears to involve different brain regions. These findings support those of previous studies of the organization of extrastriate visual cortex in human and nonhuman primate lesions, including studies of the unusual syndrome of prosopagnosia, in which the patient can recognize a face as such but cannot recognize familiar faces.

▶ This provocative study suggests that different mental operations associated with the recognition of faces require processing in substantially different regions of the cerebral cortex. The general agreement of the localization proposed with inferences derived from neuroanatomical and neurophysiologic data in nonhuman primates lends some validation to the theoretical framework used to interpret the data. This study will probably stimulate new assessments of patients with increasingly localized lesions and various disturbances of visual object recognition.

R. Kultis, M.D.

Vascular Dementia
Amar K, Wilcock G (Bristol Univ, England)
BMJ 312:227–231, 1996   13–3

Introduction.—At the turn of the century, cerebral atherosclerosis was believed to be the most common cause of dementia. Alzheimer's disease was thought to be a rare cause of dementia that only affected younger patients. By the 1950s, it was discovered that cerebral atherosclerosis could be present in normal individuals, as well as in those with cognitive impairment. The characteristics of ischemic vascular dementia were reviewed.

Mechanisms.—Vascular dementia is 1 of the 3 most common causes of dementia and may be caused by multiple infarcts, a single strategically placed infarct, or white matter ischemia. Infarcts can be in the cerebral cortex, in subcortical regions, or in both cortical and subcortical areas. The site of the infarction has more effect on resulting dementia than does the volume of tissue lost. Multiple cortical infarcts often result from thromboembolic disease or cerebral vasculities. Dementia can also result from multiple lacunar infarcts. Angular gyrus syndrome is a dementia that results from infarction of the angular gyrus in the inferior parietal lobule.

This syndrome was often misdiagnosed as Alzheimer's disease. White matter ischemia may be the most common mechanism of vascular dementia. White matter lesions are seen in 70% to 90% of patients who have vascular dementia, in 10% to 20% of those who have early onset Alzheimer's disease, and in 70% to 80% of those who have late onset Alzheimer's disease.

Risk Factors.—Stroke and age are the most significant risk factors for dementia, and stroke alone increases the risk 9 times. Other risk factors include older age, low education, history of stroke, diabetes, and left-sided lesions.

Evaluation and Differential Diagnosis.—Evaluation of a patient who has possible cognitive impairment should include assessment of vascular risk factors, examination of the cardiovascular system, and neurologic examination. It is important to determine whether the cause of dementia is treatable. Such causes include hypothyroidism, neurosyphilis, vitamin B12 deficiency, normal pressure hydrocephalus, frontal lobe tumors, cerebral vasculitis, and even hyperviscosity syndromes and severe bilateral carotid stenosis. Computed tomography or MRI is necessary to exclude some of these possible causes; MRI is more sensitive that CT, as it shows more white matter lesions (Fig 4). Vascular dementia must be differentiated from Alzheimer's disease, Lewy body type dementia, progressive supranuclear palsy, corticobasal degeneration, Parkinson's disease dementia, and frontal lobe tumors.

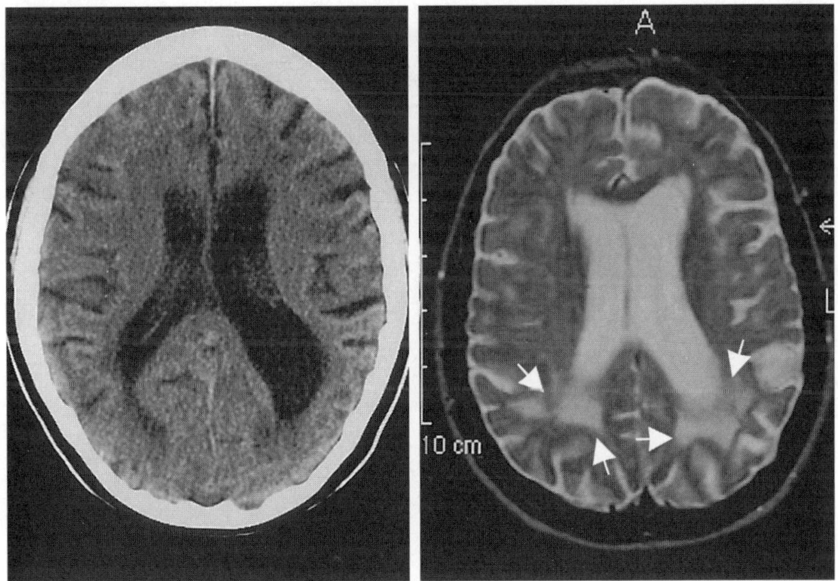

FIGURE 4.—**Left,** CT of brain showing moderate degree of low attenuation of white matter. **Right,** MRI of brain of same patient showing more extensive white matter hyperintensities (*arrows*). (Courtesy of Amar K and Wilcock G: Vascular dementia. *BMJ* 312:227–231, 1996.)

Discussion.—Vascular dementia is preventable, and cognitive functioning may be improved by controlling risk factors, such as hypertension and diabetes, and by using an antiplatelet drug. There is ongoing research into the role of white matter disease in dementia. Further research is needed on the relation of structural pathologic changes to signs and symptoms in vascular dementia subtypes. The use of thrombolytic drugs to treat acute stroke may also have implications for vascular dementia.

▶ The authors have provided a useful review of a complex and often confusing subject, with a cogent analysis of recent trends in the thinking about the mechanisms involved in dementia produced by cerebrovascular disorders. Perhaps more emphasis is needed on the study of mechanisms and on methods of assessment for functional impairments of cerebral blood flow that do not produce strokes. This remains an area of speculation, which is only tangentially addressed in reviews of the subject.

R. Kuljis, M.D.

14 Demyelinating Disease

Accumulation of Hypointense Lesions ("Black Holes") on T_1 Spin-Echo MRI Correlates With Disease Progression in Multiple Sclerosis
Truyen L, van Waesberghe JHTM, van Walderveen MAA, et al (Free Univ, Amsterdam; Univ Hosp St Radboud, Nijmegen, The Netherlands)
Neurology 47:1469–1476, 1996   14–1

Introduction.—In trials of treatment for multiple sclerosis (MS), MRI findings are increasingly used as primary outcome measures. New MRI lesions are generally considered to represent a relapse. However, the extent of lesions on conventional T2 MRI is not necessarily related to the clinical condition of the patient. As a result, the MRI findings cannot be used as a marker of disability. There is some evidence to suggest that hypointense lesions on T1 MRI—sometimes called "black holes"—are correlated with disability. This relationship was studied in detail.

Methods.—The study included 46 patients with clinically definite MS. At baseline and again after a median of 40 months' follow-up, the patients were studied by T2- and T1-weighted MRI. The MRI findings were correlated with the patients' clinical condition, as evaluated on the expanded disability status scale.

Results.—At baseline, the load of hypointense lesions on T1-weighted spin-echo MRI was significantly correlated with the disability score. There was a nonsignificant trend toward a relationship between T2 and disability score. The ratio of T1 to T2 lesion load was significantly correlated with baseline disability score (Fig 4). In patients with secondary progression of MS, there was a significant relationship between the rate of accumulation of hypointense T1 lesions and disability score.

Conclusion.—The load of hypointense lesions on T1-weighted spin-echo MRI may be a useful marker of disability in patients with MS. As these T1 "black holes" accumulate, the rate of disease progression increases. The appearance of black holes may be an MRI indicator of failure of remission.

▶ Multiple sclerosis clinical trialists remain concerned that clinical outcome measures are insensitive, unresponsive, and unreliable, yet MRI outcome measurements are imperfectly correlated with disability progression. Parallel studies performed elsewhere suggest that MR spectroscopy and the measurement of brain and spinal cord atrophy may be predictive of disability progression. It is crucial to determine which of these measures correlates

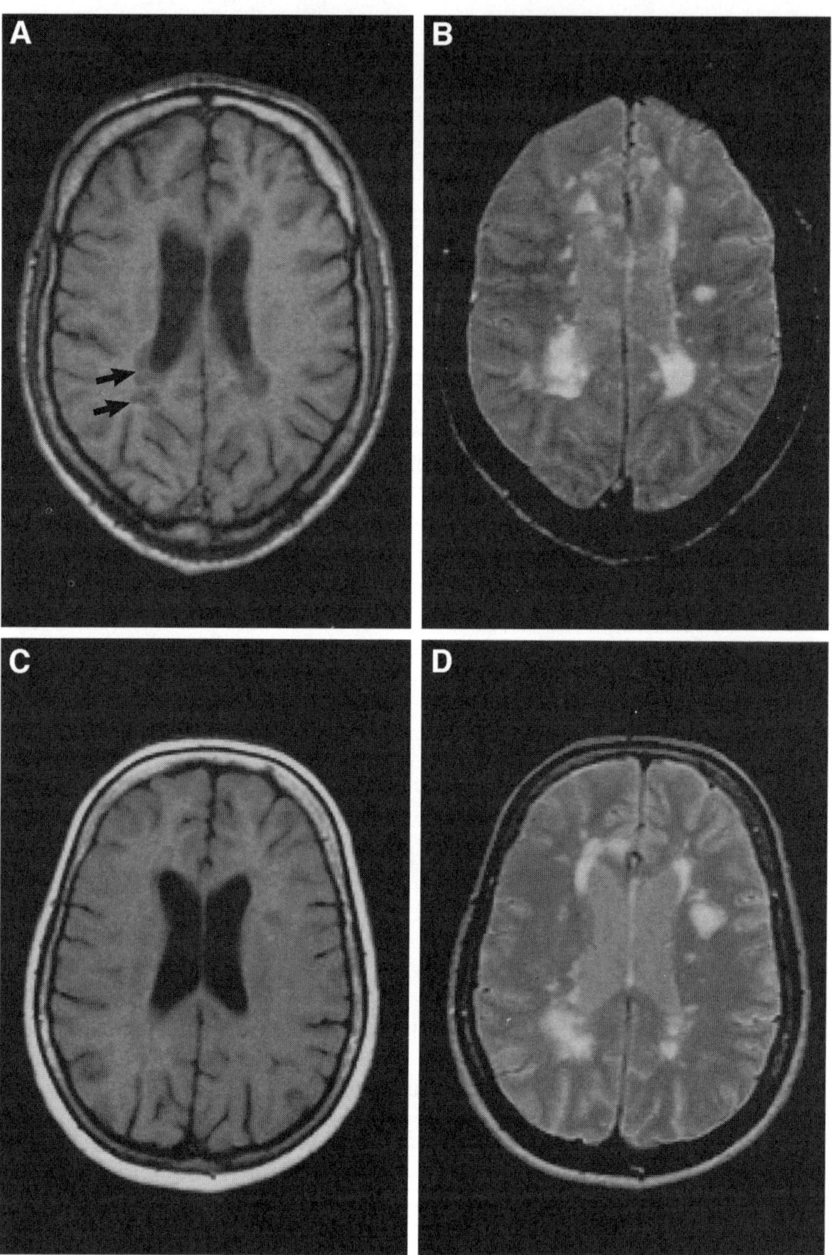

FIGURE 4.—Two patients, 1 with secondary progressive multiple sclerosis (SPMS) (**A, B**), the other with relapsing-remitting multiple sclerosis (RRMS) (**C, D**). T1-weighted images are represented on the left side, T2-weighted images on the right side. Note that the lesion load on T2 is nearly identical, whereas the T1 lesion load is clearly higher in the SPMS patient (example of a hypointense lesion is indicated by the *arrow*). The expanded disability status scale (EDSS) for the SPMS patient was 6 at the time of the scan; the EDSS of the RRMS patient was 3. (Reprinted from *Neurology*, courtesy of Truyen L, van Waesberghe JHTM, van Walderveen MAA, et al: Accumulation of hypointense lesions ("black holes)" on T_1 spin-echo MRI correlates with disease progression in multiple sclerosis. *Neurology* 47:1469–1476, 1996, by permission of Little, Brown and Company, Inc.)

best with disability progression and to determine whether these indices are sensitive to treatment effects. The promising results from this serial follow-up study need to be validated in blinded, randomized, controlled trials in patients with relapsing-remitting, secondary progressive, and primary progressive MS.

J.H. Noseworthy, M.D.

Linomide Reduces the Rate of Active Lesions in Relapsing-Remitting Multiple Sclerosis

Andersen O, Lycke J, Tollesson PO, et al (Univ of Göteborg, Sweden; Pharmacia Oncology Immunology, Lund, Sweden)
Neurology 47:895–900, 1996

14–2

Introduction.—In multiple sclerosis trials, several immunomodulatory agents, including naturally occurring cytokines, are currently being investigated, and Linomide, a synthetic agent with immunomodulatory effects, is one such agent. Linomide facilitated T-cell responses in a screening program for anti-inflammatory drugs through an effect on macrophages. In the development of several experimental autoimmune diseases, Linomide also had a profound inhibitory influence; the diseases included systemic lupus erythematosus, autoimmune insulin-dependent diabetes mellitus, experimental virus-induced myocarditis, and experimental autoimmune myasthenia gravis. The results of a trial of Linomide in relapsing-remitting multiple sclerosis were reviewed.

Methods.—Thirty-one patients with relapsing-remitting multiple sclerosis were randomly assigned to a placebo or an oral dose of 2.5 mg Linomide once a day for 6 months in this double-blind trial. The trial was completed by 14 patients receiving placebo and 14 receiving Linomide.

Results.—In the patients receiving Linomide, there were 1.37 active lesions per monthly MRI scan; there were 4.22 lesions in those receiving placebo (Fig 1). In the Linomide-treated group, the percentage of scans with active MRI lesions was lower than in the placebo group (Fig 2). The Linomide group showed an improvement of 1% of the maximal Regional Functional Scoring System range, but there was a deterioration of 0.2% in the placebo group. Six relapses occurred in the placebo group and 3 relapses in the Linomide group. In the Linomide group, there was a slightly decreased proportion of natural killer cells in CSF and peripheral blood. One Linomide-treated patient had a severe adverse event of pleuropericarditis. Musculoskeletal pain, of mild to severe degree, was the most frequent adverse event; it diminished after 3 months on Linomide treatment.

Conclusions.—The development of multiple sclerosis–related active MRI lesions was significantly suppressed in the Linomide group, and there also was a positive clinical effect in relapsing-remitting multiple sclerosis.

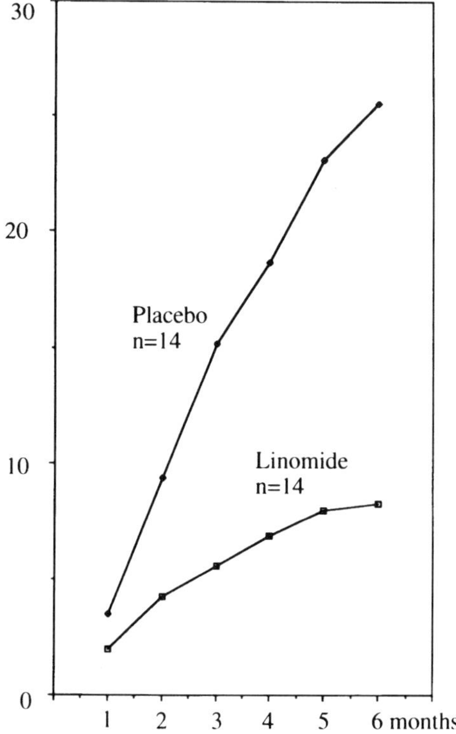

FIGURE 1.—Cumulative number of active (new or enlarged) T2 lesions per 4-week period in the Linomide and placebo groups. (Courtesy of Andersen O, Lyeke J, Tollesson PO, et al: Linomide reduces the rate of active lesions in relapsing-remitting multiple sclerosis. Reprinted from *Neurology*, vol. 47, pp 895–900, 1996, by permission of Little, Brown and Company, Inc.)

It still must be determined what is the optimal dose of Linomide, and further studies are warranted.

▶ Linomide belongs to a new class of immunosuppressant molecules that have marked effects in the treatment of a number of human autoimmune diseases. The immunosuppression appears to affect mainly macrophages and spare the T- and B-cell compartment. A multicenter phase III Placebo Controlled Study in secondary progressive multiple sclerosis is currently under way. If proven efficacious, Linomide, along with the β-interferons and Copolymer 1, will be the third class of compounds that will "put the brakes" on multiple sclerosis.

S. Sriram, M.D.

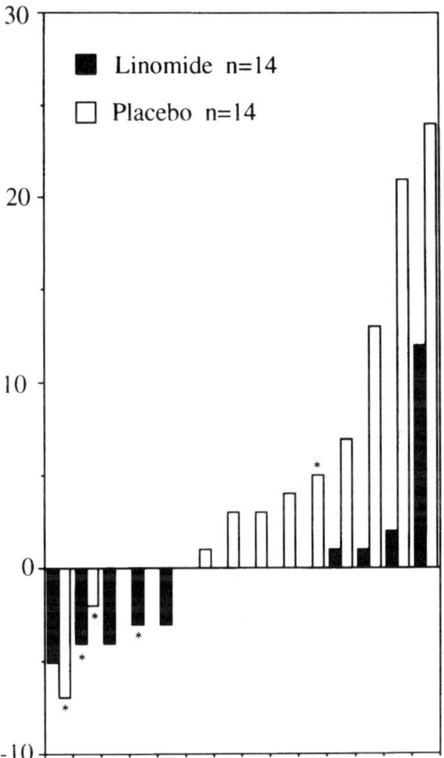

FIGURE 2.—Net result (number at week 24 minus number at baseline) of new and disappeared T2 lesions: increased or decreased number of T2 lesions in individual patients, 14 receiving placebo and 14 receiving Linomide. *Asterisks* indicate patients who had more than 1 contrast-enhancing lesion at baseline scan, as an indication of relatively high disease activity before treatment. (Courtesy of Andersen O, Lycke J, Tollesson PO, et al: Linomide reduces the rate of active lesions in relapsing-remitting multiple sclerosis. Reprinted from *Neurology*, vol. 47, pp 895–900, 1996 by permission of Little, Brown and Company, Inc.)

15 Neuro-Oncology

Neurologic Disorders in 203 Consecutive Patients With Small Cell Lung Cancer
van Oosterhout AGM, van de Pol M, ten Velde GPM, et al (Univ Hosp Maastricht, The Netherlands)
Cancer 77:1434–1441, 1996
15–1

Background.—Neurologic complications in patients with small-cell lung cancer (SCLC) are a major cause of morbidity and mortality. The incidence and course of the various metastatic and nonmetastatic neurologic disorders in such patients were studied prospectively.

Methods.—Between 1983 and 1994, 203 patients underwent regular neurologic examinations before, during, and after therapy. Routine CT or MRI of the brain was done before treatment and after 2 years of survival.

Findings.—One hundred seventy-four neurologic disorders were diagnosed in 132 patients. Most of these disorders were associated with metastases. Brain metastases developed in 79 patients. Two years after diagnosis, the cumulative risk of brain metastases was 47% in patients

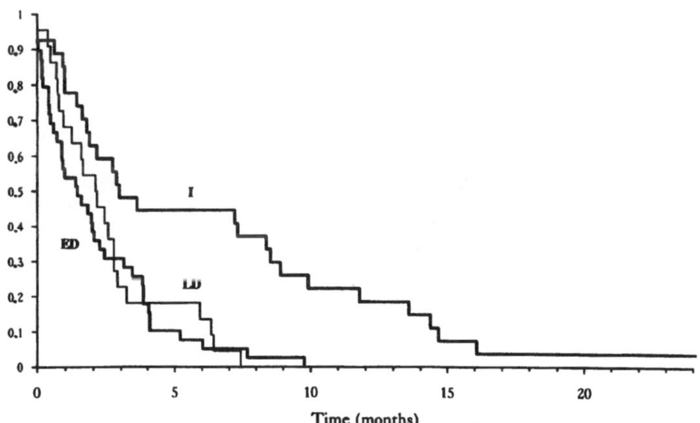

FIGURE 2.—Proportion of survivors after a diagnosis of brain metastases for patients with initial brain metastases diagnosed before therapy (*I*), and for patients with limited (*LD*) and extensive disease (*ED*) who had delayed brain metastases diagnosed during or after therapy. (Courtesy of van Oosterhout AGM, van de Pol M, ten Velde GPM, et al: Neurologic disorders in 203 consecutive patients with small cell lung cancer. *Cancer* 77:1434–1441, copyright © 1996. Reprinted by permission of Wiley-Liss, Inc., a division of John Wiley & Sons, Inc.)

with limited disease and 69% in patients with extensive disease. Patients with brain metastases at the initial SCLC diagnosis had a significantly longer survival than did patients with delayed brain metastases (Fig 2). The most common paraneoplastic syndrome with neurologic symptoms was inappropriate secretion of antidiuretic hormone (SIADH), which occurred in 11 patients. Five patients were found to have antibody-mediated paraneoplastic neurologic syndromes. In most patients, chemotherapy for SCLC caused a regression of SIADH. In contrast, SCLC treatment did not affect antibody-mediated syndromes. Adverse treatment effects included peripheral neuropathy, which was reversible, and encephalopathy, radiation plexopathy, and steroid myopathy, which were not reversible.

Conclusions.—The neurologic complications of SCLC are diverse. Central nervous system metastatic involvement is common. The high frequency of brain metastases indicates that prophylactic cranial irradiation should be reappraised in these patients.

▶ This report describing a prospective analysis of the neurologic complications of 203 patients with SCLC demonstrates how frequently neurologic complications develop in such patients. The complications are usually related to metastases and neurotoxicity of therapy. The major *paraneoplastic* syndrome was that of hyponatremia; 5 patients suffered other paraneoplastic syndromes (2 Lambert-Eaton syndromes, 2 cerebellar degeneration, 1 limbic encephalitis). When this paper is considered in light of the precious paper by Erlington et al.,[1] who found that neuromuscular and autonomic deficits occurred in up to 44% of 150 patients with SCLC prospectively analyzed, neurologists should recognize that they have an important role to play in the evaluation of patients with SCLC. Most neurologic complaints are related to metastases or therapy, but 1% to 3% of patients acquire Lambert-Eaton syndrome, a treatable paraneoplastic disorder that should be identified and treated.

J. Posner, M.D.

Reference

1. Earlington GM, Murray NM, Spiro SG, et al: Neurological paraneoplastic syndromes in patients with small cell lung cancer: A prospective survey of 150 patients. *J Neurol Psychiatry* 54:764–767, 1991.

Non-Hodgkin Malignant Lymphomas and Peripheral Neuropathies—13 Cases
Vallat JM, De Mascarel HA, Bordessoule D, et al (Univ Hosp, Limoges, France)
Brain 118:1233–1245, 1995   15–2

Background.—Non-Hodgkin's malignant lymphomas (NHML) are currently classified as malignant lymphoid proliferations of B or T lymphocytes. The reported incidence of peripheral neuropathy (PN) in patients

Subscribe to the related journal in your field!

Yes! Begin my one-year subscription to
Journal of Vascular Surgery (12 issues).

Name ___________________________________

Institution ______________________________

Address _________________________________

City _____________________ State _________

ZIP/PC __________ Country _______________

Specialty _______________________________
  (Students/residents, please list Institution)

Subscription prices (through 9/30/98)

		USA	Canada*	Int'l
Individuals	❏	$148.00	$196.88	$184.00
Institutions	❏	279.00	337.05	315.00
Students, residents	❏	74.00	117.70	110.00

Method of payment

Enclose payment (check or credit card number)
and we'll send an extra issue FREE!

❏ Check (in U.S. dollars, drawn on a U.S. bank, and
  payable to *Journal of Vascular Surgery*)

❏ VISA   ❏ MasterCard   ❏ Discover

❏ AmEx   ❏ Bill me   Exp. date__________

Card #___________________________________

Signature ________________________________

*Includes Canadian GST

Individual/student subscriptions must be in the name of,
billed to, and paid for by the individual.

Airmail rates available upon request.
Prices subject to change without notice.

J024983YA

Reservation Card for the Year Book

Yes! I would like my own copy of *Year Book of Neurology and Neurosurgery*® at the price of
$78.00 plus sales tax, postage, and handling. Please begin my subscription with the current edition
according to the terms described below.* I understand that I will have 30 days to examine each
annual edition.

Name ____

Address ____

City ____ State ___________ ZIP____________

Method of Payment

Check (in U.S. dollars, drawn on a U.S. bank, payable to *Year Book of Neurology and Neurosurgery*®)

❏ VISA   ❏ MasterCard   ❏ Discover   ❏ AmEx   ❏ Bill me

Card number ____ Exp. date: ___________

Signature ____

Prices are subject to change without notice.

PMC-020

Your Year Book service guarantee:

When you subscribe to the *Year Book*, you will receive advance notice of future annual volumes
about two months before publication. To receive the new edition, you need do nothing—we'll send
you the new volume as soon as it is available. If you want to discontinue, the advance notice allows
you time to notify us of your decision. If you are not completely satisfied, you have 30 days to
return any *Year Book*.

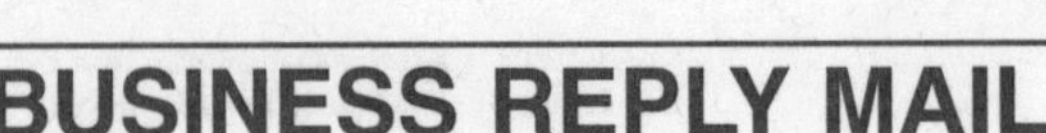

NO POSTAGE
NECESSARY
IF MAILED
IN THE
UNITED STATES

SUBSCRIPTION SERVICES
MOSBY–YEAR BOOK, INC.
11830 WESTLINE INDUSTRIAL DRIVE
ST. LOUIS   MO 63146-9988

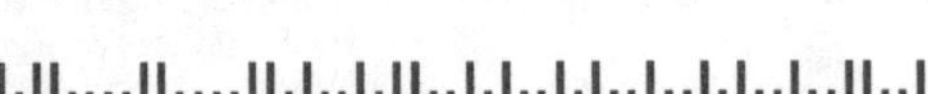

NO POSTAGE
NECESSARY
IF MAILED
IN THE
UNITED STATES

PAT NEWMAN
11830 WESTLINE INDUSTRIAL DRIVE
PO BOX 46908
ST. LOUIS   MO 63146-9934

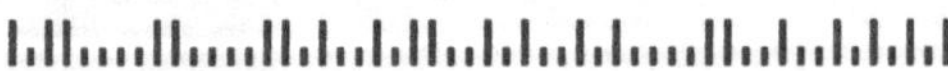

Want to speed up the process?

To order the *Year Book*,
you also may call 1-800-426-4545

To subscribe to the journal today,
call toll-free in the U.S.:
1-800-453-4351
or fax 314-432-1158
Outside the U.S., call: 314-453-4351

Visit us at:
www.mosby.com/Mosby/Periodicals

Mosby–Year Book, Inc.
Subscription Services
11830 Westline Industrial Drive
St. Louis, MO   63146 U.S.A.

Mosby

with NHML varies greatly, dependent on whether patients with electro-physiologic evidence of PN but an absence of clinical symptoms are included. Thirteen patients initially seen with clinical signs of PN at some time during the course of NHML were described.

Case Series.—All had an association between PN and B type NHML, but none showed evidence of meningeal propagation or neurotoxicity from chemotherapy. The mechanisms of PN were divided into 4 broad categories. Four patients in group 1 had peripheral nerve lesions linked directly to a propagation of malignant cells into the peripheral nervous system, which were identified with autopsy and/or nerve biopsy. Three of these patients had malignant B cell proliferation as demonstrated by immunolabeled infiltrates. Three patients in group 2 had a monoclonal immunoglobulin (IgM) with antimyelin activity in serum, and another 2 had pathologic IgM deposits in endoneural connective tissue. In group 3, which consisted of 2 patients, immune dysfunction of the NHML was responsible for a Guillain-Barre syndrome in 1 and for a chronic inflammatory demyelinating polyneuropathy in the other. In the 2 patients in group 4, the mechanism of the PN, though probably directly associated with the NHML, could not be definitively established. The PN may have resulted from a paraneoplastic process or an undetected lymphomatous invasion of nervous tissue.

Conclusions.—Peripheral neuropathy may reveal or complicate any type of NHML. The neurologic symptomatologies range from isolated or multiple mononeuropathies to polyneuropathies and meningoradiculoneuropathies. The lesional mechanism of the peripheral nerve trunks varies and can be unclear.

▶ Non-Hodgkin's lymphoma is the cancer that has most rapidly increased in incidence throughout the world. Particularly striking increases of extranodal lymphomas are evident, especially those in the stomach and central nervous system.[1,2] As this review describes, PN of varied pathogenesis can accompany NHML. (1) B cells may directly invade peripheral nerves and cause mononeuropathy multiplex or polyneuropathy. At times, lymphomatous involvement may be restricted to peripheral nerves (neurolymphomatosis).[3] (2) Malignant B cells may produce an IgM with anti-myelin activity that secondarily affects the peripheral nerve. (3) Peripheral nervous system damage may result from a paraneoplastic syndrome without an identifiable IgM. Not included in the group of patients reported in this article are those with (4) paraneoplastic vasculitic neuropathy,[4] or (5) peripheral nervous system infiltration by intravascular lymphomatosis.[5] Severe and subacute polyneuropathy of undetermined cause demands a search for an underlying cancer. As this report demonstrates, nerve biopsy and immunohistochemistry of any observed lymphocytes can be extremely helpful to establish a diagnosis.

J. Posner, M.D.

References

1. Devesa SS, Fears T: Non-Hodgkin's lymphoma time trends: United States and international data. *Cancer Res* 52(Suppl 19):5432S–5440S, 1992.
2. Lutz J, Coleman MP: Trends in primary cerebral lymphoma. *Br J Cancer* 70: 716–718, 1994.
3. Schoenfeld Y, Aderka D, Sandbank U, et al: Fatal peripheral neurolymphomatosis after remission of histiocytic lymphoma. *Neurology* 33:243–245, 1983.
4. Hawke SH, Davies L, Pamphlett R, et al: Vasculitis neuropathy: A clinical and pathological study. *Brain* 114:2175–2190, 1995.
5. Roux S, Grossin M, DeBandt M, et al: Angiotropic large cell lymphoma with mononeuritis multiplex mimicking systemic vasculitis. *J Neurol Neurosurg Psychiatry* 58:363–366, 1995.

Multifocal Leukoencephalopathy Associated With 5-Fluorouracil and Levamisole Adjuvant Therapy for Colon Cancer: A Report of Two Cases and Review of the Literature
Luppi G, for the Intergruppo Nazionale Terapia Adiuvante Colon Carcinoma, Italy (Univ of Modena, Italy)
Ann Oncol 7:412–415, 1996   15–3

Introduction.—The standard postoperative adjuvant therapy for patients with stage B2-C colon cancer is 5-fluorouracil plus levamisole. Since 1992, 14 cases of multifocal leukoencephalopathy have been reported in patients receiving this chemotherapy regimen. Two new cases are reported. In addition, to assess the possibility that levamisole plays a specific role in this rare but severe neurologic syndrome, the literature was analyzed.

Patients.—Two cases of multifocal demyelinating leukoencephalopathy were found in a series of 1,827 patients received 5-fluorouracil, levamisole, and L-leucovorin after resection of stage B2-C colon cancer. The patients were referred for neurologic evaluation after the second or third cycle of chemotherapy. The cumulative levamisole dose was 1.8 g for the second cycle and 2.7 g for the third. Neurologic signs included confusional syndrome, behavioral disorders, and aphasia but no fever. Neither patient had evidence of metastases or infection.

In 1 patient, MRI scan revealed widespread, nearly symmetric hyperintensity of the periventricular and hemispheric white matter, consistent with multifocal demyelination of possible inflammatory origin (Fig 1). The patient remained in stable clinical condition without specific therapy. She had tetraplegia and required nasogastric feeding. The MRI scan in the second patient showed diffuse, bilateral hyperintensity of the hemispheric white matter, consistent with leukoencephalopathy (Fig 2). This patient

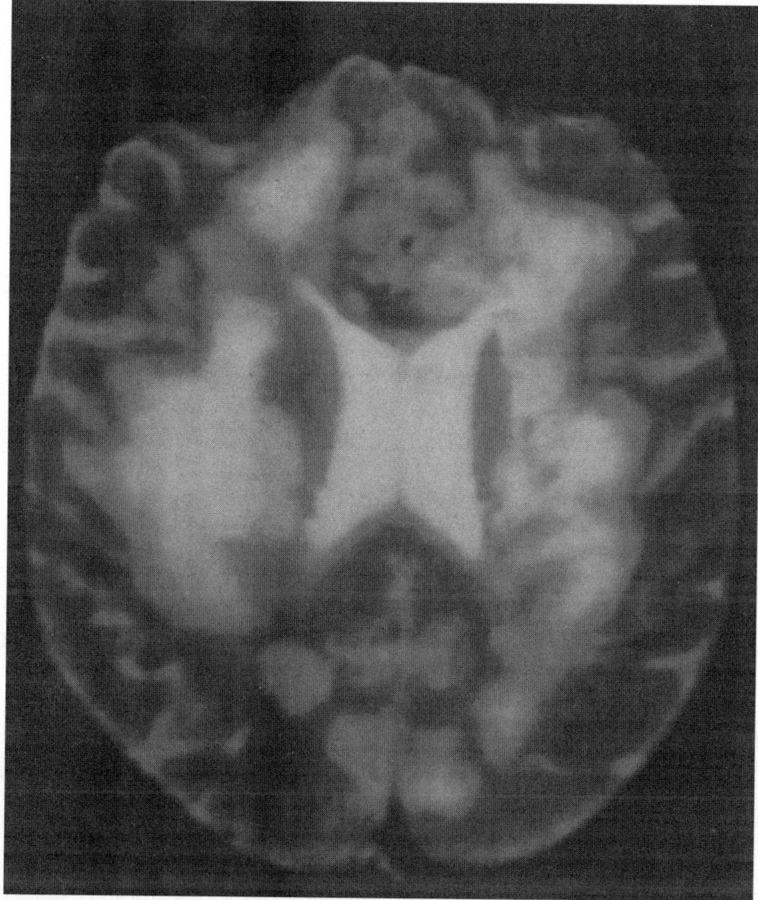

FIGURE 1.—Axial T2–weighted images show extensive white matter abnormalities in a symmetric fashion, which cause no mass effect. (Courtesy of Luppi G, for the Intergruppo Nazionale Terapia Adjuvante Colon Carcinoma, Italy: Multifocal leukoencephalopathy associated with 5–fluorouracil and levamisole adjuvant therapy for colon cancer. A report of two cases and review of the literature. *Ann Oncol* 7:412–415, 1996. Reprinted by permission of Kluwer Academic Publishers.)

improved with high-dose dexamethasone therapy, but she still had slight neurologic impairment at 6 months.

Discussion.—Patients receiving adjuvant 5-fluorouracil for colon cancer are at risk for multifocal leukoencephalopathy. No clear causal relationship can be established. However, because there are no reports of 5-fluorouracil causing any such syndrome, levamisole may play a crucial pathogenetic role. The clinical and statistical relevance of the reported cases cannot yet be determined. Still, all patients who show neurologic symptoms during treatment with 5-fluorouracil and levamisole should be examined for multifocal leukoencephalopathy, including an MRI scan of the brain.

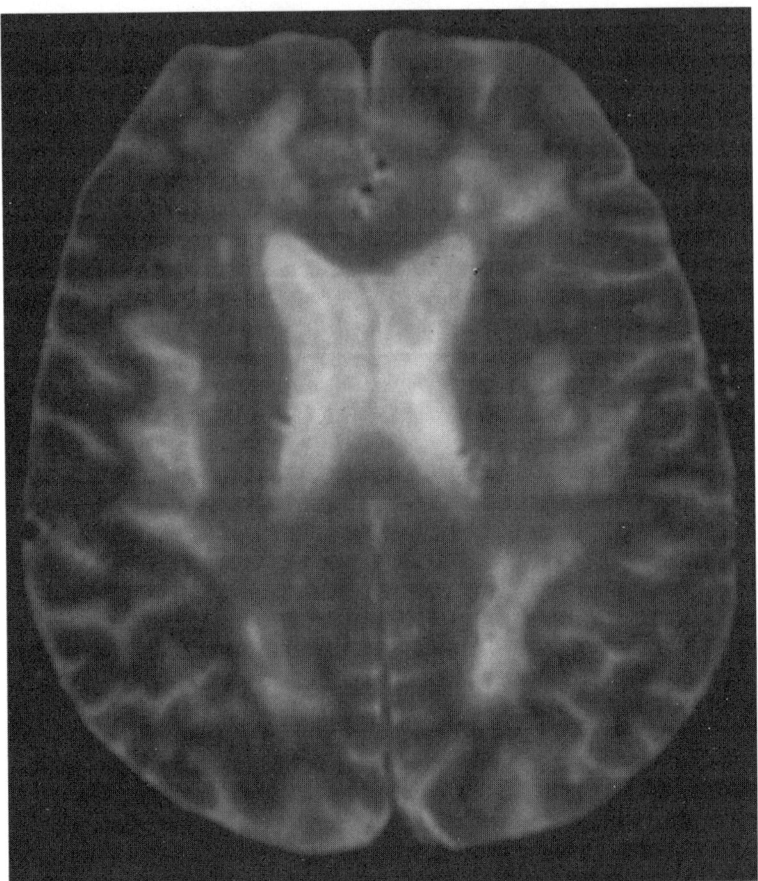

FIGURE 2.—Axial T2–weighted images show bilaterally symmetric and confluent hyperintensities throughout white matter, mostly affecting the frontal and parieto-occipital subcortical regions. No mass effect is present. (Courtesy of Luppi G, for the Intergruppo Nazionale Terapia Adjuvante Colon Carcinoma, Italy: Multifocal leukoencephalopathy associated with 5–fluorouracil and levamisole adjuvant therapy for colon cancer. A Report of two cases and review of the literature. *Ann Oncol* 7:412–415, 1996. Reprinted by permission of Kluwer Academic Publishers.)

▶ The disorder described by Luppi and colleagues, although rare, is probably more common than their report of 2 cases and review of the literature (14 additional cases) would indicate. Five additional reports (6 cases) bring the total number to 22.

The clinical picture of confusion and multifocal neurologic signs associated with multiple contrast-enhancing lesions on MR scan[1] can lead to a misdiagnosis of metastatic lesions. If an incorrect diagnosis is made, not only may toxic drugs continue to be administered but the patient also may receive inappropriate brain radiation therapy, which worsens and probably makes irreversible the demyelinating lesions.[2] Savarese et al. have suggested that single photon emission CT imaging may assist in noninvasive diagnosis: increased uptake of thallium suggests metastatic disease, whereas the demyelinating lesion did not take up thallium. The pathogenesis of the disorder is unknown, although contrary to the statement in the discussion by Luppi et al., both levamisole[3] and 5–fluorouracil, or its derivatives,[4] have been reported to cause leukoencephalopathy.

J. Posner, M.D.

References

1. Savarese DM, Gordon J, Smith TW, et al: Cerebral demyelination syndrome in a patient treated with 5-fluorouracil and levamisole: The use of thallium SPECT imaging to assist in noninvasive diagnosis—A case report. *Cancer* 77:387–394, 1996.
2. Peterson K, Rosenblum MK, Powers JM, et al: Effect of brain irradiation on demyelinating lesions. *Neurology* 43:2105–2112, 1993.
3. Kimmel DW, Wijdicks EFM, Rodriguez M: Multifocal inflammatory leukoencephalopathy associated with levamisole therapy. *Neurology* 45:374–376, 1995.
4. Aoki N: Reversible leukoencephalopathy caused by 5-fluorouacil derivatives, presenting as akinetic mutism. *Surg Neurol* 25:279–282, 1986.

Frequency and Severity of Central Nervous System Lesions in Hemophagocytic Lymphohistiocytosis
Haddad E, Sulis M-L, Jabado N, et al (Hôpital Necker Enfants Malades, Paris; Hôpital Bicêtre, France)
Blood 89:794–800, 1997

15–4

Introduction.—The cause of hemophagocytic lymphohistiocytosis (HLH) remains unknown, but most reported cases suggest an autosomal recessive inheritance. Patients exhibit a nonmalignant diffuse infiltration by lymphocytes and macrophages into visceral organs, lymph nodes, bone marrow, and the CNS. A review of 34 consecutive patients considered the frequency, features, and influence on outcome of neurologic manifestations of HLH.

Methods.—Patients were 19 girls and 15 boys who were hospitalized at the study institution from 1981 to 1993. In 25 cases, the diagnosis of HLH was based upon family history. The remaining cases were the first in the family, and diagnosis was based upon occurrence of a hemophagocytic syndrome without concomitant infection which recurred after complete remission. All patients received chemotherapy, and those treated in more recent years also underwent bone marrow transplantation. The patients' clinical, radiologic, and CSF cytology data were analyzed according to treatment modalities.

Results.—Twenty-nine of 34 patients had CNS involvement; in all but 4 of 29, CNS disease was present at diagnosis of HLH. Initial CNS manifestations were meningitis in 20 patients and neurologic symptoms (seizures, coma, brain stem symptoms, or ataxia) in 9. In all cases, CNS involvement was associated with a systemic hemophagocytic syndrome, and all had the same CSF abnormalities. The most frequent lesions in those with initial neurologic symptoms were focal neurosis with parenchymal

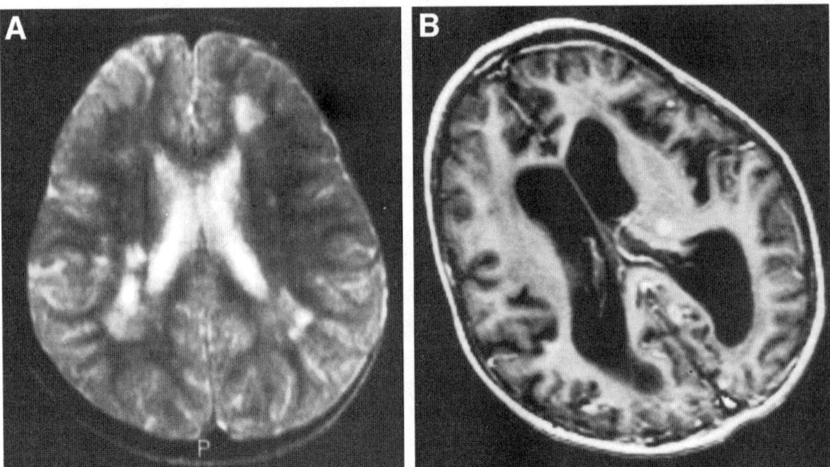

FIGURE 3.—Evolution of brain lesions during hemophagocytic lymphohistiocytosis. **A,** MRI of a 4½-year-old girl showing focal white matter hypersignal on T2–weighted images. **B,** MRI of the same child 1 year later with an important atrophy of both the white matter and the cortices. (Courtesy of Haddad E, Sulis M-L, Jabado N, et al: Frequency and severity of central nervous system lesions in hemophagocytic lymphohistiocytosis. *Blood* 89:794–800, 1997.)

volume loss and atrophy and white matter abnormalities. Chemotherapy led to complete remission in the 20 patients with initial meningitis and in 3 of 9 patients with initial neurologic symptoms. Nineteen of these 23 patients, however, had primary severe CNS disease progression or CNS relapse. Imaging showed severe brain atrophy (Fig 3) in 3 patients with progression of CNS disease. All 16 patients treated exclusively by systemic and intrathecal chemotherapy and/or immunosuppression died after relapse or disease progression. Seven of 9 patients who underwent bone marrow transplantation are long-term survivors, including 3 who received an HLA partially identical marrow. All 7 have normal neurologic function and cognitive development and are not receiving treatment.

Conclusion.—The optimal strategy for treatment of patients with HLH is to perform a bone marrow transplant as early as possible after remission induction. In this series, no patient survived without a bone marrow transplant.

▶ It is important for neurologists to recognize this rare, but lethal, autosomal recessive disorder of infants and children for 2 reasons. The first is that although it is usually characterized by high fever, hepatosplenomegaly, and pancytopenia, the disorder can sometimes begin with neurologic symptomatology characterized by a progressive encephalopathy with a variety of neurologic symptoms including seizures, focal neurologic signs, nuchal rigidity, and signs of increased intracranial pressure.[1] The second reason is that if a diagnosis is made early, chemotherapy with bone marrow rescue appears to be effective treatment. Most patients with the disorder have a

CSF pleocytosis early in the course of the disease, often—but not always—with the characteristic hemophagocytosis.

The neuropathologic findings are variable and consist of leptomeningeal infiltration with lymphocytes, and macrophages sometimes associated with perivascular parenchymal infiltrates, and, in the most severe cases, with massive tissue infiltration of lymphocytes and macrophages.[2] The last can often be identified in life by white matter lesions on CT or MR scans. The paper abstracted here, together with the 2 recent papers referenced below, represent valuable additions to our understanding of this rare but important pediatric neurologic disorder.

J. Posner, M.D.

References

1. Henter J-I, Elinder G: Cerebromeningeal haemophagocytic lymphohistiocytosis. *Lancet* 339:104–107, 1992.
2. Henter J-I, Nennesmo I: Neuropathologic findings and neurologic symptoms in twenty-three children with hemophagocytic lymphohistiocytosis. *J Pediatr* 130:358–365, 1997.

Intravenous Immunoglobulin Treatment in Paraneoplastic Neurological Syndromes With Antineuronal Autoantibodies

Uchuya M, Graus F, Vega F, et al (Hôpital de la Salpêtrière, Paris; Hosp Clinic i Provincial, Barcelona; "Principes España", Hospitalet del Llobregat, Spain)
J Neurol Neurosurg Psychiatry 60:388–392, 1996   15–5

Background.—Patients with paraneoplastic syndromes of the nervous system have specific autoantibodies against neuronal antigens in the serum and cerebrospinal fluid. The effect of IV high-dose human immunoglobulin (IVIg) treatment on the autoantibody titers and clinical course of patients with such syndromes was investigated.

Methods.—The study included 22 patients with paraneoplastic encephalomyelitis and sensory neuronopathy syndrome associated with anti-Hu antibodies or paraneoplastic cerebellar degeneration with anti-Yo antibodies. Treatment consisted of 1 to 26 cycles of IVIg.

Findings.—Serious toxicity occurred in only 1 patient, in whom hemolytic anemia developed. Therapeutic response could be evaluated in 21 patients. One with subacute sensory neuropathy (SSN) showed improvement for at least 15 months. Ten patients remained stable, and 10 deteriorated. Of the 10 patients whose conditions stabilized, 7 had a plateau in the syndrome when treatment began. The other 3, who had progressed, were stable for 6, 8, and more than 48 months, respectively. Another patient with SSN and an initial stable response worsened when IVIg was decreased and improved when it was increased. No significant predictive factors of outcome could be identified, but patients with isolated involvement of the peripheral nervous system improved or stabilized more commonly than patients with evidence of CNS damage at treatment onset. In patients with CNS involvement, stabilization was only achieved when the neurologic dysfunction was already severe. Autoantibody titers did not change significantly.

Conclusions.—High-dose IVIg was not effective in patients with paraneoplastic CNS syndromes associated with antineuronal antibodies. However, further study of the value of this treatment approach in patients with SSN is warranted.

▶ Certain paraneoplastic syndromes are known to respond to immune manipulation. Plasma exchange and intravenous immunoglobulin are effective in the treatment of the Lambert-Eaton myasthenic syndrome and corticosteroids control opsoclonus/myoconus associated with neuroblastoma. Occasional enthusiastic case reports also describe improvement in some patients with paraneoplastic syndromes that affect neurons such as encephalomyelitis, sensory neuronopathy, and cerebellar degeneration after immune manipulation. Because occasional patients with these disorders also experience spontaneous remissions, individual case reports are hard to interpret. Uchuya and colleagues have now indicated, in a series of 22 patients with established paraneoplastic syndromes associated with well-characterized autoantibodies, that IVIg is generally ineffective in the treatment of these disorders. This, in addition to their previous study (which indicated that plasma exchange and antineoplastic treatment is equally ineffective),[1] indicates that at least at the time the autoantibodies are identified and treatment is begun, these modalities are unlikely to work. Whether such immunosuppression is intrinsically ineffective, or whether irreparable damage has already been done to neurons so that even effective treatment cannot reverse the symptomatology, is not certain, but the authors observation of continued progression, despite IVIg, suggests it is the former.

J. Posner, M.D.

Reference

1. Graus F, Vega F, Delattre JY, et al: Plasmapheresis and antineoplastic treatment in CNS paraneoplastic syndromes with antineuronal autoantibodies. *Neurology* 42:536–540, 1992.

16 Neuro-Ophthalmology

Hyperbaric Oxygen Therapy for Nonarteritic Anterior Ischemic Optic Neuropathy
Arnold AC, Hepler RS, Lieber M, et al (Univ of California, Los Angeles; Santa Monica Hosp, Calif; Northridge Hosp, Calif)
Am J Ophthalmol 122:535–541, 1996   16–1

Background.—The most common cause of acute optic neuropathy in patients older than 50 years is nonarteritic anterior ischemic optic neuropathy. Although many patients have some spontaneous improvement in visual function after the initial visual loss, most have visual loss, and some experience progressive deterioration. The efficacy of hyperbaric oxygen treatment in decreasing optic nerve injury in patients with acute nonarteritic anterior ischemic optic neuropathy was investigated.

Methods.—Twenty patients with 22 affected eyes were studied. Treatment consisted of hyperbaric oxygen administered in 2 90-minute inhalation sessions per day for 10 days. Twenty-seven untreated patients with acute nonarteritic anterior ischemic optic neuropathy composed a control group. Changes in mean visual acuity and sensitivity loss in the 2 groups were compared.

Findings.—In both groups, mean visual acuity values were increased at the final assessment. Although this increase was higher in the control group, the difference was nonsignificant. A minimal increase was noted in mean visual field sensitivity. Although this increase was smaller in the control group, the between-group difference was again nonsignificant. The proportions of patients with change in acuity score or mean sensitivity loss were comparable in the 2 groups. Treatment initiation within 9 days did not appear to improve visual outcomes compared with later treatment initiation or no treatment.

Conclusions.—Hyperbaric oxygen treatment with 100% oxygen and 2 absolute atmospheres of pressure did not significantly improve visual acuity or visual field in patients with acute nonarteritic anterior ischemic optic neuropathy. At the final assessment, only 13.6% of patients in the treatment group and 14.8% of those in the control group showed improvement in mean visual acuity levels—proportions substantially lower than the spontaneous improvement rates reported recently by others. The measured improvement in acuity documented in the current study was probably limited by the mildness of the initial loss.

▶ All sorts of treatments have been described as having some benefit in restoring visual function in nonarteritic anterior ischemic optic neuropathy. The natural history of the disease was only recently described. Spontaneous improvement rates have varied from 15% to 42.7%.

The speculation that hyperbaric oxygen might be of benefit may not be sound. This study is well done, and the conclusion that 100% oxygen at 2.0 absolute atmospheres of pressure does not produce significant improvement in visual acuity of field is helpful in excluding this as another useless form of therapy.

N.J. Schatz, M.D.

Benign Episodic Unilateral Mydriasis: Clinical Characteristics

Jacobson DM (Marshfield Clinic, Wisconsin)
Ophthalmology 102:1623–1627, 1995

16–2

Objective.—Most cases of neurologically isolated unilateral mydriasis result from benign causes, such as an Adie tonic pupil or exposure to a topical mydriatic agent. Some patients have recurrent episodes of unilateral mydriasis; the cause of these episodes is unknown, although a parasympatholytic process has been proposed. The clinical features of patients with neurologically isolated episodic unilateral mydriasis were evaluated.

Methods.—Twenty-four patients with this syndrome were identified for review. Seven were treated by the author and 17 were identified by a survey of other neuro-ophthalmologists. To be included in the study, the patients had to be older than 10 years and could have no other focal neurologic signs or symptoms, such as lid retraction, diplopia, or ophthalmoplegia; no exposure to topical mydriatics; no signs of "tadpole-shaped" pupil, indicating segmental spasm of the iris dilator; no history of tonic pupil, Horner syndrome, or oculomotor nerve palsy; and no spinal cord injury or myelopathy.

Findings.—The patients were 19 women and 5 men (median age, 31 years). Fourteen had migraine. Three patients linked a specific event, such as a motor vehicle accident, with the onset of the episodes. Five reported specific precipitating factors, such as rapid head movement, descent during airplane travel, or emotional stress. Sixteen records included information on how the mydriasis was first recognized. Thirteen patients saw the pupil was dilated when blurred vision prompted them to look in the mirror; 2 others noted the dilation incidentally, without symptoms; and 1 was seeing an ophthalmologist for eye pain. Blurring was reported by 15 patients, whose symptoms varied depending on near or distance viewing. Nine patients reported headaches, but these were typical migraine headaches in only 5 cases. In 11 patients examined during an actual episode of mydriasis, 3 had impairment of near visual acuity. In 6 patients, the degree of anisocoria was greater in light than in darkness. When they were not having an episode, 19 patients had equal-sized pupils and 5 had simple anisocoria of less than 0.5 mm.

Conclusion.—These episodes of neurologically isolated unilateral mydriasis typically occur in young women and are commonly associated with migraine. They can last for hours to days and can be associated with blurred vision, eye pain, headache, photosensitivity, or redness of the eye. No single mechanism can account for all of the presentations noted. Some cases appear to involve parasympathetic underactivity of the intraocular muscles, whereas others are more consistent with sympathetic overactivity of the iris dilator muscle.

▶ The neurologist is often faced with the diagnostic issues raised by the patient with the isolated episodic dilated pupil. This report of 24 patients helps review potential anatomical sites of involvement; ciliary ganglion dysfunction or ocular sympathetic overactivity seem the likely cause. Episodic unilateral mydriasis is a benign condition which may be secondary to underaction of parasympathetic tone or sympathetic overactivity. Neurodiagnostic studies are not recommended. Migraine is a common predisposing factor.

N.J. Schatz, M.D.

Wolfram Syndrome: Hereditary Diabetes Mellitus With Brainstem and Optic Atrophy

Scolding NJ, Kellar-Wood HF, Shaw C, et al (Univ of Cambridge, England; Addenbrooke's Hosp, England; Papworth Hosp, Cambridge, England)
Ann Neurol 39:352–360, 1996

16–3

Introduction.—In 1938, a family in which diabetes mellitus and bilateral optic atrophy developed in 4 siblings was presented by Wolfram and Wagener. These siblings later experienced deafness, incontinence, ataxia, and spinal cord signs. Diabetes insipidus developed in other patients, and the acronym DIDMOAD (diabetes insipidus, diabetes mellitus, optic atrophy, and deafness) was coined. Autosomal recessive inheritance has been considered, but there is recent interest in the mitrochondrial genome because optic atrophy, diabetes mellitus, and deafness occur in mitrochondrial disorders. Described are 4 patients from 2 families with Wolfram syndrome with previously unreported neurologic features and neuroradiologic findings.

Methods.—The patients underwent mitrochondrial analysis to determine whether a deletion spanning 7.6 kilobases of mtDNA was present in the DIDMOAD pedigrees becasue it has been detected in 1 patient with Wolfram syndrome. Magnetic resonance imaging was used to make linear measurements of the anteroposterior diameters of the midbrain, pons (at the midfourth ventricular point), and medulla to determine the degree of atrophy in brain stem structures.

Family 1: Patient 1.—Insulin-dependent diabetes mellitus (IDDM) and bilateral optic neuropathy, nocturnal enuresis, and episodes of vertigo and unsteadiness, developed in the patient at the age 9, 10, 11, and 20 years, respectively. At the age of 26 he had symptoms of startle myoclonus. When he was 27 years old, his mother found him unconscious, pulseless, and not breathing. She resuscitated him, and in the hospital he required intubation and mechanical ventilator support for laryngospasm during 2 separate episodes. He was alert and oriented. Startle myoclonus was easily produced. Visual acuity was reduced to finger counting at 3 mm bilaterally. He had low-amplitude pendular nystagmus, marked nuchal and axial rigidity with normal limb tone, and bilateral optic atrophy. No retinopathy was detected. A CT scan showed evidence of brain stem atrophy, and MRI showed stricking atrophic changes affecting the brain stem. Sleep studies revealed central apneic and hypopneic spells. Before respiratory arrest, he had been experiencing persistent noisy breathing for 6 months. It may be that vocal cord adduction caused the airway obstruction. He was given a tracheostomy tube that was capped by day to bypass the vocal cords, and he was discharged home.

Family 1: Patient 2.—Patient 2 was the older sister of patient 1. Both children with Wolfram syndrome had 3 healthy siblings. The parents were nonconsanguineous. Patient 2's history was similar to that of her brother: IDDM at age 9 and bilateral atrophy at age 14. She was blind in the following year. She was seen for primary amenorrhea at the age of 22 years. She had diurnal and nocturnal incontinence and underwent ileocystoplasty and then cecocystoplasty in the following year. She was given phenytoin at the age of 27 years for presumed "fits." At 29 years of age she was admitted to the hospital with confusion and was found to have central respiratory failure. She and her parents refused long-term respiratory support, and she died at the age of 28 years.

Family 2: Patient 3 and Patient 4.—Patient 3 had 1 healthy brother, but he and his sister Patient 4 were affected. Both were born to nonconsanguineous parents. Insulin-dependent diabetes mellitus and bilateral optic atrophy developed in Patient 3 at the age of 8 and 10 years, respectively. He was blind at 16 years of age and diabetes insipidus developed. He experienced urinary urgency, frequency, and nocturnal incontinence without bowel disturbance, and startle myoclonus was easily elicited. His findings on MRI were similar to those of Patient 1. Visual failure secondary to bilateral optic atrophy, diabetes insipidus, IDDM, and mild and nonprogressive urinary frequency and urgency developed in Patient 4 at the age of 10, 11, 12, and 13 years, respectively. Changes of atrophy were detected mainly in the brain stem on MRI.

Magnetic Resonance Imaging Findings.—All patients had striking atrophy of the brain stem, particularly the midbrain and pons. The medulla was involved to a lesser extent, the middle cerebellar peduncles were significantly thin, the optic tracts were thin, and the posterior lobe of the pituitary was conspicuously absent.

Discussion.—The suggested diagnostic criteria for Wolfram syndrome include a combination of juvenile-onset diabetes mellitus, optic atrophy, and 1 or more of the following: brain stem signs, deafness, seizures/myoclonus, ataxia, axial rigidity, neuropsychiatric/congenital abnormalities, neurogenic incontinence/dilated urinary tract, hyporeflexia or areflexia, extensor plantar responses, diabetes insipidus, and a positive family history. Additional complications include pyramidal signs, dystonic hand posturing, and breathing difficulties secondary to upper airway obstruction. The patients in this report did not have the point mutation in mtDNA that has previously been reported. It is unlikely that mutations of mtDNA provide an etiologic basis for Wolfram syndrome because autosomal recessive inheritance has been consistently observed.

Conclusion.—These findings suggest a unique neurodegenerative process that is accompanied by diabetes mellitus. The term "DIDMOAD" only partially describes the disease process. The term "Wolfram syndrome" is a more useful and impartial term.

▶ The authors present a strong case that the term "DIDMOAD syndrome" includes features that may not always be found in this disorder and excludes other important neurologic signs. Replacement by the term "Wolfram's syndrome" may allow inclusion of all features of this unique neurodegenerative disorder.

The additional features of dystonic hand posturing, axial and nuchal rigidity, mid brain tectal eye movement signs, and apnea that were described are features not usually considered part of DIDMOAD. The authors' suggested diagnostic criteria (see the table in the original article) may be helpful to the clinician.

The MRI features, in addition, are unique and demonstrate striking brain stem atrophy, extensive involvement of the medulla, thinning of the optic tracts, and a conspicuous absence of posterior lobe pituitary signal.

The mitochondrial data are less convincing but might be a promising area of investigation in the future.

N. Schatz, M.D.

17 Other Neurological Disorders

Therapeutic Potential of Neurotrophic Factors for Neurological Disorders
Yuen EC, Mobley WC (Univ of California, San Francisco)
Ann Neurol 40:346–354, 1996   17–1

Background.—Neurotrophic factors (NTFs) are growth factors that act directly on neurons, supporting their growth, differentiation, and survival. According to the NTF hypothesis, developing neurons compete with one another for a limited supply of an NTF provided by cells in their target of innervation. Many NTFs have been discovered in the past 50 years. The therapeutic potential of NTFs in the treatment of neurologic disorders was discussed.

The Therapeutic Potential of NTFs.—Research has shown that NTFs regulate many aspects of neuronal structure and function. Autocrine and nontarget-derived paracrine modes of presentation are used in addition to target-derived delivery. The production of NTF is highly regulated, with distinctive regional and developmental patterns observed. Individual populations of neurons can respond to many different NTFs. Conversely, a single factor can act on many different neuronal populations. Studies also have shown that certain NTFs can act on nonneuronal cells and that the actions of NTFs are not limited to developing postmitotic neurons. In certain animal models of injury and neurologic disease, NTFs protect against neuronal dysfunction and death.

Although research on NTFs in the treatment of neurologic disease is in an early stage, the results of insulin-like growth factor-1 studies suggest that NTFs will play a role in the treatment of human neurologic disease. However, aggressive efforts must be made to understand the most basic characteristics of the actions of NTFs in both normal and diseased neurons. Moving from animal studies to human trials has been difficult, suggesting that the use of realistic animal models should be a high priority. In addition, the pharmacology and toxicity of individual NTFs in animals and humans must be examined carefully. Continuous NTF administration may be more effective than intermittent injections. Also, more robust effects may be produced by using combinations of factors. Earlier treatment in the disease course may be beneficial, increasing the activity and efficacy of NTFs and preventing disease progression.

Conclusions.—Although the potential of NTFs in the treatment of neurologic disease is exciting, research is at an early stage. Industry and academic physicians and scientists need to work together to resolve critical questions about study design and appropriate end points to further define the therapeutic potential of NTFs.

▶ The exciting field of neurotrophic factors began with the discovery by Levi-Montalcini of nerve growth factor. The amazing breakthroughs in terms of molecular genetics now allow the production of kilogram amounts of neurotrophic factors by transfection of appropriate genes into *Escherichia coli.* Advances in neuroscience have characterized many of the neurotrophic receptors and studied their changes in chronic neurological diseases. Few such diseases result from specific abnormalities or deficiencies of the factors or their receptors, and it is possible that such defects are incompatible with nervous system development and survival. However, the possibility that such neurotrophic factors can be used for treating acute and chronic neurological diseases remains a very exciting field for research. This is an excellent review of the current status of knowledge.

W.G. Bradley, D.M., F.R.C.P.

Complications of Intravenous Immune Globulin Treatment in Neurologic Disease
Brannagan TH III, Nagle KJ, Lange DJ, et al (Columbia-Presbyterian Med Ctr, New York)
Neurology 47:674–677, 1996   17–2

Background.—Intravenous immune globulin (IVIg) has been advocated as a safe therapy for patients with immune-mediated neurologic disease. The complications of this treatment were reviewed.

Methods and Findings.—The medical records of 88 patients receiving IVIg for neurologic disease were studied for reports of complications. Four patients (4.5%) had major complications. These included congestive heart failure in a patient with polymyositis, hypotension after a recent myocardial infarction, deep venous thrombosis in a patient confined to bed, and acute renal failure with diabetic nephropathy. Other adverse effects were vasomotor symptoms in 26 patients, headache in 23, leukopenia in 4, rash in 5, and fever in 3. Proteinuria, pruritus, dyspnea, and viral syndrome occurred in 1 patient each. Fifty-nine percent of the patients had some adverse effects associated with IVIg infusion. The most common were vasomotor symptoms, headaches, fever, or shortness of breath, occurring in 45% and improving with a reduced infusion rate or using symptomatic medications. Six percent of the patients had laboratory abnormalities with no associated symptoms. Eight percent had other minor adverse effects. Treatment had to be discontinued in 16% of the patients and permanently stopped in 10% because of adverse effects. However, none of the patients died or had long-term complications.

Conclusion.—Intravenous immune globulin therapy is associated with frequent adverse effects. However, serious complications are rare, occurring mainly in patients with heart disease and renal insufficiency and in those confined to bed.

▶ Intravenous immunoglobulin therapy is frequently used because of its favorable risk/benefit ratio compared with other immunomodulating therapies. Although serious adverse effects are relatively uncommon, minor side effects are frequently encountered. Serious side effects—heart failure, stroke, renal failure, or thromboembolic disease—most often occur in predisposed patients with nephropathy, migraine, or heart disease. In such patients, the total daily dose and infusion rate should be lowered. Minor side effects (e.g., rash, headache, vasomotor complications) are difficult to anticipate. Their occurrence during the course of the infusion can sometimes be treated with aspirin or diphenhydramine or by lowering the infusion rate.

The presence of side effects during one infusion does not necessarily predict future similar reactions or new adverse reactions. In patients with pror IVIg related rashes or aseptic meningitis, we have had good results pretreating with prednisone before subsequent infusions. Although IVIg remains a reasonably safe therapy, it is likely that as higher dose infusions become more common, the incidence of major and minor side effects will increase.

A.R. Berger, M.D.

Neurologic Complications in Critically Ill Patients
Wijdicks EFM (Mayo Clinic and Mayo Found, Rochester, Minn)
Anesth Analg 83:411–419, 1996   17–3

Introduction.—Common neurologic complications of serious illnesses often seen in the ICU were reviewed.

Coma.—Coma is usually found in the ICU when illness subsides, but the patient does not awaken. The accumulation of previously administered sedative drugs is associated with altered consciousness. An anoxic-ischemic insult from an episode of hypoxemia or hypotension may produce a diffuse encephalopathy. When coma is associated with sepsis, the outcome is poor. Cholesterol embolization may be an under-reported cause of coma. Acute renal failure leading to acute uremic encephalopathy is a common cause of coma in the ICU. Ischemic strokes in multiple arterial territories or microemboli are also associated with failure to awaken. Resuscitation for cardiac or respiratory arrest can result in post-anoxic-ischemic encephalopathy. Transplant patients, particularly those receiving heart or liver transplants, are at higher risk for coma than other ICU patients. Failure to awaken after liver transplant may be caused by brain edema, neurotoxicity to cyclosporine, seizure, and central pontine myelinolysis. Central pontine myelinolysis can be confirmed by MRI (Fig 2).

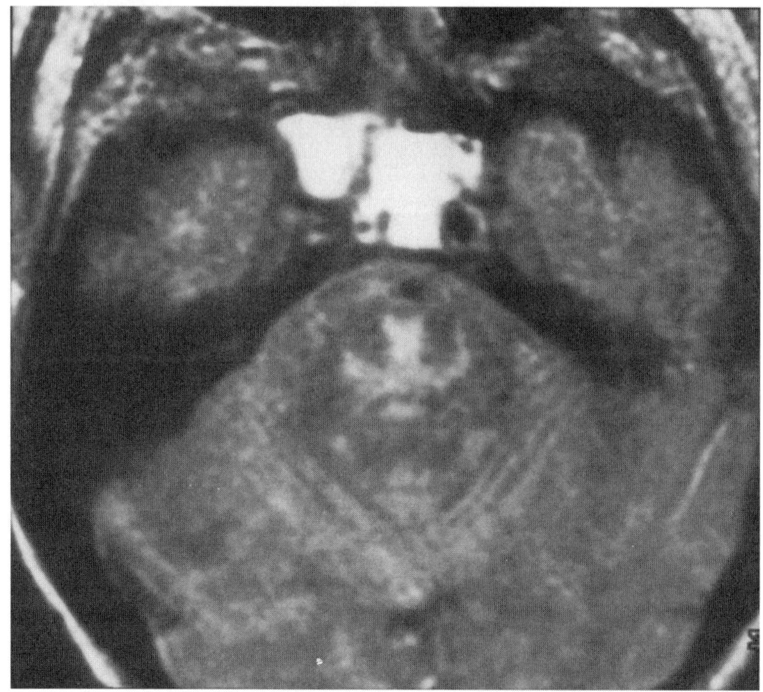

FIGURE 2.—Axial T2–weighted MR image of the pons showing typical trident-shaped high-intensity signal after liver transplantation. (Courtesy of Wijdicks EFM: Neurologic complications in critically ill patients. *Anesth Analg* 83:411–419, 1996.)

Intracranial hematomas are not common but can occur in ICU patients. There are multiple causes of coma in ICU patients. The cause is usually obvious after a review of the medical record. Computed tomography scanning and CSF analysis should be performed when patients fail to awaken.

Generalized Muscle Weakness.—There are 3 categories of muscle weakness: axonal neuropathy, usually associated with sepsis; acute steroid myopathy, which can be associated with the use of neuromuscular junction blockers; and prolonged muscle weakness after neuromuscular junction blockers, which may be a toxic myopathy. Polyneuropathy is the most common cause of generalized muscle weakness in ICU patients and is often associated with sepsis. Other factors associated with polyneuropathy include age, extended ICU stay, hypoalbuminemia, and hyperglycemia. Clinical features include normal cranial nerve findings, distal limb weakness, areflexia, muscle wasting, and diminished pinprick in a stocking-glove pattern. Outcome is usually good, with progressive resolution over several months. Use of neuromuscular blocking drugs, such as pancuronium and vecuronium, is also associated with generalized muscle weakness. Patients with renal failure, metabolic acidosis, and hypermagnesemia are more likely to accumulate blocker metabolites. Outcome is

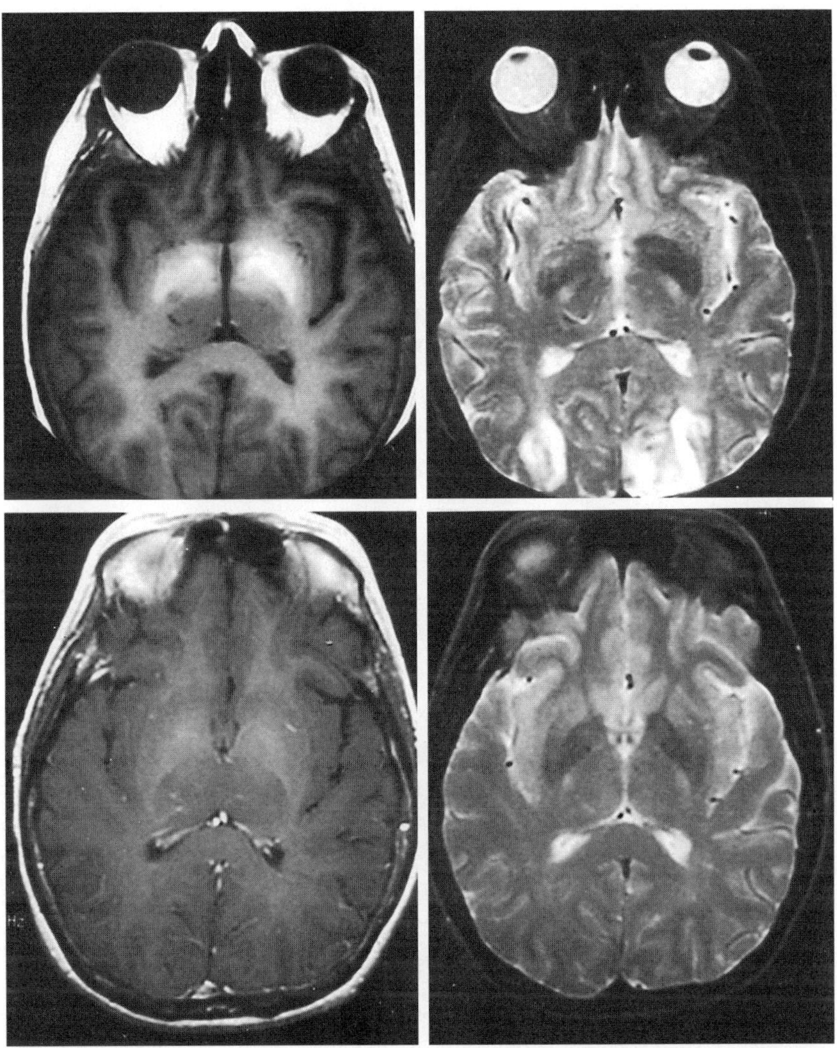

FIGURE 4.—Upper left, MRI findings in a patient with seizures and FK 506 toxicity. Note marked hyperintensity signal in the globus pallidus on T1–weighted images, typically seen in patients with advanced liver disease. **Upper right,** marked hyperintensity signal in white matter and cortex in occipital lobe appears on T2–weighted images in a patient with seizures and an impaired level of consciousness. **Lower panels,** complete resolution of both abnormalities in 1 month. (Courtesy of Wijdicks EFM: Neurologic complications in critically ill patients. *Anesth Analg* 83:411–419, 1996.)

good for this type of neuropathy. Acute necrotic myopathy can occur when a neuromuscular blocker is given by IV in combination with large corticosteroid doses. A myopathy has been described in lung transplant patients in which there is a loss of myosin. In these cases, there is no evidence of sepsis and no neuromuscular blocking agents have been used. Normal creatine kinase levels are present. The cause of this myopathy remains unknown. Rhabdomyolysis can cause muscle weakness and is usually associated with trauma, ischemia, and sepsis.

Seizure.—Generalized tonic-clonic seizure is not common in the ICU. Seizures are associated with drug toxicity, drug withdrawal, and alcohol-withdrawal. Metabolic disorders increase the risk of seizure. Most ICU seizures occur in those patients with postoperative hyponatremia. Seizures in transplant patients can indicate immunosuppressive drug toxicity. The incidence of seizures is increased by administration of cyclosporine, OKT3, and FK 506 (Fig 4).

Conclusion.—Critically ill patients are at increased risk of neurologic complications, which can have an unfavorable effect on outcome. The patient management plan must be reassessed when neurologic complications occur. This review describes neurologic complications frequently encountered in the ICU.

▶ For the neuro-intensivist and consulting neurologist seeing patients in the ICU, the neurologic sequelae of ICU care are becoming of ever-increasing interest. The cause of many of these conditions is still far from clear, although the clinical manifestations are now being increasingly recognized and characterized. There are so many "metabolic disasters" that occur in ICU patients and so many medicines used in their resuscitation that it is probable that the cause of many of these syndromes is multifactorial. More research is needed to discover the cause and pathogenetic mechanisms of these syndromes. Very little experimental research has been undertaken in these disorders, except for central pontine myelinolysis.

W.G. Bradley, D.M., F.R.C.P.

Cervical Spondylosis: An Update

McCormack BM, Weinstein PR (Univ of California, San Francisco)
West J Med 165:43–51, 1996

17–4

Background.—Degenerative disease of the cervical spine and its cartilaginous and ligamentous structures is the most common cause of cervical cord and root dysfunction in individuals older than 55 years. The pathogenesis, clinical diagnosis, and treatment of cervical spondylosis were reviewed.

Cervical Spondylosis.—Cervical spondylosis usually causes intermittent neck pain, which typically responds to modifications in activity, neck immobilization, isometric exercises, and medication. Neurologic symptoms are uncommon, usually occurring in patients with congenital spinal stenosis. The preferred initial diagnostic assessment for such patients is MRI. Neurologic structure involvement on imaging studies may be asymptomatic; thus, a neurologist should be consulted to exclude other neurologic diseases. In most patients with spondylotic radiculopathy, conservative treatment yields such good results that surgical intervention is not

Anterior Surgical Approach

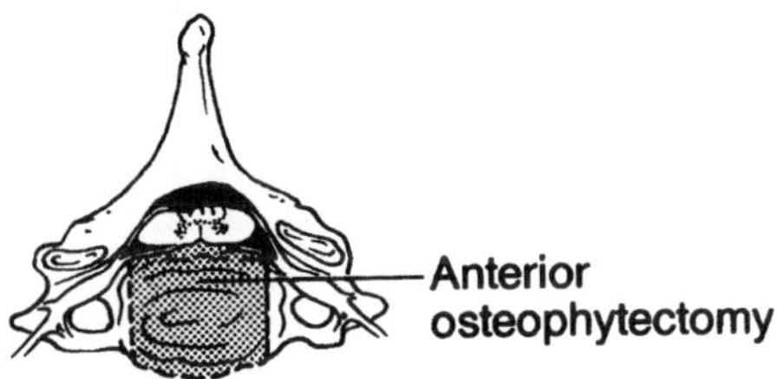

Posterior Surgical Approaches

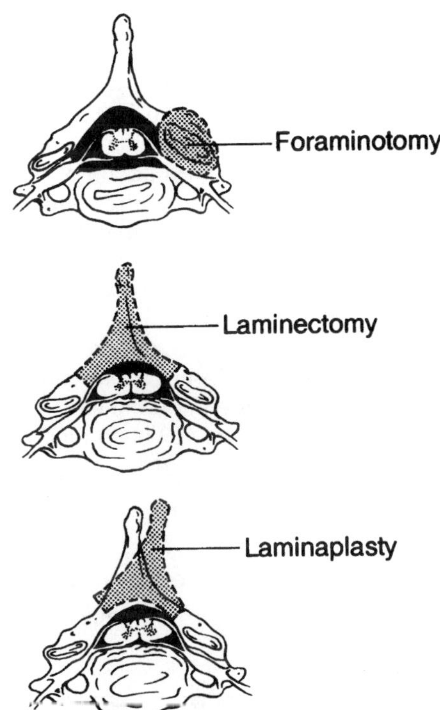

FIGURE 4.—The anterior and posterior approaches to the cervical cord and nerve roots are depicted. Three posterior procedures are illustrated: laminectomy, foraminotomy, and laminaplasty. Laminaplasty procedures expand the spinal canal by partially removing the lamina and elevating the remaining bone fragments. (Courtesy of McCormack SM, Weinstein PR: Cervical spondylosis. *West J Med* 165:43–51, 1996.)

considered unless pain persists or unless progressive neurologic deficit is present.

When indicated, surgery may be done through the anterior or posterior cervical spine. Long-term improvement occurs in 70% to 80% of patients who have surgery. The most serious and disabling condition is cervical spondylotic myelopathy. Many such patients have nonprogressive minor impairment. Thus, neck immobilization is a reasonable treatment in patients with minor neurologic findings or contraindications to surgery. Thirty to fifty percent of patients will improve with this treatment. Patients initially seen with severe or progressive neurologic deficits require surgery, generally done through anterior cervical approaches, although laminectomy is still sometimes indicated (Fig 4). The outcomes of surgery are modest, with about 70% of patients having good initial results. Functional results decline noticeably with long-term follow-up, raising the question of how surgery affects the natural course of the disease.

Conclusions.—In this article, the pathogenesis, diagnosis, and treatment of cervical spondylosis were reviewed. Further prospective randomized research is needed.

▶ More than 2 decades ago, my neurosurgical colleagues and I came to the conclusion that we did not know whether surgical or medical treatment was better for cervical spondylotic myelopathy. We initiated a randomized study to compare medical and surgical treatment, the medical treatment being immobilization in a cervical collar for a period of time, depending on symptoms. In the end, many of the referring physicians lost their nerve in terms of seeing dramatically impressive neuroimaging changes and therefore deciding that the patient should undergo surgical procedures rather than be put into the randomized study. Consequently, the trial failed because of prejudgment on the part of the physicians.

Now, more than 20 years later, we still do not know the answer to this question. This is a good review of the current knowledge concerning symptomatology and the outcome of either surgical or medical treatment. However, the review concludes that we still need randomized studies to answer the questions raised.

W.G. Bradley, D.M., F.R.C.P.

Radiculomedullary Complications of Cervical Spinal Manipulation

Padua L, Padua R, LoMonaco M, et al (Catholic Univ of Rome; CSS Hosp IRCCS San Giovanni Rotondo, Italy)
Spinal Cord 34:488–492, 1996   17–5

Background.—Spinal manipulation, used by some therapists to treat cervical pain, can cause cerebrovascular complications. Reports of adverse effects on the spinal cord and nerve roots, however, are relatively few. Cervical myelopathy and/or radiculopathy caused or aggravated by spinal manipulation in 4 patients was described.

Case 1.—Man, 67, had several years' duration of nonradiating cervical pain that was periodically treated by a chiropractor with reportedly positive results. During a first strong cervical manipulation by a new chiropractor, the man experienced a sharp pain in his left arm that was followed by parsthesia and severe weakness of the limb. An MRI scan 1 week later showed marked central narrowing of the cervical spinal canal and prolapse of the C5–C6 and C6–C7 disks, which were not present on MRI studies performed 8 months before (Fig 1). The left-arm deficits slowly improved without treatment.

Case 2.—Man, 60, showed parsthesia in the hands and generalized limb weakness 2 hours after manipulation of the cervical spine for neck pain. Computed tomography revealed a bulky median C4–C5 disk herniation. Progressive improvement occurred.

Case 3.—Man, 56, suffered sensory and motor deficits in the upper limbs and decreased deep sensation and loss of postural sense in the lower limbs after cervical manipulation for neck and arm pain. Radiography and imaging studies showed diffuse spondylarthrosis and protrusion of several cervical disks with stenosis of the cervical canal and cervical myelopathy. He was treated surgically but retained an ataxic gait 1 month later.

Case 4.—Man, 62, had suffered cervical pain and bilateral hand dysesthesia for 1 year and had an abnormal feeling in his legs when

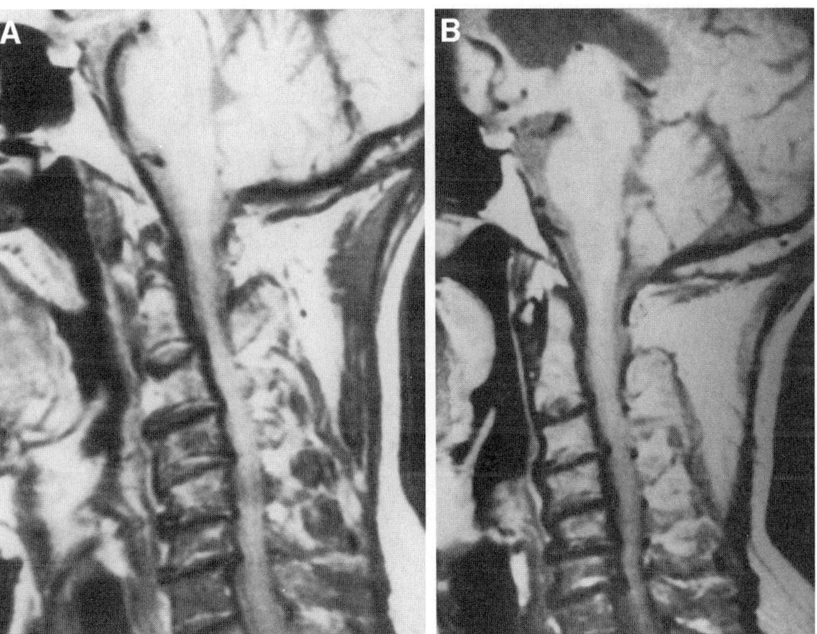

FIGURE 1.—Case 1: Premanipulation (**A**) and postmanipulation (**B**) sagittal T1–dependent MRIs. The posttreatment study shows prolapse of the C5–C6 and C6–C7 disks that was not present in the previous examination. Spondylosis at the C5–C6 level results in pressure on the ventral surface of the spinal cord. Note that the cuts (sequences) were the same in the pretreatment and in the posttreatment scans. (Courtesy of Padua L, Padua R, LoMonaco M, et al: Radiculomedullary complications of cervical spinal manipulation. *Spinal Cord* 34:488–492, 1996.)

walking during the past 3 months. After 2 chiropractic manipulations of the cervical spine, sensory deficits and weakness developed in all 4 limbs and he had difficulty walking. One month later, spinal canal stenosis and cervical myelopathy were diagnosed. Two years after surgical treatment, he walks with a crutch.

Discussion.—When the spinal cord is flexed and extended, the vertebrae slide over each other and cause a physiologic reduction in the anteroposterior diameter of the spinal canal. Spinal manipulation can cause a more significant reduction in canal diameter by provoking movements that exceed the physiologic limits of these articulations. These movements may cause or aggravate myelopathy in patients with pre-existing stenosis or vertebral instability. To screen for these problems, patients considered for spinal manipulation must first undergo a thorough neurologic examination with cervical spine films and, if necessary, MRI and/or evoked potential studies.

▶ This is one of a long series of papers in the literature describing neurologic damage resulting from cervical manipulation. Damage can result from cervical disk prolapse, spinal cord injury from vertebral instability, and vascular damage that probably results from dissection and thrombosis of either the vertebral or carotid arteries. The number of patients damaged per year by such manipulations is not known, but from my personal experience I would guess that there must be many cases that do not get reported in the literature. Chiropractors and many physical therapists still consider the neck to be an area that is susceptible to treatment by manipulation, and if one watches some of these procedures with the yanking and twisting that is involved, one becomes extremely anxious for the safety of the patient. I strongly urge all neurologists to pass on to their patients and, wherever possible, to chiropractors and physical therapists the dangers of these procedures.

W.G. Bradley, D.M., F.R.C.P.

NEUROSURGERY

SCOTT R. GIBBS, M.A., M.D.

18 Aneurysms and Intracranial Hemorrhage

Aneurysm Clips

Titanium Aneurysm Clips: Part I. Mechanical, Radiological, and Biocompatibility Testing
Lawton MT, Ho JC, Bichard WD, et al (St Joseph's Hosp, Phoeniz, Ariz; Wichita State Univ, Kan)
Neurosurgery 38:1158–1164, 1996   18–1

Objective.—Aneurysm clips are generally constructed of nonferromagnetic, cobalt-based alloys. However, these clips may still produce troublesome artifacts on MRI scans. Titanium has several important advantages for use in spinal instrumentation systems, including lack of interference with postoperative imaging. A new titanium aneurysm clip was tested for its mechanical, radiologic, and biocompatibility characteristics.

Methods.—The clips tested were constructed of chemically pure titanium metal, and had blade lengths ranging from 5 to 30 mm and widths from 1.1 to 1.2 mm. Fifty-five different shape and size configurations were tested. In vitro mechanical tests were performed, followed by biocompatibility tests in rabbits and radiologic tests in greyhound dogs.

Results.—The clips' average closing forces, which ranged from 151.6 to 181.8 g, were unaffected by repeated sterilization or stress. The clips did not open, and their closing force was not reduced, even after more than 20 million cycles of high-pressure and high-frequency pulsations. When implanted into the subarachnoid space of rabbits for 1–6 months, titanium aneurysm clips produced a mild gliosis identical to that produced by cobalt-alloy clips. The titanium clips did not corrode while implanted, according to the results of preoperative and postoperative weighing and electron microscopic scanning. In greyhound dogs, titanium clips placed on the internal carotid artery produced 2–3 times less artifact on CT and MRI than identical cobalt-chrome clips.

Conclusions.—Tests suggest that titanium aneurysm clips have many favorable characteristics for clinical use. Their mechanical performance is comparable to that of conventional cobalt-alloy clips. The titanium clips are biocompatible and resistant to corrosion. They also have superior radiologic characteristics, which reduce CT and MRI artifacts and permit better resolution of anatomical structures than cobalt-alloy clips. Titanium clips promise a substantial improvement in the quality of postoperative imaging studies in patients undergoing aneurysm clipping.

Titanium Aneurysm Clips: Part III. Clinical Application in 16 Patients With Subarachnoid Hemorrhage

Lawton MT, Heiserman JE, Prendergast VC, et al (St Joseph's Hosp, Phoenix, Ariz)
Neurosurgery 38:1170–1175, 1996   18–2

Background.—Titanium aneurysm clips have the same opening and closing forces as cobalt alloy clips without any increased epileptogenic activity. Titanium clips also produce fewer artifacts on MRI in experimental animals. However, they have not been tested in human research subjects. These authors used titanium aneurysm clips in patients with subarachnoid hemorrhaging, with excellent results.

Methods.—Titanium aneurysm clips were used in 16 patients (12 women and 4 men; average age, 61 years) with aneurysmal subarachnoid hemorrhaging. According to the Hunt and Hess classification, the status of 3 patients was grade I, the status of 6 was grade II, the status of 5 was grade III, and the status of 2 was grade IV. A control group of 11 patients (6 women and 5 men) with similar aneurysms was treated with conventional cobalt-alloy clips. Craniotomies and aneurysm clipping occurred within 24 hours of hospital admission. Imaging studies included angiograms and CT scans immediately after surgery, and MRI and MR angiography 3 months after surgery.

Findings.—Because some patients had multiple aneurysms, 22 titanium clips were used in the 16 patients. Postoperative imaging revealed no residual filling of the aneurysms, and no complications or clip malfunctions occurred. The outcome was good in 13 patients, 1 patient had moderate deficits, and 2 patients died (both had grade IV status). In the 12 patients in whom MRI was performed, the average artifact area ranged from 0.96 cm^2 on T1–weighted images to 1.36 cm^2 on T2-weighted images. Corresponding values for the cobalt clips in controls were 3.13 cm^2 on T1-weighted images and 3.70 cm^2 on T2-weighted images. Furthermore, the average volume of artifact on gradient echo images was only 1.70 cm^3 in the patients with titanium clips, compared with 10.13 cm^3 in the patients with cobalt clips. Results with MR angiography were just as striking: the artifact gaps in the patients with titanium clips were only one third of those in the controls (0.86 vs. 2.58 cm).

Conclusions.—Titanium clips safely and completely stopped aneurysm filling in these patients with aneurysmal subarachnoid hemorrhaging. Furthermore, because titanium is a nonferromagnetic metal, it caused much less distortion in MRI and MR angiographic studies. Given their comparable safety and better advantage in MR studies, titanium clips should be considered for clipping aneurysms in patients undergoing aneurysm surgery.

Titanium Aneurysm Clips: Part II. Seizure and Electroencephalographic Studies in Implanted Rabbits

Fisher RS, Ehsan T, Smith K, et al (St Joseph's Hosp, Phoenix, Ariz)
Neurosurgery 38:1165–1169, 1996   18–3

Background.—In experimental animals, many metal brain implants cause interictal spikes. Whether titanium clips would cause seizures and, if so, at what threshold are not known. Thus, the threshold for seizures in normal rabbit brains and after treatment with pentylenetetrazole (PTZ, a γ-aminobutyric acid antagonist that induces epileptic activity) was determined using titanium implants.

Methods.—New Zealand rabbits (15 males and 15 nonpregnant females) were split into 3 groups. In the 2 test groups, either cobalt-alloy ($n = 12$) or titanium ($n = 12$) clips were placed into the subarachnoid space next to the brain. In the control group ($n = 6$), no clip operations were performed. Electroencephalographic (EEG) electrodes were placed in all animals, and EEG recordings were made at 1 month for 12 animals and monthly for 6 months for 18 animals. One month after insertion of the clips, 6 animals from each of the 2 tests group were administered PTZ, and ECG recordings were made until the end point was reached. For the other 18 animals (6 from each of the 3 groups), PTZ was administered 6 months after implantation, and ECG recordings continued until the end point was reached. The end point was the occurrence of an epileptiform burst or a tonicoclonic seizure.

Findings.—No rabbits developed seizures for up to 6 months before the administration of PTZ. In fact, all 24 animals in the 2 test groups had grade 0 or 1 EEGs before PTZ dosing. The administration of PTZ caused spiking in all the animals, at a mean time after dosing of 327 sec for the controls, 389 sec for rabbits with cobalt clips, and 216 sec for rabbits with titanium clips (no significant differences between groups). Seizure latencies did not differ significantly between the 3 groups either (1031 sec for controls, 1267 sec for rabbits with cobalt clips, and 875 sec for rabbits with titanium clips).

Conclusions.—The titanium implants did not have epileptiform activity, either spontaneously or as induced by PTZ, for 6 months after implantation. Although a longer period of implantation might show different results, most studies have shown that any seizures that occur will do so within this time frame. Furthermore, rabbits are not the same as humans, and results might differ in the clinical setting. Nonetheless, based on these results, titanium aneurysm clips should not cause any seizure activity in humans.

Economic Issues

Predicting Length of Hospital Stay and Cost by Aneurysm Grade on Admission

Elliott JP, Le Roux PD, Ransom G, et al (Univ of Washington, Seattle)
J Neurosurg 85:388–391, 1996   18–4

Background.—Outcome prediction for subarachnoid hemorrhages (SAHs) and for the management of cerebral aneurysms has been increasingly emphasized. The length of hospital stay (LOS) offers an estimate of resource use. The relationship of aneurysmal SAH clinical grade on admission to LOS and cost was determined.

Methods and Findings.—The LOS and total hospitalization cost (excluding professional fees) were determined for 543 patients admitted for aneurysm surgery between 1983 and 1993. The overall median LOS was 18 days, ranging from 1 to 165. An increased median LOS was associated with Hunt and Hess grades 0 to IV on admission. The median LOS among patients with grade V aneurysms was decreased, partly because of early mortality. Increased cost was also correlated with worse clinical grade on admission. For patients in all clinical grades, a significant proportion of total expenditures were incurred early in the course of hospitalization.

Conclusions.—In patients with cerebral aneurysms, the Hunt and Hess grade on hospital admission is correlated with LOS and cost. Thus, the clinical grade on admission will be useful when considering issues of hospital resource management. Because a high percentage of treatment costs are incurred early in the course of management, factors that may reduce perioperative LOS in the ICU without jeopardizing outcomes need to be identified.

▶ Worse clinical grade portends longer hospital stays and greater hospital charges. The worst clinical grade portends attenuated survival rates, and lesser hospital charges. Although these issues seem intuitive, supporting data have not been previously available. This study serves to complete an initial step in the logic stream by linking the clinical and financial aspects of aneurysmal SAHs. These efforts move toward finding a place for financial efficiency alongside rapidly advancing clinical knowledge in the evaluation and treatment of this challenging process.

C.P. Bondurant, M.D.

Hospital Resource Utilization in the Treatment of Cerebral Aneurysms
Yundt KD, Dacey RG Jr, Diringer MN (Washington Univ, St Louis)
J Neurosurg 85:403–409, 1996   18–5

Background.—The cost of cerebral aneurysm treatment is among the highest incurred by neurosurgical patients. The effects of the severity of illness, indicated by Hunt and Hess scores and Fisher grades, and the clinical course on resource use were determined.

Methods.—The clinical and financial data for all patients treated for nontraumatic subarachnoid hemorrhages (SAHs) and unruptured cerebral aneurysms at 1 center between June 1993 and December 1994 were analyzed. Twenty-eight patients had surgically treated unruptured aneurysms (group 1), 42 had acute SAHs (group 2), 32 had SAHs with vasospasms (group 3), and 10 had SAHs with negative angiograms (group 4).

Findings.—The total cost per patient was greatest for group 3 and was associated with the hospital length of stay, the Hunt and Hess grade, and the Fisher grade. Patient charges did not always reflect areas of the greatest hospital cost. The 3 areas of greatest cost were ICU room, arteriography, and ICU medicosurgical supplies, together accounting for 48.5% of the total cost.

Conclusions.—Cost-containment efforts should be based on cost rather than charges. Novel approaches are needed to decrease the cost of treating SAHs. Such approaches may include preventing vasospasms, decreasing ICU stays, selective use of arteriography, and decreasing the expenditure on supplies.

▶ Nontraumatic SAHs, especially those complicated by vasospasms, remain a daunting neurosurgical challenge. Although morbidity and mortality remain significant, outcomes have improved in recent decades. The pathophysiologic characteristics and the natural history are better understood; surgical skill and medical management have advanced; and supporting technology has kept pace. The improved prognosis, however, has brought higher cost. Financial pressures are now more a part of medical decision making. As cost becomes a more important issue in medicine and its supporting research, improved guidelines for level of care, evaluation, and intervention are emerging. These data will add security to decisions aimed at avoiding overuse of resources. Local efforts though, remain important: the surgeon who periodically reviews a patient's bill is often quite enlightened.

C.P. Bondurant, M.D.

Genetics

Familial Cerebral Aneurysms: A Bias for Women
Leblanc R (McGill Univ, Montreal)
Stroke 27:1050–1054, 1996   18–6

Background.—Up to 20% of patients with aneurysmal subarachnoid hemorrhages (SAHs) may have familial histories of cerebral aneurysms. Familial cerebral aneurysms appear to be more common in women and may rupture at a younger age and at a smaller size (especially in women) than sporadic cerebral aneurysms. Fourteen families with 2 or more members with documented cerebral aneurysms were studied prospectively.

Methods and Findings.—The 30 affected family members were compared with patients with sporadic aneurysms. Eighty percent of the familial aneurysms and only 59% of the sporadic aneurysms occurred in women, which was a significant difference. Among patients younger than 50 years, 78% with familial aneurysms and 45% with sporadic aneurysms were women. The incidence did not differ significantly between the sexes among patients older than 50 years. Fifty-nine percent of the familial aneurysms in women ruptured before 50 years of age, compared with 31% of sporadic aneurysms. Aneurysms ruptured within 10 years of each other in sisters in 4 of 5 families. Although the occurrence of multiple aneurysms was equal in both groups (17%), multiple familial aneurysms occurred primarily in women.

Conclusions.—Compared with patients with sporadic aneurysms, women are overrepresented among those with ruptured familial aneurysms. In most cases, familial aneurysms rupture in women before the age of 50 years, in the same decade, and at the same site within families.

▶ The information gleaned from 14 families with 30 ruptured and 3 unruptured aneurysms attempts to clarify some issues surrounding the pathogenesis and treatment of familial and sporadic aneurysms. The familial clustering and, moreover, the clustering by sex support a genetic (likely multifactorial), an environmental, and perhaps a hormonal influence in familial aneurysms that could possibly apply, in some part, to the understanding of sporadic aneurysms as well. The suggested tendency for earlier rupture in smaller aneurysms in women with familial aneurysms justifies a more aggressive approach to treatment of such women with unruptured aneurysms. More importantly, the clustering by sex refines support for screening with regard to the frequent family question, "Should I have an angiogram?"

C.P. Bondurant, M.D.

Alpha-$_1$-antitrypsin Phenotypes Among Patients With Intracranial Aneurysms

Schievink WI, Katzmann JA, Piepgras DG, et al (Mayo Clinic, Rochester, Minn)
J Neurosurg 84:781–784, 1996   18–7

Background.—The pathogenesis of intracranial and other arterial aneurysms may involve a deficiency of α_1-antitrypsin. The highly polymorphic α_1-antitrypsin gene is located on chromosome 14. The allele is designated protease inhibitor (Pi). Severe α_1-antitrypsin deficiency develops in patients who are homozygous for the allelic variant PiZ allele; however, heterozygous patients usually remain asymptomatic throughout life. Different phenotypes of α_1-antitrypsin deficiency were prospectively assessed in patients with intracranial aneurysms.

Methods.—The study included 100 consecutive patients with confirmed intracranial aneurysms. Their α_1-antitrypsin phenotype was determined and compared with that of the general population, based on a previously reported study of blood donors—mainly of German or Scandinavian heritage—from the same state. Fisher's exact test was used for comparisons.

Results.—The combined heterozygous α_1-antitrypsin states—PiMS and PiMZ—were found in 16% of patients with intracranial aneurysms vs. 7% of the general population. Odds ratio was 2.56, with a 95% confidence interval of 1.32–4.75. Among the patients, men were more likely to have α_1-antitrypsin deficiency.

Conclusions.—α_1-Antitrypsin deficiency is a genetic risk factor for intracranial aneurysm. The mechanism of this effect may be interference with the protease/antiprotease balance, leading to degradation of the arterial wall. Patients with intracranial aneurysm have high rates of the heterozygous α_1-antitrypsin deficiency states, especially men.

▶ The search for a possible genetic influence on the development of cerebral aneurysms remains compelling. The strongest evidence to date that genetically determined influences may operate on the development of cerebral aneurysms is epidemiologic: cerebral aneurysms develop in association with well-described, genetically determined conditions, such as adult polycystic kidney disease; they occur in identical twins, usually at the same sites and rupture at roughly the same age; and they can cluster in families. To date, no specific biochemical defect or marker has been identified in patients with cerebral aneurysms. The characterization of such a lesion would provide a better understanding of the etiology and evolution of cerebral aneurysms, as well as serve to identify individuals at risk, such as family members, who may harbor an asymptomatic cerebral aneurysm, which could then be diagnosed and treated before rupturing.

The report by Schievink et al. makes a significant contribution to the first of these concerns by demonstrating a deficiency in one or more of the numerous α_1-antitrypsin phenotypes in a small proportion of patients with cerebral aneurysms, mainly males. The presence of such a deficiency in at least 7% of the general population, and in a relatively small fraction (16%) of patients with a cerebral aneurysm, makes the demonstration of α_1–antitrypsin deficiency a poor marker for the presence of cerebral aneurysms in asymptomatic individuals, such as might be encountered in familial cases. The fact that others were not able to identify such a deficiency in a large number of patients with cerebral aneurysms, and the poorly controlled studies showing a deficiency of α_1–antitrypsin in patients with aneurysm that preceded that of Schievink et al. should compel others to try to replicate their results in a well-controlled setting, and within familial cases.

Of special interest is the demonstration that the deficiency in question need not reside necessarily within the arterial wall itself but, by resulting in a dysinhibition of circulating proteolytic enzymes, would secondarily affect the cerebral arterial wall. This supports a genome linkage analysis strategy rather than a candidate gene approach based on the constituents of the cerebral arterial wall, especially in the elucidation of a possible genetic influence in familial cerebral aneurysms.

R. Leblanc, M.D., M.S.C., F.R.C.S.C.

Intracranial and Subarachnoid Hemorrhage

Computed Tomographic Criteria and Survival Rate for Patients With Acute Subdural Hematoma
Zumkeller M, Behrmann R, Heissler HE, et al (Medizinische Hochschule, Hannover, Germany)
Neurosurgery 39:708–713, 1996   18–8

Introduction.—Prognosis is poor and mortality rates are high among patients with acute subdural hematoma. On admission, patients usually have been intubated, sedated, and placed on artificial ventilation. Because neurologic examination is not possible in this setting, CT scan criteria are crucial for determining prognosis and choice of therapeutic interventions. A retrospective study of CT data from 174 patients sought to identify parameters that could be evaluated independently of clinical and neurologic status to estimate outcome.

Patients and Methods.—The patients had isolated head injury and unilateral acute subdural hematoma. The following 2 parameters were determined morphometrically from the CT data: (1) thickness of the hematoma, and (2) midline shift. The difference between these parameters yielded a third parameter—the displacements or brain swelling factor. At admission, patients were categorized according to the Glasgow Coma Scale. The Glasgow Outcome Scale was used for postoperative evaluation.

Results.—Postoperative data were incomplete for 10 patients, leaving 164 available for analysis. Of these, 78 (48%) survived, and 86 (52%) died. Among the survivors, 27 had a good outcome with complete recovery, 24 achieved moderately good outcomes with slight handicaps, 14 were severely handicapped, and 13 remained in a vegetative state. Hematoma thickness ranged from 5–35 mm in surgically treated patients, and midline shift ranged from 0–33 mm. The hematoma thickness was greater than the midline shift in 81 (46.6%) patients, and the midline shift exceeded the hematoma thickness in 69 (39.6%). These 2 parameters were similar in the remaining 24 patients (13.8%). The median survival rate was at a hematoma thickness of approximately 18 mm, and the interquartile range was between 13 and 25 mm. Survival fell to 10% when the hematoma was 30 mm thick. The median survival rate was at midline shifts of 19 mm, and the interquartile range was limited by 13 and 26 mm. Calculation of displacement by brain swelling showed that negative differences of up to –5 mm were associated with a high survival rate. A displacement of +3 mm was associated with 50% mortality, and the interquartile range was between 0 and 6 mm. Glasgow Outcome Scale scores correlated significantly with these parameters.

Conclusion.—The CT parameters of hematoma thickness, midline shift, and the difference between the 2 (displacement) allow survival and outcome to be estimated in patients with acute subdural hematoma. Indications for surgery could thus be assessed without a neurologic examination of the patient.

▶ In intubated and paralyzed patients harboring traumatic hematomas, meticulous assessment of CT parameters is very important. The article highlights the prognostic value of the "brain swelling index;" that is, the difference between hematoma thickness and midline shift. A relevant CT parameter that should be taken into account is the degree of brain atrophy on the contralateral hemisphere (brain atrophy index). An atrophic brain can accommodate a larger hematoma with less associated midline displacement. This can "shift" favorably the survival rate of patients with bigger hematomas and/or bigger brain swelling index. Nevertheless, there is a limit to the predictive ability of CT. This is particularly true in patients who have a hematoma thickness or midline shift in the middle of the range of values (16–25 mm). In such patients, the neurosurgeon can mainly rely on the pupillary reactivity. If this has been lost, then the primary remaining predictive variable is the length of time from injury to scanning or operation. Prolonged displacement of the brain may affect the outcome negatively.

D.E. Sakas, M.D.

Effects of a Hydroxyl Radical Scavenger on Delayed Ischemic Neurological Deficits Following Aneurysmal Subarachnoid Hemorrhage: Results of a Multicenter, Placebo-controlled Double-blind Trial
Asano T, Takakura K, Sano K, et al (Saitama Med Ctr/School, Japan; Tokyo Women's Med School; Teikyo Univ, Tokyo)
J Neurosurg 84:792–803, 1996
18–9

Introduction.—A growing body of evidence suggests that treatment with free-radical scavengers can reduce the incidence of delayed ischemic neurologic deficits (DINDs) in patients with aneurysmal subarachnoid hemorrhage (SAH). Experimental and clinical studies have demonstrated the benefits of a water-soluble, novel synthetic compound, AVS ([±]N,N'–propylenedinicotinamide; nicaraven) in scavenging hydroxyl radicals and ameliorating vasospasm. The clinical applications of AVS were evaluated in a study of patients with SAH.

Methods.—The multicenter study enrolled 162 patients between May 1992 and December 1993; 147 met all entry criteria. All had experienced SAH from aneurysmal rupture within the previous 120 hours and had Glasgow Coma Scale scores between 7 and 15. Eighty patients were randomized to AVS and 82 to placebo. Treatment (4 g AVS- or glucose-infused IV for 6–8 hours once a day) was started within 5 days post-SAH and continued for 10–14 days. The primary end point of the double-blind trial was the amelioration of DINDs. Patients were required to undergo repeat CT scans on completion of treatment and at approximately day 30. Detailed neurologic assessments were performed at enrollment and at 1 and 3 months post SAH.

Results.—The 2 treatment groups were similar in demographic and clinical data at study entry. The overall incidence of DINDs, defined as an exacerbation of impaired consciousness and/or focal neurologic deficits, was 35.5% in the AVS group and 54.2% in the placebo group. This reduction in the incidence of DINDs with AVS treatment (34.5%) was significant. Treatment with AVS also led to significant improvement in the Glasgow Outcome Scale (GOS) score at 1 month and a tendency toward greater improvement in the GOS score at 3 months. Compared with placebo, AVS significantly reduced the cumulative incidence of death. The global safety rating scores were almost the same between AVS and placebo groups, confirming the safety of AVS treatment.

Conclusion.—The incidence of DINDs was significantly reduced in these patients with aneurysmal SAH who were treated with AVS. Treated patients also showed marked improvement in the GOS scores at 1 month, and had a significantly lower cumulative incidence of death at 3 months than patients randomized to placebo. The safety and efficacy of AVS recommend its use in this setting.

▶ Delayed ischemic neurologic deficits attributable to cerebral vasospasm develop in about 50% of all patients treated for a ruptured intracranial aneurysm. Despite decades of research, vasospasm remains the leading cause of severe disability, vegetative state, or death after otherwise successful aneurysm treatment. The cause of vasospasm remains obscure and the treatment unknown. That is why this multicenter Japanese study of the influence of AVS, a novel hydroxyradical scavenger, on the outcome of patients after bleeding from an intracranial aneurysm is of great value. It presents a successful, *pathophysiologically* targeted treatment for DINDs. Moreover, prospective randomized studies are rare, despite their unquestionable immediate usefulness in clinical settings, because of their costs and logistical difficulties. It is, for those 2 reasons, that this study has significant potential for changing the contemporary standard of treatment for patients at risk of cerebral vasospasm.

This study is the result of Dr. Asano's devotion to an idea he proposed many years ago; his admirable patience and perseverance have changed theory into a successful prospective study. There are, however, 2 small flaws in this study that should be drawn to the reader's attention. First, in Europe and the United States, nimodipine is a standard of care; therefore, leaving the use of calcium channel blockers to the neurosurgeon's discretion seems to weaken the study's conclusion. Second, the lack of arteriographic confirmation of cerebral vasospasm makes it difficult to accept the conclusion that AVS effectively prevents vasospasm, particularly because the number of patients with low-density areas on the CT scan, a marker of vasospasm, was not different between the treatment group and the placebo group. Arteriographic confirmation of vasospasm is important because many experimental agents (e.g., nimodipine, trilizad, and papaverine) have been claimed to prevent vasospasm, a claim that has not been confirmed by clinical studies, even these agents unquestionably improved the outcome (e.g., nimodipine).

R.M. Pluta, M.D., Ph.D.

An Audit of Aneurysmal Subarachnoid Haemorrhage: Earlier Resuscitation and Surgery Reduces Inpatient Stay and Deaths From Rebleeding
Whitfield PC, Moss H, O'Hare D, et al (Addenbrooke's Hosp, Cambridge, England)
J Neurol Neurosurg Psychiatry 60:301–306, 1996   18–10

Background.—Delayed surgery for an aneurysmal subarachnoid hemorrhage (SAH) has been associated with a lower operative morbidity and mortality than surgery done within 10 days of the event. However, surgical delay is accompanied by a high incidence of rebleeding, which is usually fatal. Earlier surgery to secure the aneurysm neck decreases the occurrence of rebleeding, but increases operative morbidity. Factors that may contribute to the pathogenesis of delayed ischemia include hypotension, hypovolemia, increased intracranial pressure, metabolic disturbances, and hypoxia. With improvements in neuroanesthesia and operative microsurgical methods, the morbidity associated with early surgery may be reduced.

Methods.—A retrospective analysis of patients with SAHs occurring during 20 months (phase 1) was followed by a prospective analysis of patients seen in the next 20 months (phase 2). In phase 2, the patients underwent a protocol-driven management regimen of immediate IV fluid resuscitation and earlier surgery. Patients in phase 2 were grouped according to the timing of their surgery.

Findings.—Surgical morbidity and mortality in the 2 phases were comparable. However, the rebleeding rate was significantly reduced in patients undergoing surgery within 4 days of the SAH in phase 2, and there was a related trend toward a decreased incidence of postoperative ischemia and mortality. Earlier surgery in phase 2 resulted in a decreased length of hospital stay.

Conclusions.—In this study, surgical morbidity and mortality appeared to be independent of the timing of aneurysm surgery. Surgery performed within 4 days was associated with a very significant decrease in the rebleeding rate and the length of hospital stay.

▶ There has long been controversy over the timing of aneurysm surgery. Cogent arguments have been presented by the proponents of early surgery (i.e., generally less than 4 days after ictus) and late surgery (i.e., generally 10–14 days after ictus or longer).

Those who favor early surgery argue that, if successful, this virtually eliminates the mortality from rerupture, which is generally estimated to be 40% during the first week.[1] In addition, early surgery facilitates combating vasospasms, which generally peak between 6–8 days after an SAH. In addition, for those who use thrombolytic agents to remove a subarachnoid clot, theoretically this will allow removal of potentially vasospasmogenic factors.

Some prefer late surgery because brain inflammation and edema are less severe with the passage of time after an SAH. This provides for easier brain retraction and potentially less brain retraction injury. In addition, some of the subarachnoid clot has had time to lyse, thereby improving visibility and reducing the intraoperative risk of aneurysm rupture. Late surgery also theoreticlly reduces the probability of vasospasms from manipulation of the cerebral vessels.

The authors' data reveal that early surgery is associated with a significant reduction in the rate of aneurysm rerupture and in the length of inpatient stay.

Although posterior circulation aneurysms comprised 6% of the study population, the authors did not state how many of these were basilar artery aneurysms. Because of the deep location, limited visibility, and relatively high importance of the perforating vessels of the basilar artery, I would reserve late surgery for this subset and for patients with Hunt and Hess grade IV and V SAHs.

S.R. Gibbs, M.A., M.D.

Reference:

1. Weir B: *Aneurysms affecting the Nervous System.* Baltimore, Md, Williams and Wilkins, 1987.

19 Brain Tumors

Acoustic Tumors

Management of 1000 Vestibular Schwannomas (Acoustic Neuromas): Clinical Presentation
Matthies C, Samii M (Nordstadt Hosp, Hannover, Germany)
Neurosurgery 40:1–10, 1997   19–1

Objective.—The last few decades have seen major advances in the surgical treatment of vestibular schwannomas, also known as acoustic neuromas. Surgery can now provide a cure, with a completely normal quality of life and life expectancy. However, questions remain about how the symptoms, duration, and sequence of symptoms correlate with tumor size or extension or damage to the cranial nerves. These epidemiologic aspects must be understood before an optimal diagnostic and treatment protocol can be realized. The clinical findings of vestibular schwannoma were analyzed in a review of a large surgical experience.

Methods.—The experience included 962 patients undergoing surgery for a total of 1,000 vestibular schwannomas from 1978 to 1993. All operations were performed by 1 surgeon. The patients were 522 women (mean age, 47.6 years) and 440 men (mean age, 45.2 years). The clinical evaluation included the patient's general state of health, cranial nerve involvement, cerebellar and cerebral involvement, and symptom duration and sequence. Subjective disturbances were analyzed in terms of objective morbidity. The duration and pattern of symptoms were compared with the size and extension of the tumor.

Results.—Ninety-five percent of patients had disturbances of the acoustic nerve. Other symptoms included disturbances of the vestibular nerve (61% of patients), the trigeminal nerve (9%), and the facial nerve (6%). Hearing loss had been present for a mean of 3.7 years, facial paresis had been present for 1.9 years, and trigeminal disturbances had been present for 1.3 years. There was no clear relationship between the incidence and duration of symptoms and the size of the tumor. The diagnosis was made when symptoms resulted from tumor extension, such as trigeminal disturbances caused by large tumors with brain stem compression, or tinnitus caused by smaller neuromas. Patients with symptoms related to the trigeminal or facial nerve had a shorter duration of symptoms. The patients subjectively noticed only one third to two thirds of nerve disturbances identified. Twenty-three percent of patients had become deaf over a long period of time, and 3% had sudden deafness. Sudden deafness sometimes occurred even in patients with long-lasting moderate hearing deficits. Although patients who could hear were more likely to have tinnitus than patients who could not hear, nearly half of patients with preoperative deafness had tinnitus. Vestibular disturbances usually manifested as unsteady walking or vertigo. Vestibular symptoms tended to fluctuate, rather than being constant.

Conclusions.—The clinical findings of a large series of patients with vestibular schwannomas are reviewed. Clinical characteristics do not always reflect differences in the biological characteristics of the tumor, which do not appear on imaging studies. The duration of symptoms may be similar for small intrameatal tumors—which often cause vestibular symptoms and tinnitus—as for larger tumors. Patients with large tumors causing brain stem compression may have a shorter duration of symptoms at a younger age. Both large tumor size and young age may be associated with faster tumor growth. The findings suggest the need for a new look at the dynamics of both tumor growth and the affected neural tissues.

Management of Vestibular Schwannomas (Acoustic Neuromas): Radiological Features in 202 Cases—Their Value for Diagnosis and Their Predictive Importance

Matthies C, Samii M, Krebs S (Nordstadt Hosp, Hannover, Germany)
Neurosurgery 40:469–482, 1997   19–2

Purpose.—In patients with vestibular schwannomas, the tumor's biological characteristics and clinical findings may be reflected by the tumor-induced bony and soft-tissue findings. The influence of the individual anatomical conditions of the posterior fossa is also of obvious interest. Vestibular schwannomas usually cause a typical displacement of the cranial nerves: the cochlear nerve is pushed downward and the facial nerve is pushed anteriorly and upward. Because of these changes, the extent of the caudal and anterior tumor growth could affect the extent of the clinical deficit or the chances for surgical preservation of the cochlear and facial nerves. The predictive value of bone and tumor parameters in patients with vestibular schwannoma were assessed.

Methods.—The study included 202 patients with vestibular schwannomas operated on at a single hospital. All were studied in the same CT unit and using the same technique, that is, preoperative and postoperative high-resolution CT at bone windows, preoperative contrast-enhanced high-resolution CT, and postoperative native high-resolution CT. One hundred three cases were evaluated for anatomical parameters of the petrous bone and posterior fossa cavity. In all cases, tumor-induced changes in bony structures, tumor relationships to bony and neural structures, and the postoperative bony and neural findings were assessed. The radiologic findings were evaluated for their diagnostic reliability and their relationship to postoperative outcome.

Results.—Factors related to the degree of postoperative hearing deterioration were the length of the posterior auditory canal wall and the interear difference of the maximum porus width. The likelihood of postoperative hearing preservation or hearing loss was significantly predicted by the extent of internal auditory canal widening. In patients with large tumors, the extent of tumor growth anterior and caudal to the internal auditory canal was a significant predictor of postoperative hearing function. Preoperative and postoperative facial and cochlear nerve function were significantly correlated with tumor extension in all directions and with the extent of cystic tumor components. For surgical planning, the danger of labyrinthine destruction could be assessed by the positions of the labyrinthine structures in relation to the fundus and sigmoid sinus, and thus, to the suboccipital surgical approach.

Conclusions.—Preoperative radiologic studies provide a great deal of useful information in patients with vestibular schwannomas. In addition to their value for surgical planning, they can identify the key biological traits of the tumor—such as bony destruction of the internal auditory canal, tumor shape, and cyst formation—and can provide predictive information on postoperative outcome. Although contrast-enhanced MRI is the most sensitive technique for tumor detection, high-resolution bone CT is needed to assess tumor destructiveness, to plan the microsurgical approach, and to reduce the dangers of labyrinthine destruction and CSF fistulas.

▶ The authors, based on their extensive experience with the investigation and treatment of patients with acoustic schwannomas, attempt to relate some of the radiologic features seen on CT scans to an assessment of surgical outcome. From a larger database of 1000 patients, they selected some 200 who were investigated within a standardized CT protocol. Their CT scans were analyzed for bony changes related to tumor expansion and, in half of these cases, for specific features and relationships of the petrous bone and posterior fossa.

Within this group, they analyzed a number of morphometric features, structural changes, and tumor characteristics. Extensive, absolute measurements and measurements of specific relationships were then submitted to a battery of statistical tests—an earlier reviewer counted 84 statistical tests, 47 of which were significant[1]—and significant features were retained. These included the length of the posterior auditory canal wall and the interear difference of the width of the porus acusticus, which correlated with the degree of preoperative hearing loss; the extent of widening of the internal auditory canal and the anterocaudal extension of the tumor, which were related to postoperative hearing function; the overall extension of the tumor and the presence of cystic degeneration, which correlated with postoperative facial and cochlear nerve functions; and the position and relationship of the labyrinth, which correlated with the risk of intraoperative labyrinthine damage.

Despite the statistical significance of some correlations, the biological importance of these correlations is challenged by the fact that the test population was selected from a much larger group. Thus, the absolute predictive value of the presence or absence of some of the features that they think are more pertinent is not immediately apparent and limits the applicability of some of the measurements that they have identified. Further, as the authors recognize, the investigative modality of choice for acoustic neuromas is now MRI. Although some of the features they identified could be applicable to MRI measurement, some of the very detailed measurements that they performed would be difficult to replicate by MRI. We are left, thus, with an exquisitely detailed statistical analysis of morphological and biological features related to acoustic schwannomas that may be of special interest to neuroradiologists, but whose practical importance in the assessment and treatment of the average patient with an acoustic nerve tumor remains to be demonstrated.

To this reader, the memory of 1 or 2 fine line drawings amidst a blur of measurements, angles, relationships, probabilities, confidence intervals, and statistically significant minutiae are all that remain from a reading of this paper. The illustrations are striking in their simplicity, and the incorporation of precisely measured features and relationships give them an artistic air reminiscent of D'Arcy Thompson's *On Growth and Form.*[2]

R. Leblanc, M.D., M.S.C., F.R.C.S.C.

References

1. Ojemann RG, Barker FG II: In commentary: Matthies C, Samii M, Krebs S: Management of vestibular schwannomas (acoustic neuromas)): Radiologic features in 202 cases—their value for diagnosis and their predictive importance. *Neurosurgery* 40:481, 1997.
2. Thompson D'AW: *On Growth and Form*, revised edition. Cambridge, England, Cambridge University, 1942 (reprinted 1992).

Management of 1000 Vestibular Schwannomas (Acoustic Neuromas): Surgical Management and Results With an Emphasis on Complications and How to Avoid Them
Samii M, Matthies C (Nordstadt Hosp, Hannover, Germany)
Neurosurgery 40:11–23, 1997   19–3

Introduction.—With proper training and experience on the part of the neurosurgeon, surgery for a vestibular schwannoma (VS) is a safe procedure in terms of morbidity and mortality. The senior author has used the suboccipital approach to VS, exclusively for the past 16 years. This provides a unique opportunity to analyze the importance of other variables in relationship to the results and the complication rate of VS surgery.

Methods.—The analysis included 962 patients undergoing surgery, for a total of 1,000 VSs from 1978 to 1993. Eighty-two patients had neurofibromatosis-2, and 120 bilateral tumors were treated. All operations were performed by the suboccipital transmeatal approach. Preoperative and postoperative data on each patient were analyzed, including the radiologic and surgical findings.

Results.—Complete tumor removal was achieved in 979 cases. In the remaining cases, partial tumor removal was performed for brain stem decompression in severely ill patients or in an attempt to preserve hearing in the last hearing ear. The rate of anatomical nerve preservation was 93% for the facial nerve and 68% for the cochlear nerve. The recurrence rate among patients without neurofibromatosis-2 was 0.7%. One patient was left with tetraparesis, and 10 had hemiparesis; the rate of caudal cranial nerve palsy was 5.5%. Other complications and their rates of occurrence were CSF fistula, 9.2%; hydrocephalus, 2.3%; hematoma, 2.2%; bacterial meningitis, 1.2%; and wound revision, 1.1%. Eleven patients died within 2–69 days postoperatively, which yielded a mortality rate of 1.1%. Factors associated with an increased risk of complications included pre-existing severe general morbidity and/or neurologic morbidity, cystic tumors, and major caudal cranial nerve deficits.

Conclusions.—This extensive experience shows that a suboccipital approach permits complete resection of VS, with continuing reductions in morbidity. Careful patient selection should allow reduction of the already low mortality rate to less than 1%. In their experience, the authors have developed some techniques to prevent complications. They urge close attention to patients with cystic schwannomas, which pose a greater danger to brain stem and facial nerve integrity, and are more likely to be associated with postoperative bleeding.

Management of 1000 Vestibular Schwannomas (Acoustic Neuromas): Hearing Function in 1000 Tumor Resections
Samii M, Matthies C (Nordstadt Hosp, Hannover, Germany)
Neurosurgery 40:248–262, 1997   19–4

Purpose.—It is generally accepted that vestibular schwannomas can be completely resected with low mortality and decreasing facial-nerve–related morbidity. However, the effects of surgery on the cochlear nerve are less clear. Many authors have described hearing preservation in their own experience of vestibular schwannoma surgery; this suggests that it might be possible to attempt to preserve the cochlear nerve in every case or selected cases. A surgical experience with 1,000 vestibular schwannomas was reviewed with a focus on the possibility of hearing preservation.

Methods.—The experience included 1,000 vestibular schwannomas in 962 patients, including 82 patients with neurofibromatosis-2 and bilateral tumors. All operations were performed over a 15-year period by 1 surgeon. The patients were managed by uniform principles, with efforts to preserve the cochlear nerve whenever possible. The Norstadt classification system was used to analyze the audiometric data, which were graded in 30-dB steps by audiometry and in 10% to 30% steps by speech discrimination. The hearing results were also graded by the criteria of Gardner, Shelton, and House and assessed in terms of the Hannover tumor extension grading system.

Results.—The cochlear nerve was anatomically preserved in 68% of cases. This included some patients with preoperative deafness, a very few of whom had some return of hearing. There were 732 patients with some preoperative hearing. In this group, the anatomical cochlear nerve preservation rate was 79% and the functional preservation rate 39.5%. For the most recent 200 cases, the actual preservation rate was 47%. Factors associated with a better chance of hearing preservation were male sex; small-to-medium tumor size, with extension mainly within the cerebellopontine cistern; good-to-moderate preoperative hearing, with loss no greater than 40 dB; and hypoacusis lasting less than 1.5 years or vestibular disturbances lasting less than 0.7 years. Depending on these factors, the chances of hearing preservation ranged as high as 88%.

Conclusions.—Hearing preservation is a possibility for many patients undergoing vestibular schwannoma surgery, depending on the tumor extension and preoperative hearing quality. Poor preoperative discrimination should not exclude attempts at hearing preservation. Currently used hearing classification systems do not adequately account for the real problems posed by patients with schwannomas. Functional preservation of the cochlear nerve should be attempted whenever possible in patients undergoing complete resection of vestibular schwannomas.

▶ This article describes the highly commendable work of a most distinguished surgeon over a period of 16 years. It is significant, however, that, in the last 600 of 1,000 cases operated on, there was no further improvement in the cochlear nerve's functional preservation rate, which did not exceed 47%. Is this the limit of current surgical excellence? Is further improvement possible? Advances may depend on new insights regarding how intrameatal tumor growth distorts local anatomy. First, a better understanding is needed of the cochlear nerve's directions of displacement and patterns of distortion. If displaced inferiorly as a thin, distinct bundle, the cochlear nerve is more easily separated atraumatically, compared with instances in which it is splayed out over the tumor or, even worse, intermingled with it. Second, as the tumor grows, the small intrameatal arteries supplying the cochlear and other nerves become gradually compressed, obliterated, and replaced by new vascularization. Such vascularization of the tumor and the cochlear nerve may become partially shared or even indistinguishable in many patients; hence, the nerve and the tumor become interdependent for their blood flow. In such cases, regardless of surgical skill, separation of the tumor could deprive the cochlear nerve of a substantial part of its vascularization, which could lead, in turn, to cochlear nerve ischemia and irreversible functional loss, despite preservation of the nerve's anatomical continuity.

D.E. Sakas, M.D.

Gliomas

Prognostic Factors in Low Grade (WHO Grade II) Gliomas of the Cerebral Hemispheres: The Role of Surgery
Scerrati M, Roselli R, Iacoangeli M, et al (Catholic Univ, Rome)
J Neurol Neurosurg Psychiatry 61:291–296, 1996   19–5

Background.—The value of surgical resection for low-grade gliomas has been questioned. The role of surgery in the treatment of World Health Organization (WHO) grade II gliomas of the cerebral hemispheres was further investigated.

Methods.—The outcomes of 131 low-grade hemispheric gliomas treated surgically between 1978 and 1989 were reviewed. Forty-two tumors were fibrillary, 11 were gemistocytic astrocytomas, 49 were oligodendrogliomas, and 29 were oligoastrocytomas. The median follow-up of survivors was 93 months. Forty-nine patients underwent external radiotherapy postoperatively.

Findings.—The overall survival probability was 97.1% at 5 years, 76.1% at 8 years, and 62.7% at 10 years. In a univariate analysis, survival was significantly, positively associated with age younger than 20 years, total and subtotal surgical resection, and no radio therapy. A lower survival probability was associated with gemistocytic astrocytomas and tumor extension of more than 5 cm. Karnofsky performance was not associated with survival. In a multivariate analysis, the most relevant factor affecting survival was the extent of resection, which was the only variable that remained significant.

Conclusions.—Although this study is limited by its retrospective design, the findings are consistent with those of previous retrospective studies. The current authors would be reluctant to refuse surgery to patients with grade II cerebral gliomas in a location and of a size well-suited to resection, even in the absence of a mass effect.

▶ This is another retrospective study concerning the management of low-grade gliomas of the brain. The authors have reviewed 131 cases. Their conclusions are similar to what is already known from the literature: younger patients fare much better than older ones, and gemistocytic astrocytomas have a much more aggressive behavior than the other subtypes of low-grade gliomas. Actually, gemistocytic astrocytomas should be considered malignant tumors. Radiotherapy does not seem to be effective, but because there was no systematic approach, no conclusion can be drawn from these data. Prospective randomized studies are clearly needed to answer this important question. Such a study is currently being performed by the European Organization for Research and Treatment of Cancer. The authors state very strongly that radical surgical removal is an important favorable prognostic factor. However, they do not tell us what the clinical presentation of their patients was. It has been shown that patients with epilepsy fare much better than the others, and may even be followed up for years without signs of tumor progression.[1] Thus, I would be more reluctant than they are to offer surgery to patients with epilepsy, properly controlled under medication, with grade II cerebral gliomas without mass effect.

N. de Tribolet, M.D.

Reference

1. Loiseau H, Bousquet PH, Rivel J, et al: Supratentorial low-grade astrocytomas in adults. Prognostic factors and indications of treatments. A series of 141 patients. *Neurochirurgie* 41:38–50, 1995.

Functional Cortex and Subcortical White Matter Located Within Gliomas

Skirboll SS, Ojemann GA, Berger MS, et al (Univ of Washington, Seattle)
Neurosurgery 38:678–685, 1996   19–6

Background.—Current thinking holds that primary intra-axial tumors displace or obliterate functional tissues; thus, tumor resection will not affect functionality. This report suggests otherwise, in that these patients had functional tissue within the margins of infiltrative gliomas.

Methods.—Intraoperative brain mapping was performed in 413 patients with supratentorial neoplasms near or within cortical areas associated with language, motor, or sensory functions. Functional tissue within the margins of the tumor was found in 28 patients (6.8%), who form the basis of this report. Tumors and functional tissues in these 28 patients were identified by CT, MRI, intraoperative ultrasound, gross appearance, histologic examination, and direct cortical and subcortical stimulation mapping. Presenting symptoms included seizures (21 patients), motor deficits (11 patients), sensory deficits (5 patients), and speech deficits (6 patients). The extent of resection was based on functional considerations.

Findings.—Most patients (20 of 28, or 72%) had motor tissue within the tumor, and some had multiple tissue types within the tumor. For patients with speech arrest ($n = 4$) or language function ($n = 6$) tissues within the tumor, the tumor was resected to within 1 cm of the functional area. For patients with motor ($n = 20$) or sensory ($n = 6$) tissues within the tumor, the tumor was resected to within 5–10 mm of the functional area. Complete resection was performed in 3 patients, despite the presence of functional tissues within the tumor. Near-total resection (90% to 99% removal) was achieved in 9 patients, subtotal resection (50% to 90% removal) was achieved in 9 patients, and partial resection (less than 50% removal) was achieved in 5 patients. In 2 patients, the tumors were so full of functional tissue that no resection was performed. Most of the patients (19, or 68%) had new or worse neurologic functioning immediately after resection. However, by 3 months of follow-up, only 6 continued to have deficits, 19 had no deficits, and 2 showed improvement.

Conclusions.—Functional motor, language, and sensory tissues can be located within the tissue margins; thus, a complete resection of the tumor might well cause irreparable damage. Even partial glioma resection provided improvement of neurologic deficits in these patients after 3 months of follow-up. Thus, intraoperative brain mapping should be used to identify functional tissues within an infiltrative glioma, and the extent of the resection should be based on the functional tissues identified.

▶ Glial tumors are highly infiltrative. In contrast with brain metastases that produce well-defined tumor boundaries, gliomas spread through fiber pathways that funnel tumoral cells through normal tissue, thus producing "tongues" of tumor plunging into functional areas of the brain. This complex geometric pattern creates a surgical predicament: if radical resection is attempted, the ablation of functional tissue trapped within the tumor is possible; if, on the other hand, preservation of all functional tissue is tried, the risk of leaving residual tumor cells is also possible. In both circumstances, the therapeutic outcome is at stake. The study of Skirboll et al. shows that, by careful identification of functional tissue through stimulation mapping during surgery, a better result can be obtained in minimizing postoperative deficits. This is particularly important in patients with tumors located near motor or language areas. This study reminds us that the main problems for successful treatment of gliomas, especially malignant gliomas, lie in the transitional zone between the tumor and the normal tissue, where no clear-cut limits are easily found with existing technologies. The ideal approach would be one that has the potential for selective identification and destruction of malignant cells at the confines of the abnormal mass, while carefully avoiding functional tissue. It seems that the tools to aid surgery for complete removal of neoplastic cells will be provided by those at work in the fields of immunology and molecular biology, whose participation in the therapy of cancer is growing fast.

J. Sotelo, M.D.

Gamma Knife for Glioma: Selection Factors and Survival
Larson DA, Gutin PH, McDermott M, et al (Univ of California, San Francisco; Univ of Pittsburgh, Pa; Presbyterian Hosp, Dallas; et al)
Int J Radiat Oncol Biol Phys 36:1045–1053, 1996   19–7

Background.—For selected patients with malignant gliomas, a conformal interstitial brachytherapy boost can improve survival time. Such a conformal boost can be delivered noninvasively and on an outpatient basis using radiosurgery; this approach is often used as an alternative to brachytherapy or for patients ineligible for brachytherapy protocols. Selection factors may account for reported variations in survival time among patients with gliomas treated by radiosurgery. Factors associated with survival in patients undergoing radiosurgery for gliomas were analyzed.

Methods.—The study included 189 patients undergoing Gamma Knife radiosurgery for World Health Organization grade I–IV primary or recurrent gliomas. All information was obtained from a centralized computer database. Univariate and multivariate analyses were performed to identify factors associated with improved survival time.

Findings.—The patients received a median minimum tumor dose of 16 Gy for a median tumor volume of 5.9 cc. Sixty-five percent of patients met selection criteria for brachytherapy. Surviving patients were followed up for a median of 65 weeks after radiosurgery. Among patients with primary glioblastomas, the median survival time after pathologic diagnosis was 86 weeks for those meeting brachytherapy selection criteria and 40 weeks otherwise. Factors associated with an increased survival time on multivariate analysis were lower pathologic grade, younger age, increased Karnofsky performance status, smaller tumor volume, and presence of a unifocal tumor. Radiosurgery parameters such as dose, number of isocenters, prescription isodose percent, and inhomogeneity did not influence the survival time, nor did the extent of surgery before radiosurgery. A hazard ratio model, not including the technical details of radiosurgery, was constructed and applied to reported series of patients with gliomas treated by radiosurgery and brachytherapy. This model showed a significant correlation between survival and hazard ratio in the various series.

Conclusions.—In patients undergoing radiosurgery for gliomas, survival is strongly related to 5 patient selection variables: pathologic grade, age, Karnofsky performance status, tumor volume, and number of tumor foci. Differences in these variables explain much of the variation in survival times in previous series of patients with gliomas, whether treated by radiosurgery or brachytherapy. Future trials should incorporate these selection factors into the study design. The hazard ratio model does not include the technical details of treatment, which suggests that the treatment delivered may be more important than the modality by which it is delivered.

▶ The role of stereotactic radiosurgery in the management of gliomas is not known, despite numerous small studies. This paper is based on data from 8 Gamma Knife facilities and is an attempt to study a larger patient cohort; however, it still does not answer the question as to the real value of radiosurgery in patients with gliomas. Nonetheless, the importance of this study is that it does identify 5 factors that have a positive predictive value in terms of survival, and the authors have developed a hazard ratio model that seems independent of the technical details of radiosurgery; this model might help in quantifying survival expectations for patients being considered for radiosurgery.

The 5 factors possibly associated with improved survival time include pathologic grade, age, Karnofsky performance status, tumor volume, and a single tumor focus (rather than multiple tumors). The first 3 survival predictors are well known, and this study is useful in showing the possible influence of tumor size and unifocal tumors. However, some caution is necessary because the study involves multiple centers in different countries. The methodology used to classify the tumors as being primary, persistent, or recurrent is flawed. The authors acknowledge that no attempt was made to relate survival time to the use of chemotherapy. I also have concerns regarding the target for the radiotherapy, as the radiosurgery target volumes were determined from scans performed on the day of radiosurgery and this was performed within 16 weeks of the surgical procedure. Scans performed more than 2 days after surgery and before 12–16 weeks from the time of operation or radiotherapy cannot be relied on to differentiate residual or recurrent tumor tissue from changes associated with the operation or radiotherapy.

I agree with the authors' conclusion that the possibility that radiosurgery may increase survival times in some subgroups of patients with gliomas should be tested in prospective clinical trials.

A.H. Kaye, M.D.

Interstitial Chemotherapy With Carmustine-loaded Polymers for High-grade Gliomas: A Randomized Double-blind Study

Valtonen S, Timonen U, Toivanen P, et al (Turku Univ, Finland; Helsinki Univ; Tampere Univ, Finland; et al)
Neurosurgery 41:44–49, 1997   19–8

Background.—Biodegradable polymer combined with a biodegradable polymer wafer and implanted in the tumor resection cavity perioperatively is an easy, safe, and effective means of local application in patients with recurrent gliomas. The efficacy and safety of carmustine combined with a biodegradable polymer placed in the tumor resection cavity at the time of the first operation were determined in a placebo-controlled, double-blind study.

Methods.—Thirty-two patients with high-grade gliomas were enrolled in the study between March, 1992 and March, 1993. Sixteen patients were assigned randomly to receive active treatment, and 16 were assigned to receive placebo.

Findings.—The median time to death after surgery was 58.1 weeks among patients given active treatment and 39.9 weeks among those given placebo. For the 27 patients with grade IV tumors, these times were 53.3 weeks for those in the active treatment group and 39.9 weeks for those receiving placebo. By the end of the study, 6 patients were still alive, 5 of whom had received active treatment.

Conclusions.—The application of carmustine-loaded polymers at the time of surgery in patients with high-grade gliomas appears to positively affect the life span of these patients. Additional studies of larger numbers of patients are needed to fully determine the value of this treatment.

▶ Carmustine (bischloroethyl-nitrosourea [BCNU]) is a nucleic acid alkylating agent that, combined with surgical resection, significantly improves the survival time of patients with malignant gliomas compared with surgical resection alone.

Intra-arterial and IV delivery methods have been tried; however, intra-arterial administration of BCNU is not a safe treatment for malignant gliomas, and it is no more effective than IV administration.[1]

A slowly biodegradable polymer loaded with BCNU, in the form of a wafer, has been developed for implantation in the tumor resection cavity for patients undergoing surgery for malignant gliomas. This drug delivery system has been tested in patients with recurrent glioblastoma multiforme, and it has proved to be an easy, safe, and clinically effective method for local interstitial chemotherapy.

This prospective, randomized, placebo-controlled study was, unfortunately, terminated prematurely for economic reasons and not for scientific or ethical reasons. Despite the relatively low number of patients enrolled, the numbers were sufficient, by statistical power analysis, to demonstrate a significant improvement in the median survival time among the treatment group as compared with the randomized control group. However, the confidence intervals for the median survival estimates were wide, and the number of patients enrolled was relatively small. Consequently, as the authors stated, a larger study is needed to confirm these encouraging early findings. In addition, a larger is needed so that the results can be compared with the results of IV BCNU therapy. This biodegradable polymer, loaded for time-release delivery of interstitial chemotherapy, looks promising as a way to achieve high-target dosage.

S.R. Gibbs, M.A., M.D.

Reference

1. Shapiro WR, Green SB, Burger PC, et al: A randomized comparison of intra-arterial versus intravenous BCNU, with or without intravenous 5-fluorouracil, for newly diagnosed patients with malignant glioma. *J Neurosurg* 76:772–781, 1992.

Radiosurgical Treatment

Stereotactic Radiosurgery for the Treatment of Brain Metastases: Results of a Single Institution Series
Breneman JC, Warnick RE, Albright RE Jr, et al (Univ of Cincinnati, Ohio; Chiang Mai Univ, Thailand)
Cancer 79:551–557, 1997

19–9

Background.—Increasing numbers of patients with metastatic neoplasms to the brain are being treated with stereotactic radiosurgery. There are many unanswered questions about this treatment, including the optimal patient selection and treatment factors. A review of an experience with radiosurgery for the treatment of brain metastases identified factors useful for patient selection and treatment.

Methods.—The experience included 84 patients with brain metastases treated with stereotactic radiosurgery during a 6-year period. The patients were 58 women and 26 men (median age 55 years). The survival analysis included a total of 177 lesions, and 1–6 lesions occurred per patient. The median minimum tumor dose was 1,600 cGy, decided mainly on the basis of lesion size. Forty-five percent of patients had active extracranial disease when radiosurgery was performed. The patients were followed up with MRI scans every 3 months.

Results.—The overall median survival time was 43 weeks after radiosurgery and 71 weeks after the original diagnosis of brain metastases. The survival time was 44 weeks for patients with 1 or 2 metastases, compared with 35 weeks for those with 3 or more lesions. The survival time was also longer for patients without extracranial disease: 45 vs. 35 weeks. Local control analysis was possible in 73 patients with 145 lesions. The median time to failure in these lesions was 35 weeks. The time to failure was 52 weeks in patients receiving a radiation dose of 1,800 cGy or greater vs. 25 weeks in those receiving a lower dose. There were no local failures among 12 melanomas treated.

Conclusions.—In the authors' experience, the results of stereotactic radiosurgery for brain metastases are comparable to those of surgical resection and are better than those of whole-brain radiotherapy. Stereotactic radiosurgery appears to be a safe and effective technique for extending the survival time of patients with recurrent brain metastases. The best results are achieved for patients with 1 or 2 lesions and without active extracranial disease; however, patients who do not meet these criteria may benefit as well.

▶ This is 1 more study demonstrating that radiosurgery is a very safe and effective method with a high rate of local control capable of extending the survival time in selected patients with no more than 2 cerebral metastases and no active extracranial disease. The problem of what is indicated for patients with more than 2 cerebral lesions and/or active extracranial disease is real, and the authors gave clear arguments for this discussion.

Unfortunately, 2 major questions are not addressed: (1) is there a major benefit in terms of the quality of life for the patient? and (2) what is the role of radiotherapy before, combined with, or after radiosurgery?

The effectiveness of conventional radiotherapy alone is well known to be very poor (survival time, 18 weeks), which is why 93% of these patients, who were good candidates for radiosurgery, had previous whole-brain radiotherapy here. Whole-brain radiotherapy is suspected of deteriorating the "quality" of survival. Its efficiency in preventing the development of new cerebral lesions is low and has been demonstrated only for lung cancer. Does it make sense for the patient to suffer through whole-brain radiotherapy for a single melanoma or site of cerebral metastases, a condition that is histologically very well known to be highly radioresistant? Is it not important now to evaluate the role of radiosurgery and how we must modify our general management of cerebral metastases in the field of neurosurgery so that this new method can be integrated?

J. Regis, M.D.

Pineal Region Tumors and the Role of Stereotactic Biopsy: Review of the Mortality, Morbidity, and Diagnostic Rates in 370 Cases

Regis J, Bouillot P, Rouby-Volot F, et al (Universitaire la Timone, Marseille, France)
Neurosurgery 39:907–917, 1996

19–10

Purpose.—Patients undergoing stereotactic biopsies of tumors in the pineal region are generally believed to experience greater morbidity and mortality than those with tumors in other regions. However, there are insufficient data to support this impression. A national survey examined the mortality, morbidity, and diagnostic yield of pineal tumor biopsies.

Methods.—The analysis included data on 370 stereotactic biopsies of tumors of the pineal region performed at 15 French neurosurgical centers. The tumors represented about 5% of stereotactic biopsies performed during a 17-year period. Morbidity and mortality directly attributable to the biopsy procedure were assessed, along with the diagnostic yield of the biopsies.

Results.—The data showed no difference between the various centers in terms of morbidity, mortality, and diagnostic yield. This finding was in contrast to the heterogeneous results seen for large stereotactic biopsy series reported in the literature. The mortality of pineal tumor biopsies was 1.3%, and postoperative CT scans showed hematomas in each case. The rate of severe neurologic complications (i.e., long-term coma and akinetic mutism) was 0.8%. Slight, transient neurologic complications developed in 7% of patients. There was 1 case of a tumor seeding along the biopsy trajectory. The pineal tumor biopsy procedure had a diagnostic yield of 94%. No diagnoses were made in 5% of cases, and the initial histologic diagnoses appeared incorrect in 1%. In 93.5% of cases, the biopsy results affected the management strategy. Morbidity was unrelated to the probe trajectory, which was most often orthogonal lateral or oblique anterolateral.

Conclusions.—The morbidity, mortality, and diagnostic yield of stereotactic tumor biopsies in the pineal region do not appear significantly different from those in other regions. Stereotactic biopsy of pineal region tumors is a safe and effective way to achieve a histologic diagnosis and make treatment decisions. Prospective studies are needed to clarify the factors associated with complications of pineal tumor biopsies, and to detail the technical issues associated with the biopsy procedure.

▶ This article comprising an aggregate 17-year experience of 15 French centers shows that the mortality, morbidity, and diagnostic rates for stereotactic biopsies of pineal region tumors are not different from those for stereotactic biopsies of tumors in other regions. However, more than 60% of tumors in the pineal region consist of germ-cell tumors, and more than one third of the latter are so-called mixed germ-cell tumors composed of 2 or more neoplastic elements.[1] Therefore, small specimems taken by biopsy may not tell us the true nature of the tumor. From findings on MRI and tumor marker examinations, besides the age and sex of the patients (in the pineal region, germ-cell tumors are rare in females), one can guess the nature of the tumors to a considerable degree. In my opinion, stereotactic biopsy of pineal region tumors is useful in cases with suspected germinomas or gliomas because, in these cases, radiotherapy or chemotherapy, or both, will be the main therapeutic modalities. For cases with other kinds of tumors suspected, open microsurgery followed by chemotherapy or radiotherapy should be indicated.

K. Sano, M.D., D.M.Sc., F.A.C.S. (hon)

Reference

1. Matsutani M, Sano K, Takakura K, et al: Primary intracranial germ-cell tumors: A clinical analysis of 153 histologically verified cases. *J Neurosurg* 86:446–455, 1997.

Miscellaneous Tumors

Manganese Superoxide Dismutase Expression in Human Central Nervous System Tumors
Cobbs CS, Levi DS, Aldape K, et al (Univ of California, San Francisco)
Cancer Res 56:3192–3195, 1996   19–11

Background.—The generation of hydroxyl- and superoxide-free radicals is one mechanism by which ionizing radiation is believed to kill tumor cells. Superoxide production is critical in the cytocidal pathways of tumor necrosis factor (TNF) α, ionizing radiation, and some chemotherapeutic agents in the treatment of brain tumors and other cancers. Manganese superoxide dismutase (MnSOD), a mitochondrial enzyme, catalyzes the conversion of superoxide to oxygen and hydrogen peroxide. Increased mitochondrial MnSOD expression has been shown to play a central role in protecting various cell types, including tumor cells, from the lethal effects of interleukin-1 and TNF, cell-mediated immune responses, certain anticancer drugs, and ionizing radiation. Hypothesizing that MnSOD may be expressed by glial tumors, the authors determined whether MnSOD was produced in human brain tumors.

Methods and Findings.—Forty-two specimens of human brain tumors and tissue from 3 normal brains were analyzed by immunohistochemical staining with a polyclonal antibody recognizing human MnSOD. In addition, MnSOD was measured by enzyme-linked immunosorbent assay (ELISA) in CSF from 14 patients with brain tumors and 7 control patients. Malignant CNS tumors, including those metastatic to the brain, showed marked immunoreactivity to MnSOD intracellularity, in the extracellular matrix, and in the tumor endothelial cells. By contrast, MnSOD was not readily detected in normal brain. Grade IV astrocytomas, grade III astrocytomas, and medulloblastomas were strongly immunoreactive. Grade II astrocytomas had far less immunoreactivity. In patients with malignant tumors, ELISA analysis of CSF samples also showed high levels of MnSOD protein—up to 45-fold greater than the level of control CSF samples.

Conclusion.—In brain tumors expressing MnSOD in vivo, this enzyme may work to evade host antitumor immune mechanisms and resist such conventional treatments as radiotherapy and chemotherapy. Modulating MnSOD induction or expression may enhance the efficacy of available treatments.

▶ This nice short study demonstrates that a variety of brain tumors, including gliomas, and especially malignant gliomas, express MnSOD. The enzyme can also be identified in the CSF of patients with malignant gliomas. The authors hypothesize that this enzyme may help the tumor cells to escape the immune response and resist the effect of radiotherapy and chemotherapy. This adds to a list of well-known factors helping glioma cells to evade immune attack, including tumor growth factor-2, prostaglandin E_2, interleukin-10, and Fas-Ligand. It, thus, becomes increasingly clear that immunotherapy for the treatment of malignant gliomas can be considered only in terms of combining a stimulation of the immune response with a suppression of the inhibiting factors. The identification of this enzyme in the biopsy specimens and in the CSF of the patients, especially those with glioblastomas, might also help in deciding whether radiotherapy and chemotherapy should be given. Indeed, certain patients show a recurrence during the treatment and receive no benefit from it. It should, however, be noted that benign tumors like schwannomas, juvenile pylocytic astrocytomas, and capillary hemangioblastomas also showed a high expression of the enzyme. This shows that this is not a feature specific to malignant tumors, and that one should be very careful about using it as a tumor marker.

N. de Tribolet, M.D.

Variations in the Natural History and Survival of Patients With Supratentorial Low-grade Astrocytomas

Piepmeier J, Christopher S, Spencer D, et al (Yale Univ, New Haven, Conn)
Neurosurgery 38:872–879, 1996   19–12

Background.—Because of its unpredictable behavior and the lack of a clearly defined treatment, the prognosis of low-grade astrocytoma is highly variable. Treatment for patients with low-grade astrocytoma should seek to prevent or delay evolution to a more anaplastic tumor. The authors have been collecting data on patients with low-grade astrocytoma since 1982. The outcomes of patients treated for low-grade astrocytoma between 1982 and 1990 were reported.

Methods.—The database included 55 consecutive patients with low-grade supratentorial astrocytoma. All had at least 5 years' follow-up to allow time for evaluating the outcomes of treatment. At a median follow-up of 8 years, the end points assessed included time to recurrence, incidence of anaplastic transformation, and survival.

Results.—Outcomes were unaffected by sex, type of symptoms, presence of contrast enhancement, or timing of radiation therapy. Time to recurrence and survival were significantly increased for patients who had symptoms longer than 2 years and had gross total resection of their tumor, with age considered as a continuous variable. The prognosis was best for patients with chronic epilepsy—none of 27 patients with this diagnosis died or had a tumor recurrence. This was so, regardless of the extent of surgery and the use of radiotherapy. Thirty-one patients with gross total resection had a 10-year survival of 100%, independent of the duration of preoperative symptoms. Giving radiotherapy before surgery rather than later on did not increase time to recurrence, reduce the chances of transition to a more malignant tumor at recurrence, or increase survival. Ninety-two percent of the deaths in this series were caused by high-grade recurrence.

Conclusions.—The outcomes of treatment for low-grade astrocytoma are reviewed. These tumors have a highly variable natural history, which strongly affects survival. Recurrence risk and survival are improved for patients with aggressive surgery, compared with patients with less-than-total resection. Patients who have chronic epilepsy and low-grade astrocytoma have a better prognosis, with a much lower chance that the tumor will become more malignant over time.

▶ This is a useful study correlating a number of clinical and surgical parameters with the prognosis of patients with supratentorial low-grade astrocytomas. Although it suffers from many of the inherent limitations of a retrospective analysis, the study has been undertaken carefully and in an expert fashion. The authors acknowledge the selection bias associated with which patients are selected for tumor resection and, in addition, there remains the problem of stereotactic tissue sampling not being a true representation of the whole tumor. The study has again shown the obvious favorable effect of age on the outcome of patients with low-grade gliomas as previously reported, and it has seemingly confirmed the importance of an aggressive tumor resection for patient survival. However, it would have been helpful if the authors had given more information on the timing of postoperative radiologic investigations in their assessment of the extent of tumor resection, and a more quantitative approach to the description of tumor resection would have been useful.

It is well known that a long preoperative history of seizures (or other symptoms) is associated with prolonged survival, and this is confirmed in this study. The finding that contrast enhancement in the tumor was not a significant feature in patient prognosis is particularly intriguing; almost all other studies have shown this radiologic finding to be important, because it usually signifies at least some degree of higher tumor grade within the tumor.

This study also confirms previous reports that radiation therapy is unlikely to be of benefit for patients with low-grade astrocytomas, and it is my practice to save this treatment until there is evidence of tumor progression.

A.H. Kaye, M.D.

Prognostic Factors and Treatment Results for Supratentorial Primitive Neuroectodermal Tumors in Children Using Radiation and Chemotherapy: A Childrens Cancer Group Randomized Trial

Cohen BH, Zeltzer PM, Boyett JM, et al (Cleveland Clinic Found, Ohio; Rainbow Babies and Children's Hosp, Cleveland; Univ of California Irvine, Orange, Calif)
J Clin Oncol 13:1687–1696, 1995

19–13

Introduction.—Supratentorial primitive neuroectodermal tumors (S-PNETs) are histologically identical to medulloblastoma and account for about 2.5% of brain tumors in children. Because S-PNETs are rare, there are few data about their response to treatment. The Childrens Cancer Group started a randomized trial of treatment for high-stage medulloblastomas and other PNETs in 1986. The clinical characteristics and response to treatment in children with S-PNETs were studied.

Methods.—Fifty-five children aged 1.5 to 19 years underwent surgery and staging for S-PNET. In 17 patients, the pineal region was the primary tumor site. The patients were then randomizly assigned to 1 of 2 groups. One group received standard treatment with craniospinal radiotherapy, followed by 8 cycles of chemotherapy with 1-(2-chloro-ethyl)-3-cyclohexyl-nitrosurea, vincristine, and prednisone. The other group received 2 cycles of 8-in-1 chemotherapy, followed by radiotherapy, then 8 more cycles of 8-in-1 chemotherapy.

Results.—As estimated by the Kaplan-Meier method, the 3-year survival was 57% and the 3-year progression free survival was 45%. For patients with PNETs located in the pineal region, survival was 73% and progression free survival, 61%. Toxicity was greater for patients receiving 8-in-1 chemotherapy than for those receiving standard treatment. There was no significant difference in the distribution of progression free survival. Progression free survival was 50% for patients with M_0 metastases vs. 0% for those with M_{1-4} metastases. By age, progression free survival was 25% for patients aged 2 years or younger vs. 13% for those aged 3 years or older.

Conclusions.—This randomized trial of treatment for pediatric S-PNET finds no significant difference in outcome with standard treatment vs. 8-in-1 chemotherapy. Factors independently associated with a better outcome are absence of metastases and a pineal site of involvement. The survival results in this series are better than in previous reports.

▶ The importance of this study is that it is the first prospective randomized therapy trial for patients with S-PNET, and it will provide a useful comparison for future studies. The study failed to show any significant difference in survival or time to progression between the 2 treatment arms, and the only independent predictor of outcome was the M stage and site, with the pineal site of involvement being more favorable.

The authors acknowledge that there is insufficient evidence to confirm that adjuvant chemotherapy prolongs survival in S-PNET, and there was more toxicity in those children treated with the 8-in-1 chemotherapy protocol. This study failed to show a statistically significant difference in outcome in patients with total tumor resection, but the authors acknowledge that the study had limited power to detect a difference with progression free survival as the outcome measure.

A.H. Kaye, M.D.

Functional Anatomic Relationship Between Brain Stem Tumors and Cranial Motor Nuclei
Morota N, Deletis V, Lee M, et al (New York Univ)
Neurosurgery 39:787–794, 1996   19–14

Background.—Magnetic resonance imaging can demonstrate the anatomical location of brain stem tumors, but it cannot show the functional anatomy or the tumor's relationship to underlying functional pathways and cranial nuclei. Cranial motor nuclei (CMN) are at risk for injury via the initial incision of the floor of the fourth ventricle. Brain stem mapping has recently been used to locate and avoid damage to the CMN. This study mapped motor nuclei on the floor of the fourth ventricle to gain insight into patterns of CMN displacement in patients with intramedullary brain stem tumors.

Methods.—Twenty patients participated in the study, including 18 with brain stem tumors—7 pontine, 9 medullary, and 2 pontomedullary tumors—and 2 with spinal cord tumors located in the cervicomedullary junction. Each patient underwent neurophysiologic mapping of CMN VII, IX/X, and XII. In the mapping procedure, a handheld probe was used to apply electric stimuli over the exposed fourth ventricular floor during surgery. Electric activity in the corresponding cranial muscles was then recorded. Patterns of CMN displacement were assessed.

Results.—The tumor site determined the pattern of CMN distortion. The type 1 pattern consisted of CMN located around the tumor on the floor of the fourth ventricle, the type 2 pattern consisted of 1 or more CMN located ventrally to the tumor, and the type 3 pattern consisted of CMN in their original anatomical position. For 6 of 7 patients with pontine tumors, the type 1 pattern was apparent. Medullary tumors were associated with the type 2 pattern in 7 of 9 cases and with the type 1 pattern in 2 cases. The type 2 pattern was found in both patients with pontomedullary tumors. The pattern of CMN distortion in patients with cervicomedullary junction tumors depended on the tumor extension into the fourth ventricle: type 1 in 1 patient and type 2 in the other.

Conclusions.—Neurophysiologic studies of the motor nuclei in patients with intramedullary brain stem tumors suggest that pontine tumors push the CMN to the area around the tumor edge. Thus, the CMN must be precisely localized to avoid damaging them during surgery. With medullary tumors, growth can occur more exophytically, which can compress the CMN in a ventral direction. Surgeons should understand the specific patterns of CMN distortion associated with brain stem tumors in different locations to facilitate surgical planning and to minimize risks.

Radiosurgery for Hemangioblastoma: Results of a Multiinstitutional Experience

Patrice SJ, Sneed PK, Flickinger JC, et al (Univ of California, San Francisco; Univ of Pittsburgh, Pa)
Int J Radiat Oncol Biol Phys 35:493–499, 1996   19–15

Background.—Hemangioblastoma, a benign vascular tumor, may invade critical neurologic structures, which may preclude gross total resection. After subtotal resection, recurrence is common and can be neurologically devastating. Thus, the use of radiotherapy for unresectable or subtotally resected disease has been advocated. A multicenter experience with radiosurgery for hemangioblastoma was reported.

Methods.—Thirty-eight hemangiomas were treated with stereotactic radiosurgery (SR) at 3 centers between 1988 and 1994. A ^{201}cobalt source unit or a dedicated SR linear accelerator was used. Of the 18 primary tumors treated, 16 had not been previously operated on, and 2 had been subtotally resected. Twenty lesions were treated with SR after prior surgical failure or failure after previous surgery and conventional radiotherapy. Eight patients underwent SR for multifocal disease. The volume of SR-treated tumors ranged from 0.05 to 12 cc. Minimum tumor doses were 12–20 Gy. The median follow-up after SR was 24.5 months.

Findings.—Actuarial survival at 2 years was 88%, and freedom from progression at 2 years was 86%. The median tumor volume of lesions uncontrolled by SR was 7.85 cc, compared with 0.67 cc for those responding to SR. Lesions uncontrolled by SR received a median minimum tumor dose of 14 Gy, compared with 16 Gy for controlled lesions. Seventy-eight percent of the survivors remained stable neurologically or improved clinically. No significant permanent complications could be attributed directly to SR treatment.

Conclusions.—This is the largest reported experience of SR use in the treatment of hemangioblastomas. Radiosurgery appears to control most primary and recurrent hemangioblastomas and enables the treatment of multiple lesions in a single treatment session, which is especially important for patients with von Hippel-Lindau disease. Better control rates appear to be associated with higher doses and smaller tumor volumes.

▶ Even if microsurgical resection is the gold standard, it seems logical to evaluate the capability of radiosurgery to control hemangioblastomas. These tumors are benign slowly progessive lesions. From previous experiences with radiotherapy has emerged the evidence that more aggressive time–dose fractionation is required. In addition, the existence of recurrence after microsurgical resection and the existence of a multifocal form (von Hippel-Lindau disease) have motivated the search for alternative therapeutic methods. In this study, an interesting contribution to the body of knowledge on this subject is that better control rates appear to be associated with higher doses and smaller tumor volumes.

From the methodological point of view, the cases reported are very heterogeneous. Sometimes the cystic portion is treated, and sometimes it is not. Maximal doses ranged from 16.25 to 45 Gy, and the marginal isodose ranged from 40% to 90%. The second major problem with this paper is the very short follow-up period (only 12 of 22 patients had a follow-up of 24 months or longer). The very long natural history of these tumors requires that a longer observation period (10–20 years) take place before accurate conclusions on efficiency can be reached.

However, this work reports the largest experience with radiosurgery for treatment of hemangioblastomas and will be of very great practical help in the proper selection and treatment of patients.

J. Regis, M.D.

20 Carotid Occlusive Vascular Disease

Post-operative Care and Early Discharge Issues

Feasibility and Safety of 1-day Postoperative Hospitalization for Carotid Endarterectomy

Kaufman JL, Frank D, Rhee SW, et al (Baystate Med Ctr, Springfield, Mass)
Arch Surg 131:751–755, 1996   20–1

Background.—As health care cost containment continues to be a worrisome issue, physicians are searching for ways to minimize health care costs without settling for inadequate patient care. At one time, these authors hospitalized patients for 3–5 days after carotid endarterectomy, including 1 postoperative day in the ICU. Now their goal is a 1-day postoperative stay. This report shows how they have achieved this goal in a large proportion of patients, the safety of this protocol, and the associated morbidity.

Methods.—Over 21 months, 163 carotid endarterectomies were performed in 152 patients on either an elective ($n = 124$) or an emergent ($n = 39$) basis. Those undergoing concurrent coronary revascularization were excluded from the study. Patients undergoing elective surgery were admitted to the hospital at 6 AM on the day of the procedure. Patients undergoing emergency surgery were operated on within 48 hours of hospital admission. After surgery, patients remained in a recovery area for 2–6 hours until hemodynamics stabilized; then they were returned to surgical floors. Patients with persistent postoperative hypertension or hypotension or cardiac dysrhythmias, or who required invasive monitoring, stayed in an ICU until stable, then they, too, were moved to a surgical floor.

Findings.—Surgical indications were strokes ($n = 14$, or 9%), transient ischemic attacks ($n = 50$, or 30%), amaurosis fugax ($n = 36$, or 22%), and stenosis ($n = 63$, or 39%). General anesthesia was used in all but 4 procedures. For the patients who did ($n = 60$, or 37%) and did not ($n = 103$, or 63%) go to the ICU, the operative times averaged 2.5 and 2.6 hours and the recovery times averaged 3.9 and 4.3 hours, respectively. The mean hospital stay was 3.8 days; 82 procedures (50%) required only 1 day of postoperative hospitalization, 49 (30%) required 2 days, 12 (7%) required 3 days, and 20 (12%) required more than 3 days. Complications occurred in 21 procedures, including 3 deaths (1 stroke, 1 vein patch blowout, 1 myocardial infarction), 5 nonlethal strokes, 4 cervical hematomas, 4 cases of congestive heart failure or cardiac dysrhythmia, 2 cases of hypoglossal nerve weakness, 1 case of worsened renal failure, and 2 infections at the vein patch donor site. Readmission within 30 days occurred for only 14 procedures (8.6%), and none of the readmissions was related to a factor that could have been avoided with ICU entry or to discharge on the first or second postoperative day.

Conclusions.—Up to 80% of patients undergoing carotid endarterectomy can be safely discharged within 1–2 days after the procedure. Furthermore, postoperative admission to an ICU was unnecessary in the majority (63%) of procedures. Readmissions are not common and are not associated with either the ICU protocol or the quickness of discharge. Thus, a shortened hospital stay after carotid endarterectomy will reduce costs without compromising patient care.

▶ This retrospective analysis chronicles the evolution of hospitalization policies for patients undergoing carotid endarterectomy at a single institution. Although the authors demonstrated the feasibility of this approach (by reducing the length of stay and ICU use), they did not demonstrate safety, as there was no comparison group. Although it is feasible to discharge patients shortly after carotid endarterectomy, additional research will be required to demonstrate the safety, cost-effectiveness, and specific parameters that determine postoperative risk.

M.R. Mayberg, M.D.

Safety and Cost-efficiency of 24-hour Hospitalization for Carotid Endarterectomy
Musser DJ, Calligaro KD, Dougherty MJ, et al (Thomas Jefferson Med College, Philadelphia)
Ann Vasc Surg 10:143–146, 1996   20–2

Background.—One of the ways to reduce health care costs is to reduce the hospitalization time—if, indeed, this can be done without detracting from patient care. An approach to carotid endarterectomy was evaluated that involved same-day admission and discharge the next day, to see whether quick discharge after carotid endarterectomy would still provide adequate patient care.

Methods.—Two groups of patients were compared. In group 1, 40 procedures were performed in 38 patients (mean age, 69 years) according to the standards used between fall 1992 and fall 1993 (i.e., patients stayed in the hospital at least overnight before the procedure, there was no dedicated vascular ward, and workups were performed on an inpatient basis). In group 2, 68 procedures were performed in 64 patients (mean age, 68 years) according to a new standard developed by critical pathway analysis (i.e., patients were admitted on the day of surgery, a dedicated vascular ward was created, and workups were performed on an outpatient basis). Patients undergoing emergency surgery or concurrent coronary artery bypass grafting, and those who required preoperative anticoagulation, were excluded from the study. Indications for surgery were similar in groups 1 and 2; 42% of group 1 patients and 43% of group 2 patients had asymptomatic high-grade stenosis, and 58% of group 1 patients to 57% of group 2 patients had symptomatic stenosis. Most carotid endarterectomies were performed with the patient under general anesthesia. Follow-up averaged 12 months (range, 2–34 months).

Findings.—Mortality rates did not differ significantly between the 2 groups (1 death in each group), nor did group 1 and group 2 differ in the frequency of cardiac events (2.9% vs. 2.5%), neurologic events (2.9% vs. 2.5%), or hospital readmission rates (1.5% vs. 0%). However, the critical analysis protocol instituted for group 2 resulted in significantly more same-day hospital admissions (5% for group 1 vs. 94% for group 2) and significantly fewer postoperative days in the hospital (5.1 days for group 1 vs. 1.3 days for group 2). These changes led to a savings of approximately $5,500 per patient in group 2.

Conclusions.—A shortened hospital stay did not detract from patient care and safety after carotid endarterectomy. It did, however, detract from the hospital bill, by an average of $5,500 per patient, or an estimated $50 million per year in the United States. Keys to the success of this approach were performance of the workup on an outpatient basis, same-day hospital admission, and early discharge through a protocol developed by critical pathway analysis and administered via a dedicated vascular ward.

▶ These authors prospectively analyzed mortality, cardiac events , strokes, readmissions, and hospital charges in carotid endarterectomy after institution of critical pathways in comparison with historical data from the prior year. In a small cohort (68 patients in the year before the change and 40 patients in the year after, they showed no difference in complications despite marked reductions in the length of stay and hospital charges. This study suffers from a type II statistical error, that is, there are not enough patients to demonstrate a true difference for outcomes with very low frequencies. It probably is reasonable to send patients home the day after carotid endarterectomy or, perhaps, the same day. However, an analysis of cost effectiveness must weigh the cost of any additional strokes as a result of this approach against the cumulative per-case savings.

M.R. Mayberg, M.D.

Criteria for Selective Utilization of the Intensive Care Unit Following Carotid Endarterectomy
Rigdon EE, Monajjem N, Rhodes RS (Univ of Mississippi, Jackson)
Ann Vasc Surg 11:20–27, 1997   20–3

Background.—Patients undergoing carotid endarterectomy (CEA) are routinely admitted to the ICU for fear of adverse postoperative events.

Some authors have questioned the value of this practice and have proposed criteria for selective admission of high-risk patients. Adverse outcomes after CEA and associated risk factors were identified in a review to develop restrictive criteria for postoperative nursing unit admission.

Methods.—The review included 365 CEAs performed over a 15-year period. The records were analyzed to identify adverse events occurring during the first 24 hours after surgery that could have been prevented or better managed if the patient had been in the ICU, such as strokes, cardiac events, reoperation for hemorrhages, and the need for intensive pulmonary care. Preoperative variables that could potentially predict these adverse events were analyzed as well. The effects of selective ICU admission on patient outcomes were then assessed.

Results.—A total of 46 events best managed in the ICU developed in 38 patients in the first 24 hours after CEA. Factors associated with an increased risk of such complications included cardiac disease within the previous 6 months, emergency CEA, and the need for postoperative anticoagulation therapy. Based on indications, 69% of patients would have been admitted to a standard nursing unit, 16% would have been admitted to a nursing unit with ECG monitoring, and 15% would have been admitted to the ICU. The rate of adverse events in patients who would have been discharged to the standard nursing unit was 1.6%, and all these events could have been managed without ICU transfer.

Conclusions.—The findings suggest some criteria to select patients for ICU admission after CEA. Patients who are undergoing emergency CEA, who require postoperative anticoagulation therapy, or who have intraoperative strokes or major cardiac complications should be admitted to the ICU. Intensive care unit admission may also be considered for patients with chronic renal failure. Otherwise, all patients can be taken to the recovery room. Patients who have strokes, major cardiac events, significant bleeding, or reintubation, and those who require vasoactive medication beyond 3 hours after surgery should be taken to the ICU. Transfer to a unit with ECG monitoring is indicated for patients who have had cardiac disease within 6 months before CEA, but who lack indications for ICU admission. All other patients may safely be observed in a standard nursing unit.

▶ Close postoperative monitoring of patients who have undergone CEA has traditionally been emphasized; however, this precept was based, in part, on retrospective and anecdotal experiences. There are 3 salient points relating to this article. First, it probably is possible to identify risk factors that would enable stratification of patients for ICU monitoring after CEA. Second, this retrospective analysis does not delineate those factors because most of the patients were monitored in the ICU and may have had complications averted by indeterminate interventions. Third, because of the immense direct and indirect societal cost for even a single stroke, it is not clear whether reduction of ICU use for CEA would really be cost-effective.

M.R. Mayberg, M.D.

Surgical Technique

Carotid Endarterectomy With Homologous Vein Patch Angioplasty: A Review of 1006 Cases

Plestis KA, Kantis G, Haygood K, et al (Baylor College of Medicine, Houston)
J Vasc Surg 24:109–119, 1996   20–4

Introduction.—The use of an autologous saphenous vein for a patch in the reconstruction of the carotid bifurcation after carotid endarterectomy can cause problems. The risk of infection is of particular concern in patients with peripheral vascular disease. Its use could render the remaining vein unacceptable for later vascular or cardiac reconstruction. The use of a homologous vein as a patch was evaluated in 837 patients who underwent 1,006 carotid endarterectomies.

Methods.—Good-quality excess veins were harvested during coronary artery bypass surgery. They were either refrigerated in saline solution or cryopreserved in a 10% solution of dimethyl sulfoxide. Vein donors were tested for transmissible infections. Harvested veins were cultured for common pathogens.

Results.—Eight patients (0.8%) died in the perioperative period. Two patients (0.2%) died of ipsilateral strokes. Of the 12 patients (1.2%) with ischemic strokes, 10 were ipsilateral. Three patients (0.3%) had transient ischemic attacks. Data were available for 482 patients (56%) at a mean follow-up of 61 months. Of 8 patients (1.7%) with ipsilateral recurrent symptoms, 7 experienced strokes and 1 had a transient ischemic attack. Of 63 late deaths (13%), 25 were attributed to complications from coronary artery disease. The ten-year overall survival rate was 76%. The 10-year overall rate of freedom from late ipsilateral morbidity was 96%. Of 220 arteries evaluated by duplex scanning, the 10-year rate of freedom from late stenosis (defined as a reduction in diameter of 20% or more) was 84%.

Conclusion.—Postoperative mortality and neurologic morbidity rates for patients who underwent carotid endarterectomy with homologous vein patch angioplasty did not differ from those of patients who underwent all other types of closure. The homologous vein may be considered to be an acceptable patch for reconstruction of the bifurcation after carotid endarterectomy.

▶ Controversy exists about whether patch angioplasty provides a benefit in carotid endarterectomy. In addition, among advocates of patch angioplasty, there is disagreement regarding the optimal patch material (synthetic material vs. autologous vein vs. homologous vein). These controversies are unresolved because no prospective comparisons among techniques have been performed. Thus, this retrospective analysis of more than 1,000 homologous vein grafts does not offer any useful data for comparison of this technique to others. The immediate and long-term complications from the use of homologous vein patches in this group seem comparable with those reported from the use of autologous veins or polyethylene terephthalate (Dacron) patches, or from not performing an angioplasty. The major advantage for homologous patch use is the avoidance of a second incision for the vein graft. The disadvantages include the potential for disease transmission, an immune reaction, or indeterminate late histopathologic changes (only 6 postmortem specimens were studied in this paper). In summary, this article shows that homologous vein grafting for carotid endarterectomy is feasible. However, I suspect that most surgeons will continue to use that technique with which they are most accustomed.

M.R. Mayberg, M.D.

Complications Resulting From Saphenous Vein Patch Graft After Carotid Endarterectomy

Yamamoto Y, Piepgras DG, Marsh WR, et al (Mayo Clinic and Mayo Found, Rochester, Minn)
Neurosurgery 39:670–676, 1996

20–5

Background.—The benefit of routine saphenous vein patch graft (SVPG) use in carotid endarterectomy (CEA) is still being debated. Although this graft may decrease early postoperative thrombosis and cerebral infarcts, as well as late stenosis, the risks and complications associated with it have not been established.

Methods.—Data were obtained from 2,888 CEAs performed with SVPG for primary carotid stenosis at the Mayo Clinic between 1972 and 1994. Postoperative complications associated with SVPG were analyzed.

Findings.—Vein ruptures occurred postoperatively in 5 patients, aneurysm formation occurred in 4, and deep infection necessitating operative intervention occurred in 3. Vein patch ruptures occurred in 4 women and 1 man (mean age, 69 years). All ruptures happened within 4 days of the primary surgery. Emergent surgery performed in these patients with ruptures demonstrated intact suture lines and tears in the middle of the grafts. Two patients recovered with no deficits, 1 patient was left with major disability, and 2 patients died. Patch aneurysms developed in 2 women and 2 men, (mean age, 71 years). In all patients, painless pulsatile neck masses developed 1–9 years after the initial surgery. Two patients also had recurrent ischemic symptoms. Surgical correction was performed without complication in all patients with aneurysms.

Conclusions.—The current data show that the use of SVPG adds a small but definite risk of serious complications associated with the inherent weakness of the venous tissue. Surgeons deciding to use a patch graft should use a synthetic material instead of veins.

▶ Dr. Sundt[1] was 1 of many proponents for autologous saphenous vein grafting for CEA and demonstrated an apparent benefit from this technique by retrospective analysis of his own results.[1] The article by Yamamoto et al. extends these observations by retrospective analysis of a larger series of

CEAs done at Mayo Clinic. Among nearly 3,000 cases in which this technique was used, the authors identified 12 early complications and 4 late complications that they attributed to the vein patch grafts. Although extremely infrequent, vein patch complications such as an acute rupture or aneurysm formation may have devastating consequences. There are no data to support or refute the benefit of patch angioplasty after CEA, regardless of the patch material. The convenience and apparent safety and efficacy of collagen-impregnated polyethylene terephthalate (Dacron) patch material has prompted many surgeons to stop using vein patches. It is unlikely that the controversy regarding the optimal closure for CEA will be resolved.

M.R. Mayberg, M.D.

Reference

1. Sundt TM Jr, Meyer FB, Peipgras DG, et al: Prevention and management of postoperative complications, in Meyer FB (ed): *Sundt's Occlusive Cerebrovascular Disease*, ed 2. Philadelphia, WB Saunders, 1994, pp 248–263.

Papers Presented at the Twenty-First Annual Meeting of the Peripheral Vascular Surgery Society: A Comparison of Angioplasty With Stenting Versus Endarterectomy for the Treatment of Carotid Artery Stenosis
Jordan WD Jr, Schroeder PT, Fisher WS, et al (Univ of Alabama, Birmingham)
Ann Vasc Surg 11:2–8, 1997   20–6

Objective.—Carotid endarterectomy (CEA) has become a standard treatment for patients with high-grade carotid stenosis. Some reports have described the use of percutaneous transluminal angioplasty for the treatment of carotid artery stenoses in various anatomical locations. A trial of percutaneous angioplasty with stenting (PTAS) for the treatment of carotid artery stenosis is reported, including a comparison with patients treated by CEA.

Methods.—The analysis included a total of 310 carotid bifurcation stenoses in 273 patients treated during a 14-month period. Treatment was by PTAS in 107 patients and by CEA in 166. Forty-one percent of patients had high-grade asymptomatic stenoses, 40% had had transient ischemic attacks, 17% had had strokes, and 3% had had syncope. The patients undergoing PTAS were prospectively followed up, whereas those undergoing CEA were studied retrospectively. The 2 techniques were compared for safety and clinical results.

Results.—The combined rate of any stroke or death was 9.3% in the PTAS group vs. 3.6% in the CEA group. The rate of a minor stroke was 6.5% with PTAS vs. 0.6% with CEA; the mortality rate was 0.9% with PTAS vs. 2.4% with CEA. Significant nonneurologic complications occurred in 5.6% of patients in the PTAS group vs. 1.2% of those in the CEA group. One hundred ninety-three patients had 6-month follow-up data. The rate of minor strokes as a late result was 6.5% in the PTAS group vs.

0.6% in the CEA group. There was 1 major stroke in each group; mortality was 3.7% in the PTAS group and 3.6% in the CEA group.

Conclusions.—In patients with carotid stenosis, PTAS is not safer than CEA. The combined rate of strokes and death is lower with CEA. In selected patients, PTAS may be a useful alternative to the treatment of carotid bifurcation lesions. With further advances in technology and technique to reduce complications of PTAS, a randomized comparison with CEA may be justified.

▶ Treatment of carotid stenosis is still a controversial subject. Nowadays, the classic techniques of open surgery are confronted with novel approaches guided by endovascular navigation. The work by Jordan et al. shows that both methods, CEA and PTAS, have similar results as measured by major complications (debilitating stroke and death). However, in the PTAS group, mild complications were more frequent; mostly, they were minor strokes with minimal permanent deficit and a high incidence of transient bradycardia with hypotension during the procedure, which can be explained by the detachment of emboli caused by the passage of the catheter through the stenotic artery and by the sudden distention of the carotid bulb caused by the balloon inflation. They seem difficult to tackle, as both are secondary to the intrinsic process of intravascular angioplasty rather than a result of technical limitations. Each method has its own pros and cons; once studies with long-term follow-up are completed, it will be possible to select patients with carotid artery stenosis whose profiles make them eligible for 1 procedure or the other. Based on this initial report, the tentative list of suitable candidates for PTAS would be those with stenosis without ulceration or thrombus, those with nonarteriosclerotic stenosis, patients with surgically inaccessible lesions, or patients with recurrent stenosis after CEA (PTAS to be used as a second intervertion). In arterial stenosis, where the choice of a therapeutic procedure among rather different approaches is disputed, it will be important in the near future to outline the features by which a given technique could be selected to obtain an optimal outcome. I would like to see an algorithm, based on longitudinal multicenter studies, that would guide the selection of each treatment and that would be charted using the individual characteristics of every patient with carotid artery stenosis.

J. Sotelo, M.D.

Carotid Artery Bifurcation Advancement: An Alternative to Patching
Perkins JMT, Hands LJ, Morris PJ (Univ of Oxford, England)
J R Coll Surg Edinb 41:170–173, 1996   20–7

Objective.—In carotid artery bifurcation advancement, the in situ external carotid artery is used to patch the internal carotid artery after carotid endarterectomy. This alternative to primary vessel closure avoids the patch rupture and pseudoaneurysm formation that can occur with vein and synthetic patches. An experience with bifurcation advancement, including a comparison with other techniques of vessel closure after carotid endarterectomy, is reported.

Methods.—Thirty-three patients underwent endarterectomy of the internal carotid artery during a 1-year period: arterial closure was achieved by bifurcation advancement in 8 arteries and by a polyethylene terephthalate (Dacron) patch in 25. Retrospective comparisons were made with 30 patients in whom simple primary closure was performed and with 13 patients in whom saphenous vein patching was performed. Doppler measurements of the internal carotid artery flow were performed before and after endarterectomy. Regular duplex scans were obtained to evaluate the patients for restenosis.

Results.—The groups were similar in terms of age, sex, and risk factors. Just 1 of 76 patients had a stroke during the 30-day postoperative period. Greater than 50% restenosis of the operated artery occurred in 6 of 30 patients in the primary closure group compared with none in the bifurcation advancement or patch angioplasty groups. Patients in the patch angioplasty and bifurcation advancement groups showed no significant difference in postendarterectomy flow increase, although both were greater than in the primary closure group. Patch closure and bifurcation advancement were associated with similar operative times. The proportion of patients with plaque ulceration was not significantly different between groups. Patients in the primary closure group were less likely to have a shunt inserted.

Conclusions.—In patients undergoing carotid endarterectomy, carotid bifurcation advancement appears to be a useful alternative for vessel closure. Compared with patch angioplasty closure, bifurcation advancement is associated with comparable rates of restenosis, postendarterectomy flow increase, and operative time. Bifurcation advancement is suitable for patients with lesions located close to the origin of the internal carotid artery.

▶ The technique, carotid arterial bifurcation advancement, was first suggested by S. Hucke, Jr. and was reported by J. Rosenmann et al. in 1984.[1] This is an excellent technique to use to avoid restenosis, as compared with simple primary closure. Patching of the endarterectomy site with autogenous veins or prosthetic material such as polyethylene terephthalate (Dacron) has been advocated for lowering the incidence of restenosis. This patching procedure, however, may lead to infections or aneurysm formation. The carotid arterial bifurcation advancement technique solves these untoward problems. The only difficulty in performing this procedure may be encountered when the original bifurcation is located too high.

K. Sano, M.D., D.M.Sc., F.A.C.S. (hon)

Reference

1. Rosenmann J, Edward S, Robillard D, et al: Carotid bifurcation advancement. *Surg Gynaecol Obstet* 159:260–264, 1984.

21 Cranial Operative Technique

The Significance of Artificial Cerebrospinal Fluid as Perfusate and Endoneurosurgery
Oka K, Yamamoto M, Nonaka T, et al (Fukuoka Univ, Japan)
Neurosurgery 38:733–736, 1996   21–1

Introduction.—There are few reports regarding distinctions of various perfusates used during endoneurosurgery. The efficacy of intraoperative perfusion of the ventricular system with artificial CSF solution was evaluated.

Methods.—Twelve patients with presumed symptomatic aqueductal stenosis were treated with percutaneous neuroendoscopic third ventriculostomy and intraoperative perfusion. Ordinary saline solution was used in 7 patients and artificial CSF was used in the remaining 5. All patients received 1 40-mg dose of gentamicin after surgery. Patients underwent daily lumbar punctures for about 1 week, and CSF samples were analyzed for protein, sugar, cells, and cultures. Patients had MRI every 6 months after surgery for a follow-up of 2–4 years. Patency of the third ventricle was confirmed by MRI.

Results.—Headaches, high fever, neck stiffness, and increased cell count in lumbar CSF were experienced in the immediate postoperative period by the 7 patients who received saline solution after surgery. A striking inflammatory reaction in the CSF was detected in the saline group. Patients who received artificial CSF experienced only slightly high fever after surgery and no other symptoms.

Conclusion.—Artificial CSF used as a perfusate was more efficacious in minimizing host reactions during endoneurosurgery than saline solution.

▶ Endoscopic procedures in neurosurgery have become commonplace with the availability of new endoscopic systems and instruments. Oka et al. give attention to an issue that has been given little consideration in the past: the effects of irrigant solutions and neuroendoscopy. Although the numbers are small ($n = 12$), they found that the use of normal saline was associated with headaches, fever, and neck stiffness. The use of an artificial CSF perfusate was not associated with any of the symptoms. Many of us who perform neuroendoscopic procedures have stayed away from normal saline solution. Either from personal experience or from anecdotal reports, it has been found that saline can be associated with untoward effects. There have been reports of bradycardia and even asystole when flushing the posterior fossa with normal saline. A careful analysis of the patients' data reveals that the symptoms were associated with greater CSF pleocystosis and higher (although not statistically significant) body temperatures in the saline group. Given the low pH (5.1–6.4) and higher osmotic concentrations (328 mmol/kg), this is not surprising. Careful attention to the irrigant used should be paid by those performing neuroendoscopic procedures.

D.F. Jimenez, M.D.

Intraoperative Brain Mapping in a Community Setting—Technical Considerations
Sartorius CJ, Wright G (Indianapolis Neurosurgical Group, Ind; St Vincent Hosp, Indianapolis, Ind)
Surg Neurol 47:380–388, 1997
21–2

Background.—Brain mapping allows a neurosurgeon to identify and preserve neurons in functionally important parts of the cortex during epilepsy surgery or lesionectomy. Although this procedure is usually performed in an academic center, an experience in a community-based neurosurgical practice is described.

Patient Preparation.—Patients undergoing intraoperative brain mapping should be able to tolerate local anesthetic infiltration and remain immobile, yet be able to respond to verbal commands. The patient is placed in the lateral position with an axillary roll, draped to allow a clear view of both sides of the face and the contralateral arm and leg. Fentanyl and droperidol are administered for general anesthesia, and bupivacaine hydrochloride is injected over the entire proposed excision, including the skull base. The only problem encountered is that 20% of patients have intraoperative seizures; these are usually self-limiting, and iced Ringer's solution applied to the involved area often ends the seizure.

Mapping Technique.—While the patient is sedated, the craniotomy is performed; then the patient awakens and evoked potential recordings begin. Once the lesion is localized by ultrasound, its margins are labeled on the cortical surface. The central sulcus is approximated by direct cortical median nerve somatosensory evoked potential recordings, with subsequent electrode strip placements and stimulation every 3 cm until it is located with confidence. Electrocorticography is used to identify and mark any epileptogenic perilesional areas for resection. If any of these areas are also identified later as being functionally important, then multiple subpial transections are used. Direct cortical stimulation is used to identify the precentral and postcentral gyrus. The patient is asked to notify the surgeon when paresthesia is experienced, and the corresponding brain area is marked. Only motor mapping is performed for patients who are asleep, and the anesthesiologist watches the exposed body areas for stimulation-evoked movements. Language mapping is performed by identifying Broca's area via stimulation-evoked counting arrest with concurrent electrocorticography. Additional language sites are identified by asking the patient to name objects while the cortical area is being stimulated. Once the brain mapping is complete, the lesion is resected according to standard microneurosurgical techniques; additional mapping may be performed during surgery to preserve essential neurons.

Conclusions.—Despite short-term hemiparesis, dysphasia, and language deficits, permanent neurologic complications because of language or proprioception have not occurred. In fact, only 1 patient in 60 (2%) has had permanent neurologic sequelae related to hemiparesis. The procedures involved in intraoperative brain mapping can be learned easily without subspecialty training, and the mapping adds 1–2 hours to the operative time. Equipment costs are not great, and results with mapping of these essential cortex areas are similar to those of lesion resection in nonessential areas.

▶ Functional neurosurgery and clinical neurophysiology are quickly entering all modes of neurosurgical practice. Identification and preservation of areas essential for movement, sensation, and language have always been a problem in routine neurosurgery when eloquent areas are involved. Many undesirable side effects of neurosurgical procedures that have taken place in nonacademic institutions could have been avoided if the surgeon had been familiar with the simple principles used intraoperatively and proposed by the authors. The authors demonstrated that evoked potential recordings, with or without ultrasound, identified the central sulcus. Electrocorticography, sensorimotor stimulation, and language mapping are not an appanage of highly sophisticated academic institutions if a skilled anesthesiologist, experienced in working with patients who are awake, is available. I believe that Penfield and Milner's findings have finally been brought to regular clinical practice; I can still hear their voices asking the awake patient questions—a patient who, is receiving the benefit of their many decades of experience studying exposed brains.

R. Marino, Jr., M.D.

22 Epilepsy Surgery

Treatment of Epilepsy With Multiple Subpial Transections: An Acute Histologic Analysis in Human Subjects
Kaufmann WE, Krauss GL, Uematsu S, et al (Johns Hopkins Univ, Baltimore, Md)
Epilepsia 37:342–352, 1996

22–1

Background.—Multiple subpial transection (MST), a new operative technique for treating seizures arising from functionally critical cortical regions, is reportedly as effective as standard temporal lobe resections. The lesions created in this procedure, placed 5 mm apart at the midlevel of the cortical gyri, may cause fiber damage that prevents horizontal synchronization and spread of epileptic discharges while preserving normal cortical functions, such as those associated with movement or speech. The acute neuropathologic features associated with MST were studied in 1 group of patients with intractable temporal lobe epilepsy.

Methods and Findings.—Just before standard lobectomy, 8 patients underwent transections placed along major temporal gyri. Tissue was studied by conventional histologic and immunocytochemical methods after resection. On macroscopic assessment, subpial transections (STs) were seen to be perpendicular to the main gyral axis with appropriate spacing. Microscopic assessment showed that most of the lesions were perpendicular at midlevel. However, many transections involved the lateral aspects of the small gyri. This resulted in oblique or deep STs, some reaching the gray-white matter junction because of the complex microscopic neocortical architecture, in which small gyri are superimposed on major lobar gyri, and to the variable cortical thickness. In addition, extensive pyknosis and tissue edema adjacent to the transections were observed. These changes were variable, extending 1–3 mm laterally as irregular columnar blocks. Myelin pallor and reduced neurofilament immunoreactivity were seen in the deep lesions in the white matter (Fig 5).

Conclusions.—Multiple subpial transection produces block-type lesions that probably disrupt the propagation of epileptogenic activity. Along with horizontal desynchronization, a deafferentiation mechanism involving different fiber systems may contribute to the MST's antiseizure effects. Preserving cortical function may be mediated by cortex remaining in the

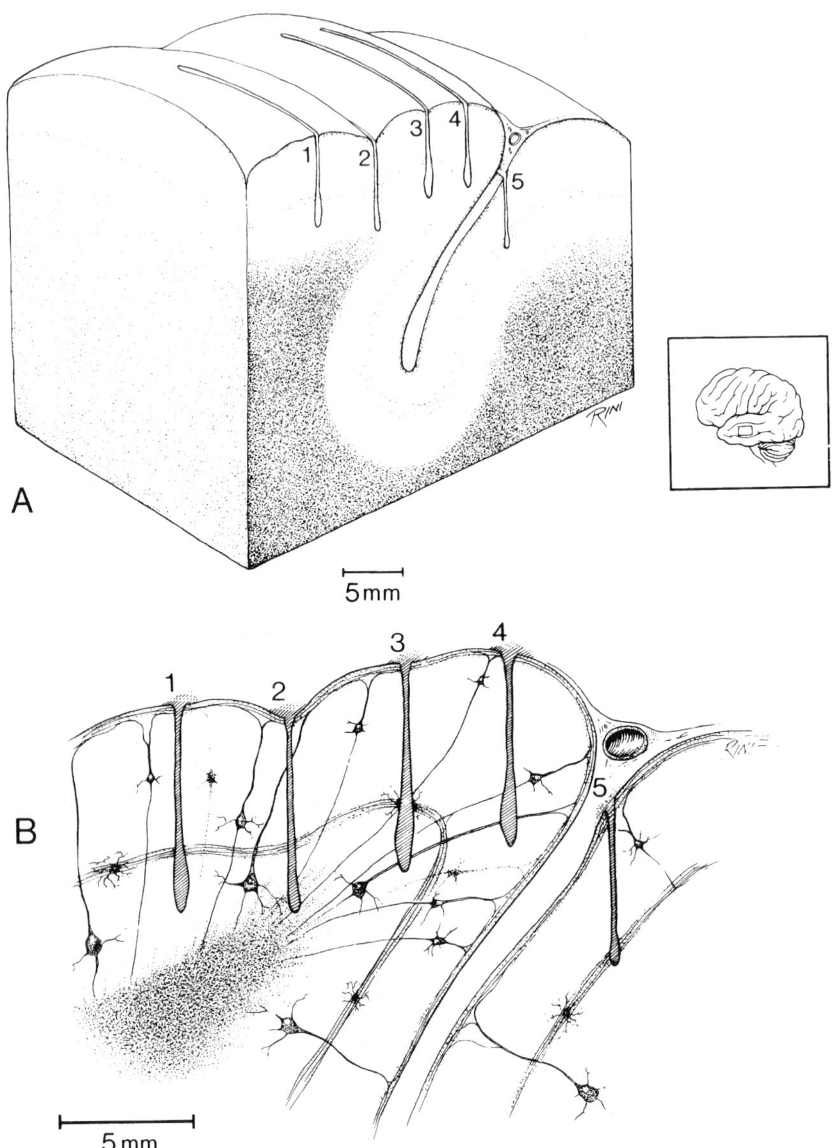

FIGURE 5.—Microscopic gyral architecture and subpial transections (STs). Three-dimensional (**A**) and bidimensional (**B**) representations of a coronal section parallel to the main axis of the middle temporal gyrus. **A**, inset shows areas of sampling in the temporal lobe. Five typical transections, taken from patients' histologic preparations, are shown in terms of orientation and location (**A**) and effects on neuronal elements (**B**). Because large temporal gyri are composed of smaller microscopic gyri and sulci, only ST 1 is ideal; that is, it reaches the midcortical level perpendicularly and disrupts layer IV horizontal fibers. By contrast, transection 2, which is placed in a gyral depression, spans the entire cortical thickness, damaging deeper neurons, as well as ascending and descending axons. Lesion 3 is similar to lesion 1; however, its deep extension horizontally disrupts layer V because of its locations on the curving plane of a small gyrus. Likewise, STs 4 and 5 result in oblique lesions that damage superficial cortex. In **A** and **B**, the bar equals 5 mm. (Courtesy of Kaufmann WE, Krauss GL, Uematsu S, et al: Treatment of epilepsy with multiple subpial transections: An acute histologic analysis in human subjects. *Epilepsia* 37:342–352, 1996.)

sulcus andgyral crown, and possibly by reorganization of tissue adjacent to transections.

▶ Multiple subpial transection is not just a new technique for the surgical treatment of focal epilepsy. It is a new concept of treatment introduced by Morrel[1, 2] in the 1960s—a contribution based on fundamental physiologic grounds and animal experimentation. It is not based on removal of the tissue containing the epileptic focus and constitutes an option of surgical therapy to a group of patients in whom the epileptic zone involves functionally critical and eloquent cortical regions, such as Broca's or Wernicke's areas, precentral or postcentral areas, cases in which resective surgery would entail the unacceptable price of loss of these important cortical functions of the human brain. Multiple subpial transection is, thus, a surgical alternative to tissue resection, with preservation of eloquent cortical function, mediated by cortex remaining in the sulcus and gyral crown and reorganization of tissue adjacent to cortical transection. It was planned to produce selective interruption of the spread of epileptogenic discharges and regional seizure propagation through the horizontal cortical connections (horizontal desynchronization) using block-type lesions (see Fig 5). This study compares its efficacy to that of standard temporal lobe resection. In their careful and detailed study, performed in 8 patients who underwent standard temporal lobectomies, the authors try to clarify the mechanism of MST by evaluating the microscopic characteristics of the acute lesions and surrounding tissue after the temporal lobe was removed. They hypothesize that disconnection of adjacent cortical areas and deafferentiation of cortical blocks are responsible for seizure control after MST.

R. Marino, Jr., M.D.

References

1. Morrel F: Secondary epileptogenic lesions. *Epilepsia* 1:558–560, 1959/1960.
2. Morrel F, Hanbery JW: A new surgical technique for the treatment of focal cortical epilepsy. *Electroencephalogr Clin Neurophysiol* 26:120, 1969.

Temporal Lobectomy for Refractory Epilepsy
Sperling MR, O'Connor MJ, Saykin AJ, et al (Univ of Pennsylvania, Philadelphia; Dartmouth Univ, Hanover, NH)
JAMA 276:470–475, 1996   22–2

Background.—Anterior temporal lobectomy, the most common operation done to treat refractory epilepsy, has been reported to abolish or markedly reduce the frequency of seizures in most patients. However, there have been relatively few long-term studies of the outcomes of this procedure. In the current study, a cohort of patients undergoing anterior temporal lobectomy for medically refractory epilepsy was followed up prospectively.

Methods.—Eighty-nine patients treated between 1986 and 1990 were included. All patients had undergone noninvasive assessments preoperatively, and 31 had had intracranial electrodes.

Findings.—At 5 years, 70% of the patients were free of seizures. Nine percent had seizures on fewer than 3 days a year or nocturnal seizures only. Eleven percent had a reduction in seizure frequency of more than 80%, and 6% had a less than 80% decrease in seizure frequency. Four percent of the patients died of causes unrelated to surgery. The proportion of patients in each outcome class was stable during follow-up. Fifty-five percent of seizure recurrences occurred within 6 months of surgery, and 83% occurred within 2 years. One-year outcomes were only moderately well correlated with 5-year outcomes. None of the patients had significant cognitive or linguistic deficits. All nonsurvivors had persistent seizures postoperatively. Significant declines in underemployment and unemployment were noted after surgery, especially among patients who were free from seizures.

Conclusions.—For most patients with medically refractory epilepsy, temporal lobectomy results in sustained seizure relief for 5 years. Freedom from seizures is associated with decreased mortality and increased employment rates. A mere decrease in seizure frequency was uncorrelated with improvement in these measures.

▶ This meticulous study of temporal lobectomy in 89 patients shows that important conclusions are not drawn only from large operative historical or individual series. The authors demonstrate that, by following a rigid protocol (their own) and by treating patients with epilepsy not only as neurologic cases with undesirable seizures but also as individuals with a disease, that is, human beings with all their medical, social, cognitive, psychiatric, and employment handicaps, the results of a surgical procedure (usually a curative one) for either a neoplasm or mesial sclerosis can be very rewarding for the patient, their family, the physician, and society (epilepsy is a common public health problem). Very few epilepsy centers are concerned with the patient with epilepsy as a whole—as a suffering human being that is prone to have depressive, suicidal, and schizophrenic tendencies, as well as other psychiatric, cognitive, and social problems. Surgery and drugs alone will not treat all these features; they must be taken care of by other specialists, social workers, and occupational therapists after surgery, under the guidance of the neurosurgeon. The important problem of mortality after 5 years, from either suicide or acute cardiac or pulmonary derangements during persistent postoperative seizures or interictal disturbances, needs to be considered: there was an impressive overall mortality rate of 4.5% in the present operative series. This is a number that we should always bear in mind in our own operative series.

R. Marino, Jr., M.D.

23 Functional Neurosurgery

Treatment of Advanced Parkinson's Disease by Posterior GPi Pallidotomy: 1-Year Results of a Pilot Study
Baron MS, Vitek JL, Bakay RAE, et al (Emory Univ, Atlanta, Ga)
Ann Neurol 40:355–366, 1996

23–1

Introduction.—Alternative treatments for Parkinson's disease (PD) are needed, given the limitations of medical therapy and thalamotomy. There is renewed interest in the surgical treatment of PD, and clinical reports have suggested that pallidotomy may be beneficial for parkinsonism and drug-induced dyskinesias. The effectiveness of posterior internal pallidal ablation (internal portion of the globus pallidus [GPi] pallidotomy) was evaluated in patients with PD in a pilot study.

Methods.—The study included 15 patients with medically intractable PD. The mean age was 57 years, and the mean duration of PD was 14 years. All patients had histories compatible with idiopathic PD, an off-medication Hoehn and Yahr score of 3.0 or greater, and a history of significant responsiveness to levodopa. Posterior GPi pallidotomy was performed in all patients, and microelectrode recording and stimulation was performed to identify the sensorimotor territory of the GPi and the adjacent optic tract and the internal capsule. The surgeon then placed radiofrequency lesions in this sensorimotor territory. Neurologic assessments were performed at intervals from 3 months before to 1 year after surgery.

Results.—All cardinal motor signs of PD—tremors, rigidity, akinesia/bradykinesia, and gait dysfunction—were significantly improved after GPi pallidotomy. Drug-induced motor fluctuations and dyskinesias were improved as well. Most of the improvements were noted contralateral to the pallidotomy lesions, although some ipsilateral improvements occurred as well. At 3 months postoperatively, the mean total United Parkinson's Disease Rating Scale scores had improved by 30%. The level of functional independence, as indicated by the mean combined "on/off" Schwab and England Scale scores, increased from 48.8% to 73.0%. Neither of these outcome measures showed any significant decline during the year after surgery. The surgical morbidity rate was low, and there were no significant abnormalities detected on neuropsychological and psychiatric testing. During the postoperative period, the patients showed significant improvement in physical and social functioning and in measures of vitality on the Medical Outcome Scale.

Conclusions.—This pilot study shows the benefits of posterior GPi pallidotomy for patients with advanced PD. Most patients achieve reduction in the cardinal motor signs of PD, as well as reduced motor fluctuations, less severe "off" states, and a greater percentage of "on" time. During on time, there are no disabling dyskinesias or dystonia and less likelihood of an unpredictable, sudden return to the off state. Surgery is associated with improved physical and social functioning without cognitive or psychiatric impairment. The 1-year follow-up results are encouraging, although longitudinal studies are needed.

▶ This report shows that posteroventral medial pallidotomy effectively controls the motor involvement features of Parkinson's disease, such as rigidity, tremors, dyskinesia, and gait dysfunction; it also reduces drug-induced motor fluctuations and dyskinesias. To identify the pallidal target, the authors used microelectrode recording as a guide so that the optic tract and the internal capsule were saved from lesioning. The pallidal target was lesioned by a radiofrequency current. In the history of stereotactic surgery for patients with recalcitrant PD, pallidotomy was first introduced as the treatment of choice, then thalamotomy became predominant. Now, again, a type of pallidotomy much more exact than the previous one has regained popularity. A more recent report[1] also showed similar good results.

K. Sano, M.D., D.M.Sc., F.A.C.S. (hon)

Reference

1. Kopyov O, Jacques D, Duma C: Microelectrode-guided posteroventral medial radiofrequency pallidotomy for Parkinson's disease. *J Neurosurg* 87:52–59, 1997.

24 Head Trauma

Pediatric/Adolescent Head Trauma

Outcome of Persistent Vegetative State Following Hypoxic or Traumatic Brain Injury in Children and Adolescents

Heindl UT, Laub MC (Behandlungszentrum Vogtareuth, Germany)
Neuropediatrics 27:94–100, 1996

24–1

Background.—With improvements in medical care, patients are surviving longer in a persistent vegetative state (PVS). This makes it increasingly important to have information on the quality of outcome and prognosis of this condition, especially in young patients. The outcomes of PVS in children and adolescents after hypoxic and traumatic brain injuries were studied.

Methods.—The retrospective study included 127 children treated at a regional specialty hospital for PVS lasting at least 30 days. Eighty-two patients had histories of traumatic brain injuries (TBI); 33 in this group were polytrauma victims. The other 45 patients had hypoxic brain injuries (HBI), from either near-drowning incidents or cardiopulmonary arrest and cardiopulmonary resuscitation. All patients were followed up for at least 19 months. The coma and functional outcomes of the 2 groups were analyzed, including possible prognostic factors. In addition, information was sought on seizures, pneumonia, myositis ossificans, kidney concretion, tracheostoma, nutritional status, home residence, and other outcomes.

Findings.—Eighty-four percent of patients in the TBI group regained consciousness, compared with just 55% of the HBI group. One patient in the TBI group died, compared with 8 in the HBI group. By 3 months, nearly two thirds of the TBI group had regained consciousness, compared with one third of the HBI group. Less than 5% of either group regained consciousness beyond 9 months after the incident. Seizures were more common among patients in the HBI group and were also more frequent. The HBI group also had higher rates of pneumonia, gastrointestinal disturbances, and myositis ossificans. In the TBI group, but not in the HBI group, posttraumatic hyperthermia and autonomic dysfunction were associated with poorer outcomes. Sixteen percent of patients in the TBI group achieved independence in everyday life, compared with just 4% of those in the HBI group. The prognosis was not significantly affected by age.

Conclusions.—The outcomes of PVS in childhood and adolescence appear worse when the cause of the brain injury is hypoxic rather than traumatic. The findings emphasize the role of hypoxia in causing severe, permanent brain injury. Even patients who remain in PVS may achieve gradual improvements. The findings may help to establish a prognosis and help to support the parents and staff, although it is not possible to perform any individual case prognostication.

▶ Presistent vegetative state is a very acute social and medical problem still poorly understood, particularly with regard to the results and the late outcome. Very few specialized institutions have sufficient experience with these patients, who, after a few months, are usually transferred to some nursing place or home. Large series are rare. The most important findings of the study are the improvement data seen after a period of up to 12 months: consciousness was regained in 84% of the children (within the TBI group) and a small number of children archieved independence in daily life. These rather encouraging results were obtained in spite of the surprisingly long time (average 8.8 months) after injury at which rehabilitation was initiated.

The striking prognostic difference between patients with traumatic vs. hypoxic brain injuries is well known. The authors present an interesting theoretical explanation, according to which the first is caused by diffuse axonal injury (DAI) and the second is caused by a more deleterious neuronal injury.

Data presented in the study may be a kind of support to parents as well as a help to the medical staff, who, often enough, is decisively pessimistic about patients in a PVS.

B. Klun, M.D., Ph.D.

Pediatric Depressed Skull Fractures: Analysis of 530 Cases
Erşahin Y, Mutluer S, Mirzai H, et al (Ege Univ, Izmit, Turkey)
Childs Nerv Syst 12:323–331, 1996   24–2

Introduction.—As many as 10% of children hospitalized for head injuries and 25% of those with skull fractures have depressed skull fractures (DSFs). These fractures can have serious complications, including posttraumatic epilepsy and infection. Compound DSFs are managed surgically, although simple DSFs may be treated conservatively. A large experience with the management of pediatric DSFs is reviewed.

Patients.—The 21-year review included 530 children undergoing surgery for DSFs. Surgery was performed in patients with compound DSF, associated intracranial hematomas, penetrating injuries, retained bone fragments, bone depression greater than the thickness of the bone, or cosmetic deformity. Two thirds of the patients were boys. The mean age was 6 years, and 52% of patients were younger than this. A fall was the most common cause of injury, followed by traffic accidents. Most patients had nausea/vomiting and headaches, and two thirds had overlying scalp lacerations. Two thirds of the fractures were compound fractures, and these became more frequent with age. The rate of lacerations was 29% with compound fractures vs. 15.5% with simple fractures. Each fracture was classified on radiographs as a true (465 cases), flat (24 cases), or ping-pong ball (41 cases) fracture.

Outcomes.—The mortality rate was 2.5%. Ninety-five percent of patients had satisfactory results. The presence of associated intracranial lesions was a poor prognostic factor. Patients with compound fractures had worse outcomes and a higher incidence of intracranial lesions and cortical lacerations. Factors associated with mortality included unilateral pupil dilation and an admission Glasgow Coma Scale score of 8 or less. Fractures with deeper depression of bone were associated with a higher risk of dural tearing and cortical laceration and a worse prognosis.

Discussion.—A large experience with the management of DSFs in children and adolescents is reviewed. Patients with simple DSFs without associated intracranial hematomas, and those with bone depression no deeper than 1 cm, can be managed conservatively. Indications for surgery include prevention of infection, improvement of neurologic deficits caused by an associated intracranial hematoma, and correction of a cosmetic deformity. Clinical factors associated with a poor prognosis are identified.

▶ The authors present an excellent review of their experience with DSFs in the pediatric population. It should be noted that this paper, coming from Turkey, represents their unique experience. Overall, a retrospective analysis of 530 patients for a 21-year period was done. They classified DSFs according to type: true, flat, or ping-pong ball. A careful analysis was done of causes of injury; presenting signs and symptoms; site, type, and depth of the DSF; associated intracranial lesions and posttraumatic seizure rate; complications; and outcome. Their management includes taking the patient to surgery within the first 24 hours. Prophylactic antibiotic treatment was used in all cases. Bone fragments were replaced unless obviously contaminated. Their outcome data indicated that 88% of the patients had an excellent recovery, only 8% had moderate deficits, and their overall mortality rate was 2.5%. Thus, this corroborates the fact that DSFs in the pediatric population, when treated appropriately, are associated with excellent recovery in the majority of patients.

D.F. Jimenez, M.D.

Management

Decompressive Bifrontal Craniectomy in the Treatment of Severe Refractory Posttraumatic Cerebral Edema
Polin RS, Shaffrey ME, Bogaev CA, et al (Univ of Virginia, Charlottesville)
Neurosurgery 41:84–94, 1997   24–3

Background.—Despite our best efforts at medical management, morbidity and mortality rates after the development of malignant posttraumatic cerebral edema remain high. Reducing the intracranial pressure

(ICP) in these patients seems the most likely factor to have an impact on outcome, but perhaps methods other than medical therapy should be considered. The results of bifrontal decompressive craniectomy to reduce and/or prevent high ICP in patients with posttraumatic cerebral edema were reported.

Methods.—All patients with head injuries were evaluated in the emergency department for ICP. Those with an elevated ICP received head elevation and mild hyperventilation to a PCO_2 value of 30–35 torr. If that failed to maintain ICP below 20 torr, then 1 g/kg mannitol was given to try to achieve an ICP of less than 20 torr. If that failed, then patients were divided into 2 groups. In the case group, 35 patients (24 males and 11 females; mean age, 18.7 years) underwent a large bifrontal craniectomy with dural expansion grafts to allow decompression. In the control group, 92 age-, sex-, and Glasgow Coma Score-matched patients received traditional drug therapy (mannitol, furosemide, and barbiturates) to reduce ICP.

Findings.—Death occurred in 8 patients in the test group (23%) and in 38 patients in the control group (31%). A good recovery or only moderate disability was achieved in 13 patients in the test group (37%) and in 15 patients in the control group (16%). In the patients undergoing decompression, the mean ICP decreased significantly from before surgery (32.1 torr) to after surgery (21.3 torr). The test group also had a significantly lower mean postoperative ICP than the controls (29.4 torr). Patients with decompression whose ICP remained above 40 torr for a sustained period and who underwent surgery more than 48 hours after admission had a significantly poorer outcome (1 of 15 [6.7%] had a favorable outcome) than patients who did not meet either criteria (12 of 20 [60%] had favorable outcomes). In the control group, a good outcome occurred in 18% of patients who did not meet either criteria. Patients in either group with a Glasgow Coma Scale of 6 or more when first seen were significantly more likely to have a good outcome (about 66% of patients) than those with a score of 3 or 4 when first seen (1 patient had a good outcome).

Conclusions.—Bilateral decompressive craniectomy provided greater reductions in ICP and better outcomes than medical management. These improvements were achieved without subsequent drug therapy, that is, patients required only head elevation and mild hypocapnia after bifrontal craniectomy. Patients with a low Glasgow Coma Score at baseline were at particular risk for a poor outcome. With decompression, patients whose ICP values remained above 40 torr and who were operated on after 48 hours or less after admission had better outcomes. Thus, careful patient selection for decompressive craniectomy can improve outcomes even further.

▶ Decompressive craniectomy for trauma is a procedure that has fallen in and out of favor over the years. In 1971, Kjellberg and Prieto[1] described a similar procedure for treatment of malignant cerebral edema. Polin et al. present their experience using a modified decompressive bifrontal craniectomy in patients with malignant posttraumatic cerebral edema. Although they have made a good attempt to do case-controlled matching, the variables in these trauma populations exceed the probability of control. Consequently, the validity of these statistics and the conclusions derived from these statistics must be carefully considered. The real value of this article lies in the observations that were made by these investigators and the advice that they share from their experience using this technique in patients with medically and pharmacologically refractory intracranial hypertension.

These authors reported a mortality rate among this patient population of 23%, and they noted that pediatric patients had a higher rate of favorable outcome than did adults. In addition, they noted that post-operative ICP was lower than pre-operative ICP, and that all patients who exhibited sustained ICP values above 40 torr did poorly if their surgery was delayed more than 48 hours after the time of their injuries.

These observations are helpful and are consistent with my own. I believe that there is a place for this operation in the management of malignant cerebral edema and elevated ICP. The circumstances leading to the decision to perform this operation are often compelling, and the decision must be made on an individual case basis. There are still times that we must trust our intuition in the face of population statistics.

S.R. Gibbs, M.A., M.D.

Reference

1. Kjellberg RN, Prieto A Jr: Bifrontal decompressive craniotomy for massive cerebral edema. *J Neurosurg* 34:488–493, 1971.

Management of Complications from 820 Temporal Bone Fractures

Brodie HA, Thompson TC (Univ of California, Davis)
Am J Otol 18:188–197, 1997   24–4

Purpose.—Temporal bone fractures occur in 14% to 22% of patients with skull fractures. Complications of these injuries may include CSF fistulas, facial paralysis, sensorineural hearing loss, vertigo, and meningitis. Temporal bone fractures have traditionally been classified as transverse or longitudinal, depending on the relationship of the fracture line to the axis of the petrous ridge and otic capsule. Involvement of the otic capsule has an important impact on whether surgery is performed and what surgical approach is used. A large series of patients with temporal bone fractures is reviewed.

Patients.—The experience included 820 temporal bone fractures in 699 patients. The patients were all treated at a level 1 trauma center during a 5-year period. Seventy-six percent of the patients were male, and 22% were less than 17 years old. Motor vehicle accidents were the most common cause of injury, followed by assault, falls, and motorcycle accidents. The fractures were open—with blood, brain, or CSF draining from the external auditory site or penetrating wound—in 62% of patients. For patients who survived beyond the emergency department, the mortality rate was about 10%. The patients' records were reviewed to determine the incidence of complications from temporal bone fractures and the outcomes of surgical and nonsurgical management.

Outcomes.—There were 58 cases of facial nerve injuries, 122 of CSF fistulas, and 15 of meningitis. The otic capsule was fractured in only 2.5% of cases. Recovery from facial paralysis occurred in all patients with incomplete paralysis and in almost all of those with delayed-onset palsies. Functional recovery was poor for 40% of patients with immediate-onset complete paralysis. For 88% of patients with spontaneous recovery of facial function, the recovery occurred within 3 months.

For 78% of patients with CSF fistulas, spontaneous closure occurred within 1 week. Twenty-three percent of patients with CSF fistulas persisting for more than 7 days went on to have meningitis, compared with 3% of those whose fistulas closed within a week. Patients with concurrent infection were also at increased risk for meningitis. Twenty-four percent of patients complained of hearing loss. In cases in which hearing loss was documented, it was conductive in 21% of cases, sensorineural in 57%, and mixed in 22%.

Conclusions.—The findings provide useful insights into the management of temporal bone fractures. Patients should undergo evaluation of facial nerve function in the emergency department. Patients with any facial motion are rarely candidates for surgery. When facial nerve decompression is indicated, it can generally be achieved by a transmastoid supralabyrinthine approach in patients with well-pneumatized temporal bones. Patients with CSF fistulas should be considered for prophylactic antibiotics; if the fistula persists beyond 7–10 days, surgical closure should be considered.

▶ Most temporal bone fractures result from head trauma sustained in a motor vehicle accident or in an assault. These fractures have traditionally been classified based on their relationship to the axis of the petrous ridge. Longitudinal fractures are the most common, running parallel to and through the external auditory canal. These usually pass between the cochlea and semicircular canals, sparing the facial and vestibulocochlear nerves. Transverse fractures are perpendicular to the external auditory canal and may injure the cochlea or geniculate ganglion, or both; vestibulocochlear nerve deficits occur when the cochlea is injured, and facial nerve deficits occur when the geniculate ganglion is injured.

These data come from a single level 1 major trauma center that saw, on average, 1 patient every 2–3 days with a temporal bone fracture! This wealth of clinical experience may serve as a benchmark for those treating temporal bone fractures and the complications that may ensue.

S.R. Gibbs, M.A., M.D.

Treatment of Traumatic Brain Injury With Moderate Hypothermia
Marion DW, Penrod LE, Kelsey SF, et al (Univ of Pittsburgh, Pa)
N Engl J Med 336:540–546, 1997   24–5

Introduction.—It has been suggested that hypothermia can limit some of the abnormal metabolic responses that can worsen the effects of traumatic brain injury. Previous trials have shown a trend toward improved outcomes in patients managed with hypothermia, compared with those maintained at a normal temperature. A randomized, controlled trial of moderate hypothermia vs. normothermia in the management of traumatic brain injury is reported.

Methods.—The study included 82 patients with severe closed-head injuries, with Glasgow Coma Scale scores of 3–7. A mean of 10 hours after injury, patients in the hypothermia group were cooled to 33°C. Their body temperature was maintained at 32°C to 33°C for 24 hours, after which the patients were rewarmed. Patients in the normothermia group were kept at normal temperatures throughout the study. Neurologic outcomes after 3, 6, and 12 months were assessed using the Glasgow Coma Scale. The outcome assessments were performed by a physical medicine and rehabilitation specialist without knowledge of the patients' assigned treatment.

Results.—The 2 groups were comparable in their demographic characteristics and causes and severity of injury. The 12-month outcomes were rated as good (i.e., moderate, mild, or no disabilities) for 62% of the hypothermia group vs. 38% of the normothermia group. The adjusted risk ratio for a bad outcome with hypothermia was 0.5, with a 95% confidence interval of 0.2–1.2. There was no difference in outcome between groups for patients with initial Glasgow Coma Scale scores of 3 or 4. Three- and 6-month outcomes were significantly improved by hypothermia for patients with Glasgow Coma Scale scores of 5–7. The adjusted risk ratio of bad outcomes for this group was 0.2, with a 95% confidence interval of 0.1–0.9. However, the risk was not significantly different at 12 months: risk ratio, 0.3; 95% confidence interval, 0.1–1.0.

Conclusions.—Moderate hypothermia may improve the outcomes of traumatic brain injury for patients with initial Glasgow Coma Scale scores of 5–7. Hypothermia of 32°C to 33°C for 24 hours, started soon after the injury, does not increase the incidence of complications. The beneficial effects of hypothermia may arise from the reduction of secondary brain injuries through suppression of the posttraumatic inflammatory response.

▶ The protective effects of hypothermia on tissues and living organisms subjected to ischemic or traumatic insults has been observed in many experimental and clinical situations, including the satisfactory survival of humans after prolonged accidental submersion in very cold water. Research during the last 30 years has established the negative effect of hypotension and hypoxia on patients with head injuries. This study suggests that hyperthermia and normothermia should be added to hypotension and hypoxia as the third condition to be prevented in the first 24 hours after trauma. Aiming the hypothermic treatment (32°C to 33°C) at a relatively small group of patients with head injuries (i.e., Glasgow Coma Scale [GCS] score, 5–7), rather than at all patients with severe head injuries, will make logistically feasible its wider acceptance and application. Further research could test (1) whether administration of cold IV fluids could facilitate earlier induction of hypothermia leading to improved outcomes, and (2) whether a wider group of patients with head injuries (GCS score, 5–9) could also benefit from either mild or prolonged hypothermia (i.e., 48 hours of 34°C to 35°C) or other refinements in the hypothermic treatment protocol. The benefit of hypothermia was less pronounced at 12 months, compared with 6 or 3 months after trauma. Hence, in addition to correct acute head injury management, rehabilitation and brain plasticity remain very important determinants of outcome.

D.E. Sakas, M.D.

Coagulopathy in Severe Closed Head Injury: Is Empiric Therapy Warranted?

May AK, Young JS, Butler K, et al (Univ of Virginia, Charlottesville)
Am Surg 63:233–237, 1997   24–6

Background.—A severe closed-head injury after blunt trauma can be complicated by the development of a coagulopathy, which can cause further blood loss and delay invasive neurosurgical procedures. Waiting for the results of coagulation studies before starting treatment causes a delay that may adversely affect outcomes. The probability of coagulopathy development in a subgroup of patients with severe closed head injuries and the value of empirical treatment with fresh frozen plasma were determined.

Methods.—Complete hospital, laboratory, and radiologic data on 26 adults who had sustained predominantly isolated, severe closed head injuries were reviewed. All had been admitted to 1 trauma center during a 9-month period and had Glasgow Coma Scale (GCS) scores of 8 or less and extracranial abbreviated injury scores of 2 or less. None had penetrating trauma or altered consciousness caused by sedation or shock. The prothrombin time and the partial thromboplastin time recorded on admission were used to determine the presence of coagulation abnormalities.

Findings.—Coagulopathies were documented in 81% of patients with GCS scores of 6 or less on admission and in all with a GCS of 3 or 4. None of the patients with a GCS of 7 or 8 had coagulopathies. The mortality tended to be greater among patients with coagulopathies than among patients without coagulopathies. In addition, patients with coagulopathies had longer ICU and hospital stays. The mean time to neurosurgical intervention was 226 minutes for the group with coagulopathies, and 84.8 minutes for the group without coagulopathies.

Conclusions.—Patients with closed head injuries with initial GCS scores of 6 or less are candidates for empirical treatment of coagulopathies to avoid the delay inherent in waiting for the results of coagulation studies. Further prospective study is needed to determine whether such therapy shortens the interval between admission and neurosurgical procedures or affects outcomes.

▶ The authors' findings are in accord with Sande and Van der Veltkamp's series,[1] which showed that almost all patients with severely impaired consciousness had abnormal coagulation tests. There have been many reports in the literature about coagulation abnormalities after head trauma. It is well known that the brain tissue has the highest concentration of thromboplastin of any body tissue; consequently, head trauma is considered an independent risk factor for disseminated intravascular coagulation (DIC), presumably because of the massive release of tissue thromboplastin from the injured brain. Clearly, the risk of coagulopathy also depends on the age of the individual and coexisting injuries.

The authors' question is interesting. Could secondary brain injury be prevented in patients with severe head injuries by empirical infusion of fresh frozen plasma on arrival to the emergency center to halt the progression of DIC and to correct the existing coagulopathy more rapidly?

Awaiting the results of coagulation studies and blood group, type, and antibody screening often results in a delay of approximately 1–1½ hours. The DIC syndrome develops within 1–4 hours after a brain injury.[2] Because the mortality rate for patients with coagulopathies and head injuries is 53% vs. 22% for those without coagulopathies, these data suggest that empirical infusion of fresh frozen plasma would be beneficial. This comes with a small risk for the rare patient who will receive it unnecessarily, although all patients in this report with GCS scores of 3 or 4 had coagulopathies.

S.R. Gibbs, M.A., M.D.

References

1. Sande JJ, Van der Veltkamp JJ: Head injury and coagulation disorders. *J Neurosurg* 94:357, 1978.
2. Hulka F, Mullins RJ, Frank EH: Blunt brain injury activates the coagulation process. *Arch Surg* 131:923–928, 1996.

Traumatic Subarachnoid Hemorrhage

Traumatic Subarachnoid Hemorrhage as a Predictable Indicator of Delayed Ischemic Symptoms
Taneda M, Kataoka K, Akai F, et al (Kinki Univ, Osaka, Japan)
J Neurosurg 84:762–768, 1996   24–7

Background.—Subarachnoid blood from a ruptured aneurysm is generally thought to give rise to vasospasm and associated ischemic symptoms. However, a causal relationship between vasospasm after traumatic subarachnoid hemorrhage and spasm-related cerebral infarction has been demonstrated in only a few case reports. The presence of traumatic subarachnoid blood and the development of delayed ischemic symptoms resulting from vasospasm were correlated.

Methods and Findings.—One hundred thirty patients with closed-head trauma were studied prospectively. All had evidence of subarachnoid blood on admission CT scans. Delayed ischemic symptoms developed in 7.7% of the patients between postinjury days 4 and 16. These symptoms occurred in 3% of 101 patients with small amounts of subarachnoid blood and 24.1% of 29 patients with massive amounts of subarachnoid blood on admission CT scans. In all 10 affected patients, severe vasospasm was shown angiographically soon after the symptoms developed. The main site of the subarachnoid blood and the location of severe vasospasm were correlated closely. Follow-up CT in 7 patients showed the development of focal ischemic regions in the cerebral territories corresponding to the vasospastic arteries.

Conclusion.—Traumatic subarachnoid hemorrhage—especially massive bleeding, predicts the delayed development of ischemic symptoms. The clinical significance of posttraumatic vasospasm has yet to be established.

▶ This study showed that even in traumatic subarachnoid hemorrhage, thick blood clots surrounding the arteries, as visualized on CT scans, may cause cerebral vasospasm in a relatively high incidence of patients, leading to development of ischemic symptoms. These ischemic symptoms appeared between days 4 and 16 after the head injury. The thickness of blood clots and the time lag before the appearance of delayed ischemic symptoms are very similar to those in cases of aneurysmal subarachnoid hemorrhage. This fact suggests that in both types of subarachnoid hemorrhage, substances produced by clot lysis (such as free radicals and lipid peroxides) may play an important role in causing cerebral vasospasm leading to delayed ischemic neurologic symptoms. The authors rightly assumed that early surgical removal of blood clots in the subarachnoid space might prove to be a prophylactic method of guarding against vasospasm and preventing or minimizing delayed ischemic symptoms.

K. Sano, M.D., D.M.Sc., F.A.C.S. (hon)

Traumatic Subarachnoid Hemorrhage and Its Treatment With Nimodipine

Harders A, Kakarieka A, Braakman R, et al (Ruhr Univ Bochum, Germany; CNS Clinical Research, Cologne, Germany; Erasmus Univ Rotterdam, The Netherlands)
J Neurosurg 85:82–89, 1996   24–8

Background.—The finding of a traumatic subarachnoid hemorrhage (tSAH) on early CT after a head injury appears to be an important, independent factor in predicting unfavorable outcomes. The value of tSAH treatment with nimodipine was assessed.

Methods.—One hundred twenty-three patients with tSAH on initial CT scans were enrolled in the prospective, randomized, double-blind, placebo-controlled study. The patients were seen at a total of 21 German neurosurgical centers between January 1994 and April 1995. All were aged 16–70 years and were enrolled within 12 hours of head injury, regardless of level of consciousness. The patients received either a sequential course of IV and oral nimodipine or placebo for 3 weeks. Close monitoring included determination of clinical, neurologic, CT, laboratory, and transcranial Doppler US parameters.

Findings.—Patients given placebo had significantly less favorable outcomes than those given nimodipine. Death, vegetative survival, or severe disability had occurred by 6 months in 25% of patients given nimodipine and in 46% given placebo. The relative decrease in unfavorable outcome in the patients treated with nimodipine was even greater (55%) when the analysis included only those complying with the protocol.

Conclusions.—Nimodipine is safe, well tolerated, and effective in patients with tSAH on initial CT scan after head injury. Consistent with previous studies, the current study found that the finding of tSAH on first CT scans helps identify patients at high risk for an unfavorable outcome.

▶ The calcium channel blocker, nimodipine has been shown to improve the outcome after an aneurysmal subarachnoid hemorrhage. Although originally speculated to be a vasodilator, it may work through multiple mechanisms, including efforts at the cellular level protecting marginal membranes from excessive calcium influx. Subarachnoid hemorrhages are a common finding in patients with traumatic brain injuries. Suspicions first raised in the pre-CT and pre-angiographic era led to the suggestion of arterial vasospasms as a component of head injuries. Recent work has since supported tSAH as a component—perhaps independent—of vasospasms and their attendant morbidity. Improved understanding and treatment of cerebral blood flow aberrations after head injuries have improved outcomes. This randomized, prospective study supports the beneficial effect of nimodipine in tSAH: thus, an additional, significant step has been taken in the treatment of this unfortunate process that is far more common than such hemorrhages from aneurysms.

C.P. Bondurant, M.D.

Monitoring

Cerebral Oxygenation Monitoring by Near-infrared Spectroscopy Is Not Clinically Useful in Patients With Severe Closed-head Injury: A Comparison With Jugular Venous Bulb Oximetry
Lewis SB, Myburgh JA, Thornton EL, et al (Royal Adelaide Hosp, Australia)
Crit Care Med 24:1334–1338, 1996   24–9

Introduction.—Jugular venous bulb oximetry is invasive, but is a useful method for continuously monitoring jugular venous oxygen saturation. Near-infrared spectroscopy has been considered as a noninvasive method for determining regional cerebral oxygenation. The findings of jugular venous bulb oximetry and those of near-infrared spectroscopy were compared in 10 patients with severe closed-head injury.

Methods and Results.—Patients were monitored continuously via jugular venous bulb oximetry, cerebral near-infrared spectroscopy, and cerebral perfusion pressure. There was poor correlation and there were wide limits of agreement between 3,691 paired measurements. When the data were grouped according to 3 clinically significant subgroups of jugular venous bulb oxygen saturation reflecting low (less than 55%), normal (less than 55% to 75%), and high (greater than 75%) saturation values, the correlation was poor and there were wide limits of agreement in all groups. Near-infrared spectroscopy values did not change significantly between groups. Fourteen episodes of jugular bulb desaturation were not detected by near-infrared spectroscopy.

Conclusion.—Determination of tissue oxygen saturation by near-infrared spectroscopy does not indicate significant changes in cerebral oxygenation, compared to jugular venous bulb oximetry. Near-infrared spectroscopy cannot be recommended for assessing cerebral oxygenation in patients with acute head injuries.

▶ The goal of this study was simple—to compare jugular venous bulb oximetry with near infrared spectroscopy in patients with severe head injury. The study was done prospectively and, although performed on only 10 patients, a total of 3,691 paired measurements were obtained for analysis. The overall findings indicated a poor correlation ($r^2 = 0.04$) between these 2 variables. These findings are not surprising, given the differences in methodology. Jugular bulb venous oximetry is a global measurement and may overlook significant regional differences. Cerebral near-infrared spectroscopy measures a regional area of cortical and subcortical cerebral oxygenation noninvasively. The authors found instances of clinically significant global cerebral desaturation detected by jugular venous bulb oximetry that were not detected by the near-infrared spectroscopy. Other sophisticated studies have shown this also to be the case. Therefore, with our current technologies, it appears that near-infrared spectroscopy does not reflect significant changes in cerebral oxygenation in patients with severe head injury. Further studies and refinement of this technology need to take place before it can be used in a clinical setting.

D.F. Jimenez, M.D., F.A.C.S.

25 Hydrocephalus

Experience With Use of Extended Length Peritoneal Shunt Catheters
Couldwell WT, LeMay DR, McComb JG (Univ of Southern California, Los Angeles)
J Neurosurg 85:425–427, 1996
25–1

Background.—Currently, the treatment of choice for diversion of CSF associated with hydrocephalus is the placement of a ventriculoperitoneal shunt. Although many possible abdominal complications can occur, they are uncommon. One experience with extended-length peritoneal shunt catheters was described.

Methods.—A total of 998 shunts were placed in 952 patients at the Children's Hospital of Los Angeles during a 14-year period. The extended-length open-ended peritoneal tubing (120 cm) was inserted primarily to avoid the need for a lengthening procedure because of patient growth. The mean patient follow-up was 6.7 years.

Outcomes.—Fifty-two distal shunt revisions were needed for malfunctions from a variety of causes. However, the distal complication rate was not increased. There were no complications related directly to the use of the extended length tubing.

Conclusion.—The use of an extended-length peritoneal shunt catheter is unassociated with an increase in complications. It also eliminates the need to lengthen the peritoneal catheter because of patient growth.

▶ The surgical implantation of any device that is to remain functional in children permanently or for several years must take into consideration the gradual growth of the child into adulthood.

An ideal prosthesis is that which can "grow" together with the child, thus preventing further surgeries. This seems to be the case with the extended-length catheter implanted in the peritoneal cavity for ventriculoperitoneal shunting in children with hydrocephalus: as the child's height increases, the catheter unwinds. Contrary to the assumption that a large tubing coiled inside the peritoneum could induce complications, such as knots or strangulated viscera, these did not occur.

Moreover, occlusion of the distal end of the shunt seems to be precluded by the slow uncoiling of the catheter as the child grows. This study clearly demonstrates the advantages of extended-length peritoneal catheters for ventriculoperitoneal shunts in children. At the same time, it reminds us that periodic shunt revisions are necessary in one third of patients and that infections develop in 10%. These data illustrate the need to both investigate the integral performance of shunts and improve the materials used in shunting devices.

J. Sotelo, M.D.

Third Ventriculostomy: A Review
Grant JA, McLone DG (Northwestern Univ, Chicago)
Surg Neurol 47:210–212, 1997

25–2

Background.—There is renewed interest in the performance of endoscopic third ventriculostomy. This procedure is performed to relieve hydrocephalus by making a hole in the floor of the third ventricle; it is almost always performed endoscopically. The definition of a successful ventriculostomy is one that avoids the need for shunting and its complications; even a "failed" ventriculostomy may make the subsequent shunt easier to manage. The current state of third ventriculostomy is reviewed.

Third Ventriculostomy.—Although traditionally regarded as an aqueductal bypass procedure for late-onset aqueductal stenosis, third ventriculostomy can be successfully performed in other forms of hydrocephalus as well. The flow of CSF through the ventriculostomy hole into the subarachnoid space is not the only factor involved the procedure's success; the rapid transmission of pulse pressure through a freely communicating CSF space plays a role as well. The authors perform third ventriculostomy in more than half of the children with hydrocephalus that they see. The success rate, in terms of freedom from shunting, ranges from 100% in children with late-onset aqueductal stenosis to 50% in older children with myelomeningocele. The main risk of third ventriculostomy consists of potential damage to the basilar tip or its perforators, which lie immediately beneath the floor of the third ventricle; however, it is not possible to judge this risk until the ventricular floor is inspected endoscopically. The ventriculostomy holes measure approximately 2.5 mm, which is approximately the diameter of a ventricular catheter.

In their experience of more than 50 procedures using simple pressure on the floor of the third ventricle, the authors have noted 1 major bleeding complication and no deaths. There has been 1 transient case of diabetes insipidus and 2 transient CSF leaks. For symptomatic patients, an external ventricular drainage chain is left in place to monitor intracranial pressure. Follow-up CT scans may or may not show a decrease in ventricular size. If symptoms continue—including neurologic signs, increasing intracranial pressure, or evidence of head growth—a shunt is placed. If not, the external ventricular drainage chain is removed.

Discussion.—Third ventriculostomy is a useful procedure for the management of hydrocephalus. More research is needed to establish the indications and long-term outcomes of this procedure. However, experience suggests that the indications are broader than currently observed and that the long-term outcomes are good.

▶ Although titled a review, this brief article simply summarizes the authors' preference with regard to third ventriculostomy. After a brief historical review, the authors appropriately address some important issues regarding this procedure, such as the size and location of the ostomy, postoperative management, and serious complications, such as basilar artery injury. They currently offer this procedure to 50% of their patients and report a success rate ranging between 50% and 100%. Although they state that "any patient with hydrocephalus is a candidate for this procedure," one must be aware that this is not a view accepted by all neurosurgeons. This is particularly true for patients with documented communicating hydrocephalus.

D.F. Jimenez, M.D.

The Value of Colour Doppler Imaging in Assessing Flow Through Ventriculo-Peritoneal Shunts

Sgouros S, John P, Walsh AR, et al (Birmingham Children's Hosp, England)
Childs Nerv Syst 12:454–459, 1996   25–3

Introduction.—There is currently no reliable, noninvasive technique for diagnosing obstructed ventricular shunts. In a patient undergoing abdominal ultrasonography, the accidental imaging of CSF emerging from the peritoneal end of the ventriculoperitoneal (VP) shunt was observed. This prompted a study of Doppler imaging for the detection of CSF flow through VP shunts in pediatric patients.

Methods.—The study included 17 young patients with VP shunts (age range, 3 months–12 years). Each was studied with a 10.5-MHz broadband linear array transducer and conventional 2–dimensional and Doppler ultrasound, both spectral and color-coded. Two patients were studied before and after VP shunt revision. The capability of Doppler imaging to detect the normally invisible flow of CSF through the shunt tubing was evaluated. Additional in vitro studies were performed using a simulated shunt–ventricular system model.

Results.—Sixty-five percent of examinations depicted CSF flow through the shunt tube, and measured flow velocities were 5–7 cm/sec. The remaining 7 examinations showed no flow; this included 3 examinations performed before revisions for a blocked shunt. The in vitro studies demonstrated that clear CSF, per se, is not visible on ultrasound. However, choroid plexus debris and other particulate matter can produce a useful Doppler signal, with the probe insonating over the length of the shunt tubing. Doppler ultrasonography can depict turbulence at the junction points of the shunt system or at the exit of the peritoneal tube, probably because of the presence of microbubbles.

Conclusions.—Color Doppler imaging may be useful for imaging of CSF flow through VP shunts. The reason why some shunts do not show

CSF flow are unknown; the CSF in these shunts may contain no particulate matter, or shunting may be intermittent through the day. This imaging technique requires training and is not suitable for small children who cannot remain still for 10–15 minutes. However, it is a noninvasive technique that uses existent technology and, therefore, warrants further investigation.

▶ Serendipitously, the authors observed CSF flow through the peritoneal limb of a VP shunt system when performing a conventional abdominal ultrasound examination. This prompted their interest in studying the application of this technology to assess VP shunts that were suspected to be malfunctioning.

Over the years since the advent of CSF shunt systems, neurosurgeons have desired a noninvasive, reliable technique for assessing CSF flow through a shunt system. The "valvogram" and other diagnostic studies, including radionuclide, ultrasonic flow meter, and telethermographic tests, were developed. Unfortunately, each of these techniques had their shortcomings and proved to have a relatively high unreliability, especially in patients whose shunts had low flow.

Insonation with color Doppler imaging is a clever use of advanced ultrasound technology. Although the sensitivity of this test is still suboptimal, the rapid advances amd forecasted developments of this technology suggest that it holds some promise in fitting the bill.

S.R. Gibbs, M.A., M.D.

Cerebral Blood Flow and Autoregulation in Normal Pressure Hydrocephalus

Tanaka A, Kimura M, Nakayama Y, et al (Fukuoka Univ, Japan)
Neurosurgery 40:1161–1167, 1997   25–4

Background.—The authors encountered a patient with normal pressure hydrocephalus after a subarachnoid hemorrhage, confirmed by clinical improvement in the response to CSF shunting. As the patient's clinical condition and CT findings improved, the cerebral blood flow (CBF) increased. The findings suggested that ischemia may have resulted from CSF diffusion, causing functional disconnection of the cortex. The CBF and vascular responses to acetazolamide were examined in patients with normal pressure hydrocephalus.

Methods.—The study included 21 patients (mean age, 69 years) with normal pressure hydrocephalus. Each patient had CSF shunting performed after showing clinical signs of dementia. The response to acetazolamide in the white matter, cortex, and thalamus was assessed, including a comparison of patients who did and did not show clinical improvement after shunting. Cerebral blood flow was measured by xenon-enhanced CT.

Results.—Global reductions in CBF were noted before shunting in both groups, although the reduction was greater in patients who did not improve after shunting. For patients who improved later, the impairment of the vascular response was noted only in the white matter. As the patients' clinical condition improved after shunting, their CBF was restored, particularly in the white matter. The recovery of the vascular response in the white matter was noted as well. Nine patients studied by CT showed reductions in ventricular dilation and periventricular lucency. Twelve of the 21 patients did not show clinical improvement; this group had a reduction in CBF after shunting.

Conclusions.—For patients with normal pressure hydrocephalus whose condition improves with CSF shunting, the underlying disease appears to be ischemia. In these patients, CSF diffusion causes loss of autoregulatory capacity in the periventricular white matter. For patients who do not improve, CBF is reduced as a result of metabolic depression; although autoregulation is preserved in this group, they have irreversible brain damage. In patients with suspected normal pressure hydrocephalus, shunting will produce clinical improvement if the preoperative hemispheric CBF is greater than 20 mL per 100 g/min and the vascular response to acetazolamide is impaired only in the periventricular white matter. If the perioperative CBF is less than this, and the vascular response to acetazolamide is not impaired, shunting will not improve the patient's condition.

▶ Normal pressure hydrocephalus has various causes, a fair proportion of which are idiopathic. Tanaka et al. show that the measurement of CBF before and after shunting is a reliable method of predicting outcome. The Evans ratio on CT scans is another: patients with a ratio below 0.40 after shunting improve in contrast to those with a ratio above 0.40 who deteriorate. Most patients with normal pressure hydrocephalus that improve after shunting are those with histories of subarachnoid hemorrhages, whereas half of those that do not improve belong to the group with idiopathic hydrocephalus. Apparently, disturbances in CSF absorption that lead to normal pressure hydrocephalus (a common sequela of subarachoid hemorrhaging) respond well to the placement of a shunting device, whereas cases attributed to homeostasis deficits in brain parenchyma (related to idiopathic hydrocephalus) do not benefit from diversion of CSF. The usual option for treatment of hydrocephalus is the placement of a shunting device. However, it is the neurosurgical condition most frequently associated with long-term complications. The functioning of all shunts are based on rather similar hydrokinetic mechanisms, thus, the use of a "universal" shunting procedure for every patient with hydrocephalus disregards different causes. Studies like this will outline the distinctive pathophysiologic characteristics of different conditions associated with hydrocephalus so that we can design rational therapies that, in some forms of normal pressure hydrocephalus, may even obviate the shunting procedure.

J. Sotelo, M.D.

26 Neuro-imaging

Tuberculosis

Imaging of Tuberculosis: III. Tuberculosis as a Mimicker of Brain Tumour
Brismar J, Hugosson C, Larsson SG, et al (King Faisal Specialist Hosp, Riyadh, Saudi Arabia)
Acta Radiol 37:496–505, 1996   26–1

Background.—Unfortunately, tuberculous infections of the CNS are becoming more common, particularly in developing countries. Tuberculosis (TB) in the brain can mimic many other intracranial lesions. An experience with the clinical and neuroimaging characteristics of intracranial TB is reported.

Methods.—The study consisted of 46 patients (24 men and 22 women; mean age, 35 years) in whom clinical and CT findings indicated an intracranial tumor of unknown cause, but in whom TB was ultimately proven be the cause. All patients underwent CT scans, 25 of 46 also underwent cerebral angiography, and 9 of 46 also underwent MRI.

Findings.—Cultures or biopsies of brain material provided the diagnosis in 23 of 46 patients (50%), and the response to anti-TB drugs provided the diagnosis in another 19 (41%). Slightly more than half of the patients (24/46, 52%) had a hilar or mediastinal mass present in the lungs. Common symptoms when patients were first seen were headaches (31/46, 67%), seizures (15/46, 33%), blurred vision (10/46, 22%), vomiting (10/46, 22%), hemiparesis (8/46, 17%), and night sweats or fevers (4/46, 9%). The TB mimicked gliomas in 23 patients (50%), posterior fossa tumors in 6 (13%), meningiomas in 7 (15%), metastases in 9 (20%), and lymphomas in 1 (2%). The TB lesions were not limited to particular lobes or areas, rather they were scattered throughout the brain. Computed tomography indicated that most single lesions (average, 3 cm in diameter) were surrounded by edema and remained homogenous after contrast enhancement. Cerebral angiography generally revealed avascular mass lesions, although, in a few cases, it did rule out vascular changes that would have been expected had a tumor been present. In 4 of the 9 patients undergoing MRI, lesions had a hyperintense rim surrounding a hypointense center on T1-weighted images.

Conclusions.—The clinical and neuroimaging findings of intracranial TB are similar to those of other brain lesions. Nonetheless, TB can be reliably confirmed by biopsy or culturing of brain tissue and/or by the response to a trial of anti-TB therapy. Tuberculosis remains an important consideration in the differential diagnosis of patients with suspected intracranial tumors.

▶ The resurgence of TB in the developed world is attributed by the authors to a number of factors, including immigration from the undeveloped world, where TB is commonplace, the increase of HIV in the population, and the use of immunosuppressive therapy in transplantation and other therapeutic regimens. The authors share their experience from the unique perspective of their institution at a crossroads between the undeveloped and developed worlds. They reviewed a large number of patients with intracranial TB masquerading as supratentorial or posterior fossa malignancies, meningiomas, metastases, and lymphomas. They provide a useful, detailed description of the CT and MRI findings in each of these categories. It is noteworthy that, in their experience, the clinical history was usually noncontributory to the diagnosis, as were the chest radiograph and evidence of TB in other organs. In contrast, a clinical presentation that appeared unusually good for the lesions imaged in a particular patient was useful as a clinical indicator, as was a rapid response to a therapeutic trial of anti-TB medication.

G. Pjura, M.D.

Imaging of Tuberculosis: IV. Spinal Manifestations in 63 Patients
Lindahl S, Nyman RS, Brismar J, et al (King Faisal Specialist Hosp, Riyadh, Saudi Arabia)
Acta Radiol 37:506–511, 1996   26–2

Background.—Tuberculous infections of the CNS are difficult to diagnose, because their symptoms and neuroimaging results can mimic so many other abnormalities. Tuberculosis (TB) of the spinal cord, which reportedly occurs in only 1% of all patients with TB, is a particular diagnostic challenge, with a slow onset of symptoms and radiologic findings and a nonspecific clinical presentation. An experience with the radiographic findings in patients with spinal TB is reported.

Methods.—Cultures and/or spinal biopsies identified spinal TB in 63 patients (37 men and 26 women; mean age, 43 years) from a total of 503 patients with TB (i.e., a spinal TB incidence of 12.5% in patients with TB). All patients underwent conventional radiography, 54 (86%) also had a CT scan, and 9 (14%) had MR images of the spine. The location of the spinal lesion was assessed, as was the involvement of bony and soft-tissue structures.

Findings.—Tuberculous lesions were evident throughout the spine: 14 cervical lesions, 24 thoracic lesions, 24 lumbar lesions, and 4 sacral lesions were identified (some patients had multiple lesions). Involvement was limited to the spine in 40 patients (63%), whereas the other 23 patients (37%) also had lesions at other body sites (typically the chest). Focal destruction was evident in the vertebral body(ies) in 57 patients (90%), and the posterior element was involved in 30 patients (48%); approximately equal numbers of vertebrae (1 or 2) were involved. Vertebral bodies contained abscesses in 38 patients (60%). Paraspinal abscesses were found in 47 patients (75%), including psoas abscesses in 17 patients (27% of total). All but 1 patient (98%) had a paraspinal soft-tissue mass, and 15 patients (24%) had a solid granulation tissue type of mass. Other findings included concomitant disk lesion(s) in 43 patients (68%), epidural lesion(s) in 39 (62%), and gibbus formation at the same level as the TB involvement in 46 patients (73%).

Conclusions.—Both CT (to visualize the lesions) and MRI (to characterize the spread of disease to soft tissues) were necessary for the characterization of TB of the spine. As in other studies, the findings were varied and nonspecific; most commonly, the findings consisted of vertebral bony destruction and a paraspinal soft-tissue mass in association with abscesses, epidural spinal canal involvement, and gibbus formation.

▶ In this and a related article (see Abstract 26–1), the authors offer a valuable reminder that, in the context of the global village, exposure to infectious processes once considered eradicated in the developed world cannot be discounted, and infectious processes such as tuberculosis, which are notorious mimics of other pathologic processes, should be given due consideration. The authors cite substance abuse, poverty, an aging population, and the HIV epidemic, as well as immigration from the third world as factors contributing to this circumstance. They remind us that vertebral bony destruction with an associated paraspinal soft-tissue mass, abscess formation, involvement of the epidural space, or focal gibbus formation are typical findings in TB but are not the only presentations possible. The authors favor conventional radiography, CT, and MRI for the radiologic evaluation of the spine and report that the radionuclide bone scan and gallium scan yield unacceptably high false-negative results. Computed tomographic fine-needle aspiration was diagnostic in the majority of cases reviewed.

G. Pjura, M.D.

Computed Tomography and 3-D Angio-CT

Three-dimensional Computed Tomographic Angiography in Detection of Cerebral Aneurysms in Acute Subarachnoid Hemorrhage
Zouaoui A, Sahel M, Marro B, et al (Hopital de la Salpêtrière, Paris)
Neurosurgery 41:125–130, 1997   26–3

Background.—Currently, digital subtraction angiography (DSA) is typically used to detect aneurysms in the circle of Willis in patients with subarachnoid hemorrhages. However, CT angiography with 3-dimensional reconstruction of the intracranial vessels (3-D CTA) is a relatively new modality that should provide accurate information in this situation also. These authors compared DSA with 3-D CTA in imaging the circle of

Willis in patients with subarachnoid hemorrhages to determine if 1 modality has advantages over the other.

Methods.—Three-dimensional CTA was used in the emergency department to image 120 patients (69 women and 51 men; 20–75 years old) with suspected subarachnoid hemorrhages. In this process, initial unenhanced CT scans were obtained, then helical acquisitions were performed with a 1-mm/sec table speed at 1 mm collimation, with a 1:1 pitch on a 512 × 512 matrix. Axial data were then transferred to a workstation and a 3-D image was rendered. Forty patients underwent surgery based solely on the images rendered by 3-D CTA, and, in 7 of these, the postoperative results were also evaluated by 3-D CTA. Digital subtraction angiography was used preoperatively in 80 patients immediately after 3-D CTA and postoperatively in 40 patients.

Findings.—All 120 patients had either subarachnoid hemorrhages or hematomas. Of these, 107 had aneurysms (total of 129 aneurysms) in the supratentorial region ($n = 121$) or the posterior cerebral fossa ($n = 8$). In each case, 3-D CTA identified the aneurysm, and DSA confirmed this identification. Furthermore, 3-D CTA identified 2 aneurysms of the middle cerebral artery that DSA did not. On the 3-D CTA views, a branch of the middle cerebral artery always masked the aneurysm. In the 40 patients who underwent surgery based on 3-D CTA findings, DSA confirmed the results in each instance. Furthermore, DSA corroborated 3-D CTA results in the 7 patients who had both imaging procedures performed postoperatively. Three-dimensional CTA could always identify the neck of the aneurysm, whereas DSA sometimes could not identify this feature because of the limited number of views possible.

Conclusions.—Both 3-D CTA and DSA accurately identified aneurysms in these patients. In fact, 3-D CTA even found 2 aneurysms that DSA had missed. The disadvantages of 3-D CTA are that it requires IV contrast injection, it cannot be used for some patients (i.e., those with pacemakers, intubated patients), and its image quality degrades when low or turbulent blood flow is present. Nonetheless, 3-D CTA offers a quick, simple, noninvasive, and reliable alterative to DSA in evaluating most patients with suspected subarachnoid hemorrhages.

▶ Three-dimensional CTA offers a noninvasive alternative to conventional DSA in the detection of cerebral aneurysms in acute subarachnoid hemorrhages. The authors report a large series of 120 patients, in which they achieved excellent sensitivity (97.3%) and specificity (100%) using CTA. All their cases were confirmed by DSA, and no aneurysms were discovered by DSA that were not detected by CTA. As CT technology continues to advance, more favorable comparisons should result, and the respective positions of CTA and DSA in the diagnostic workup of a subarachnoid hemorrhage will change accordingly. Modern spiral CT scanning technology and workstations capable of more sophisticated postacquisition image analysis and display are significant factors in this transition. The authors of this article prefer the maximum intensity projection reconstruction format for its speed and ease of use; however, advances in CT and DSA techniques and automated bone-removal algorithms may expand the spectrum of available analysis tools, which could further improve the utility of CTA in providing more realistic 3-D images of intracranial vascular anatomy in the context of surrounding structures. Digital subtraction angiography will remain a highly valuable correlative diagnostic modality and an indispensable component of endovascular therapy in those situations in which this modality is preferred to surgery.

G. Pjura, M.D.

Intracranial Aneurysm: Inner View and Neck Identification With CT Angiography Virtual Endoscopy

Marro B, Galanaud D, Valery CA, et al (Groupe Hospitalier Pitié Salpétrière, Paris)

J Comput Assist Tomogr 21:587–589, 1997

26–4

Background.—Three-dimensional CT angiography (3-D CTA) is valuable in detecting intracranial aneurysms. In 1 case, 3-D CTA and virtual endoscopy were used to identify the origin of an aneurysm.

Case Report.—Woman, 44, underwent a CT scan evaluation for severe headaches of 1 weeks' duration. Three-dimensional CTA revealed a bilobate aneurysm in the left carotid artery, and surgery was performed to clip the neck of the aneurysm. Postoperatively, digital subtraction angiography (DSA) was used to confirm that the clip was placed correctly (which it was), but DSA also revealed a second aneurysm at the distal basilar artery. The neck could not be identified, nor could the aneurysm's relationship with the right anterosuperior cerebellar artery or the basilar artery be determined. A few months later, the patient was hospitalized for treatment of this second aneurysm, at which time another 3-D CTA image was obtained. Despite high-quality data acquisition, however, the origin of the aneurysm and its relationship to adjacent vessels could not be determined.

Therefore, the authors used virtual endoscopy software to reconstruct the endovascular region. The virtual endoscope was set slightly after the origin of the left posterior cerebral artery and was pointed toward the basilar artery. This view indicated that the aneurysm had no neck and that its origin partly involved the right anterosuperior cerebellar artery. Surgery confirmed the virtual endoscopic findings, and the aneurysm was surrounded by muscle and biological glue for containment.

Conclusions.—Three-dimensional CTA is as sensitive as cerebral angiography in identifying aneurysms and their necks, yet 3-D CTA is not invasive. Nonetheless, even 3-D CTA has shortcomings in some cases, and, in this case, the addition of virtual endoscopy supplied valuable information regarding the endovascular relationships. The fact that virtual endoscopy can be performed simultaneously with 3-D CTA is an advantage that warrants further application in the evaluation of patients with intracranial aneurysms.

▶ The continued evolution of 3-D CTA has increased its utility in the non-invasive detection and evaluation of intracranial aneurysms and, potentially, other intracranial lesions.

As the authors demonstrate, the information content in the 3-D data set may exceed the capability of conventional display formats to present the information in a manner most useful to the clinical decision maker. Rapid advances in 3-D workstation hardware and software and decreasing costs are making powerful image-rendering tools developed in the computer-aided design world available for diagnostic imaging. Virtual endoscopy is 1 of these techniques currently gaining favor in a variety of areas, where it enables unique perspectives of unusual lesions or difficult-to-visualize spaces. With further advances in this technology, other applications, such as virtual ventriculoscopy or virtual cisternography, may provide new, useful perspectives for surgical planning and other diagnostic or therapeutic interventions.

G. Pjura, M.D.

Initial Clinical Experience With Spiral CT and 3D Arterial Reconstruction in Intracranial Aneurysms and Arteriovenous Malformations
Rieger J, Hosten N, Neumann K, et al (Chirurgische Universitätsklinik des Klinikums Innenstadt, Munich; Freie Universität Berlin)
Neuroradiology 38:245–251, 1996   26–5

Background.—Because of its noninvasiveness (except for contrast injection) and speed, spiral CT (SCT) seems particularly well suited for imaging cerebral aneurysms. Three-dimensional (3-D) images can be readily constructed, and 1 or 2 SCT scans typically cover the area of the circle of Willis. The effectiveness of 3-D SCT in identifying intracranial aneurysms and arteriovenous malformations (AVMs) was evaluated by comparing results of 3-D SCT with those of digital subtraction angiography (DSA).

Methods.—Patients with suspected intracranial aneurysms or AVMs underwent 3-D SCT ($n = 32$) and DSA ($n = 31$). Spiral CT was performed at a table speed of 1 mm/sec, at a slice thickness of 1 mm, and in increments of 1 mm. Up to 4 SCT procedures were performed, depending on the size of the abnormality.

Findings.—Maximally effective SCT settings were a delay time of 14–17 sec, a scan time of 24 sec, a window width of 2,700–3,100 Hounsfield units, and a window center of 750–1,100 Hounsfield units. At these settings, all 9 aneurysms (diameters from 5 to 28 mm) and all 13 supratentorial AVMs were correctly identified by 3-D SCT. Three-dimensional SCT provided valuable information about the location of the aneurysm in relation to the parent vessels and about the AVM's extent, the distribution of the embolization material, and its main feeding vessel(s), nidus, and draining veins. Results of DSA confirmed those of 3-D SCT in every case in which DSA was also performed.

Conclusions.—-Three-dimensional SCT was as effective as DSA in identifying aneurysms and AVMs. Three-dimensional SCT quickly imaged these abnormalities and provided clear information on their relationships to parent vessels and feeding and draining veins. The disadvantages of 3-D SCT were that it did not describe the blood flow characteristics within the AVM (which MR angiography can do), and it did not offer high enough spatial resolution to distinguish small feeding vessels within these abnormalities. Nonetheless, at a minimum, 3-D CST should be considered a suitable, noninvasive follow-up for surgery, radiotherapy, or embolization therapy in patients with aneurysms or AVMs.

▶ The authors provide a detailed discussion of their early use of SCT and 3-D reconstruction of intracranial vasculature in the evaluation of aneurysms and AVM that is particularly instructive in its detailed exposition of the technical considerations that they used in successfully performing both image acquisition and postacquisition reconstruction and display of intracranial vascular anatomy. Their protocol after processing includes rather sophisticated 3-D reconstruction, with a shaded surface display of thresholded data that has the advantage of allowing the accurate juxtaposition of vasculature with respect to the anatomical landmarks of the calvarium. Other authors have used the simpler and faster maximum intensity projection technique in which the landmarks are not available. Using the authors' methods, arterial and venous anatomy can be visualized simultaneously and from any arbitrary direction. Although the data processing time reported by the authors is somewhat long in a routine clinical setting, as more powerful workstations become more widely available at lower cost and software becomes more operator friendly, this type of preoperative and postoperative evaluation should become more practical for surgical planning and follow-up.

G. Pjura, M.D.

Magnetic Resonance Imaging

Neuro-endoscopic Third Ventriculostomy: Evaluation With Magnetic Resonance Imaging
Wilcock DJ, Jaspan T, Worthington BS, et al (Leicester Royal Infirmary, England; Univ Hosp, Nottingham, England)
Clin Radiol 52:50–54, 1997
26–6

Background.—Ventricular endoscopy of the CNS is often used to manage hydrocephalus. Imaging studies, particularly MRI, are useful in describing the morphologic characteristics of the third ventricle and in identifying an appropriate puncture site. The use of neuroendoscopy guided by MRI to perform third ventriculostomy for hydrocephalus was evaluated.

Methods.—Prospective MRI identified 14 patients suitable for a neuroendoscopic third ventriculostomy. A noncommunicating type of hydrocephalus was present in 11 patients, 1 had a multicompartmental hydro-cephalus, and 2 with previous treatment for postmeningitic hydrocephalus had symptoms of shunt blocking. The preoperative MR image (T2-weighted image) was used to plan the route of the endoscope and to visualize the relationship between the basilar artery and the mammillary bodies. Once the endoscope was advanced into the floor of the third ventricle, septostomy was performed. Postoperative MRI scans (T2-weighted images) were performed to evaluate the presence or absence of CSF, and to compare preoperative and postoperative ventricular size and the appearance of the third ventricle, basal cisterns, and lateral ventricles. Follow-up has extended to 2 years.

Findings.—Endoscopic third ventriculostomy was successful in all but 1 of 14 patients, in whom a small foramen of Monro prevented entry of the endoscope. All 13 patients with successful operations either had clinical improvement or became asymptomatic after the operation. In 11 of these 13, postoperative MRI revealed a CSF flow void. The other 2 patients still received clinical benefit even though their surgery did not achieve a CSF flow void. Likewise, although all patients improved after surgery, only 8 had decreases in ventricular size.

Conclusions.—Endoscopic third ventriculostomy was enhanced by the use of preoperative and postoperative MRI. Magnetic resonance images were useful in planning the surgical approach, choosing the endoscope insertion site, determining anatomical relationships, evaluating postoperative CSF flow voids, and enabling comparisons between preoperative and postoperative appearances. A CSF flow void was seen more often than a decrease in ventricular size; thus, the absence of a CSF void is a better measure of a good clinical outcome.

▶ The authors present a prospective study on 14 patients with diagnoses of hydrocephalus who underwent endoscopic third ventriculostomy. All patients were imaged before surgery on a 1.5-T MR unit using a T2-weighted fast spin-echo sequence of the cerebellum in the transverse, axial, sagittal, and coronal oblique planes. The same pulse sequencing and planes were used after third ventriculostomy. Careful patient selection allowed 13 of the 14 patients to have a successful outcome. All patients were clinically improved and asymptomatic after the operation. The longest follow-up has been 2 years. A flow void was demonstrated in 11 of the 13 patients postoperatively. The ventricular size was decreased in only 8 of the 13 patients, even though they were clinically improved. This finding is consistent with the well-known fact that ventricular size may not decrease in patients undergoing third ventriculostomies, in spite of clinical improvement. Thus, it appears that the use of the T2-weighted turbo spin-echo sequence allows fast acquisition of images and gives diagnostic evidence of patency in 85% of patients with successful third ventriculostomies.

D.F. Jimenez, M.D.

MR Parameters for Imaging Titanium Spinal Instrumentation
Wang JC, Sandhu HS, Yu WD, et al (Univ of California, Los Angeles)
J Spinal Disord 10:27–32, 1997   26–7

Background.—Magnetic resonance imaging is the gold standard in evaluating the spine after internal fixation. However, metallic internal fixation devices in the spine distort the MR image, giving a metal artifact. Some reports have indicated that this distortion is less when the implant is composed of titanium. Thus, how well MRI handles metal artifacts caused by titanium spinal screws was evaluated.

Methods.—In 2 human cadavers, the spinous processes, lamina, and facet joints from T12 to S1 were exposed and cleaned. Then, 6.5-mm titanium transpedicular screws were inserted into the 6 pedicles of L4, L5, and S1. Also, laminar hooks were placed on both sides of the T12 and L1 lamina in a claw configuration. Screws and hooks were attached to rods, and the rods were linked together. These specimens were evaluated at various settings of spin-echo T1- and T2-weighted MRI to determine the quality of bone and soft-tissue resolution.

Findings.—At all settings used, bone, neural structures, and soft tissues were well defined. Best results with the T1-weighted image were measured at an echo time (TE) of 16 and a repetition time (TR) of 500–600. Best results with the T2-weight image were measured at a TE of 60 and a TR of 1,300–1,600. Best results with a hybrid image were measured at a TE of 16 and a TR of 1,300–1,600.

Conclusions.—A metal artifact caused by titanium screws, claws, and rods was minimal and did not affect image quality substantially. Thus, with the appropriate settings, T1- and T2-weighted MRI can be used to evaluate the postoperative course in patients with titanium spinal implants.

▶ Artifacts associated with stainless steel implants have severely limited imaging of the postoperative spine by either CT or MR. The introduction of titanium alloy spinal hardware has significantly improved the MR images of the instrumented spine. To develop optimal imaging techniques for this new instrumentation, the authors used cadaveric specimens implanted with titanium pedicle screws and investigated a range of TE and TR values to determine those that provided the optimal T1- and T2-weighted images of the lumbar spine. The authors do not state the manufacturer, model, or field strength of the MR unit used for their experiment; however, the TR and TE values presented are appropriate for a 1.5-T magnet. Their findings should provide a good starting point for anyone interested in optimizing an imaging protocol with this field strength magnet. Those using other field strength magnets can make appropriate adjustments. Our institution has had similar success imaging titanium alloy fusion cages with a T1 magnet. To further minimize the interference from artifacts, one should take care to avoid using any surgical instrumentation that might implant minute ferrormagnetic particles in the bone or surrounding structures while one is installing these prosthetic devices.

G. Pjura, M.D.

Miscellaneous

Assessment of Pseudarthrosis in Pedicle Screw Fusion: A Prospective Study Comparing Plain Radiographs, Flexion/Extension Radiographs, CT Scanning, and Bone Scintigraphy With Operative Findings
Larsen JM, Rimoldi RL, Capen DA, et al (Rancho Los Amigos Med Ctr, Downey, Calif; Southwestern Orthopaedic Med Corp, Thousand Oaks, Calif)
J Spinal Disord 9:117–120, 1996   26–8

Objective.—Pseudarthrosis can be responsible for failed spinal fusion, but this is difficult to document on imaging studies. Few studies have compared the radiographic and surgical findings in this situation; the sensitivity and specificity of radiography are unknown. The situation is further complicated by the use of transpedicular instrumentation. The imaging and surgical findings of patients who had undergone lumbar fusion with stainless steel pedicle screws were compared.

Methods.—The prospective study included 25 patients who reported prolonged pain after lumbar posterolateral fusion using Selby pedicle screw instrumentation. All were to undergo surgery for removal of the fixation hardware and inspection of the fusion. Preoperatively, each patient underwent imaging studies—such as plain radiography, flexion and extension radiography, CT, and bone scanning—to rule out pseudarthrosis. Each of these studies was evaluated in blinded fashion by a radiologist, who made an interpretation of fusion or pseudarthrosis. These interpretations were compared with the surgical findings.

Results.—Sixteen patients were found to have fusion at surgery, whereas 9 were found to have pseudarthrosis. None of the imaging studies, singly or in combination, was significantly correlated with the surgical findings. Plain radiography and CT correctly predicted the surgical result in only about 62% of cases.

Conclusion.—Preoperative imaging studies—including plain radiographs, flexion and extension radiographs, CT, and bone scintigraphy—cannot reliably predict the presence of pseudarthrosis in patients with pedicle screw fixation. Such preoperative studies are inaccurate and non–cost-effective. The findings also call into question previous radiographic studies to determine fusion status.

▶ This study was done with a small but select group of patients already scheduled for hardware removal and fusion inspection. Intraoperative fusion inspection compared with the preoperative radiographic studies showed no statistically significant predictive value to these studies for determining fusion vs. pseudoarthrosis.

This is a difficult problem that most, if not all, spinal surgeons face at 1 time or another. It is especially difficult to assess fusion status when instrumentation and its associated artifact obscures the pertinent anatomy.

Nevertheless, as these tests are noninvasive and the experience of this study is small, my question to the authors is, are you confident enough of your data to propose to your patients the possibility of a straightaway reoperation with none of these tests previously performed?

Pseudoarthrosis and failed spinal fusion using transpedicular instrumentation and bone grafting are some of the main causes of long-term postoperative back pain. Before the operation, careful assessment using noninvasive tests is a rational choice for differentiating structural vs. functional causes that may ultimately modulate new surgical strategies and/or direct a patient's postoperative therapeutic plan. These tests are time consuming and expensive. However, I believe they are useful in assessing the overall architecture of the spine and the construct. In addition, it is not rare for patients who have already demonstrated degenerative changes at 1 level to have other problems develop at another level of the spine, especially at disk spaces adjacent to the level of fusion. Therefore, we must keep in mind that, although these studies may be obtained in an attempt to determine fusion vs. pseudoarthrosis, they may yield other findings that provide insight into the patient's persistent postoperative discomfort. Although the study included only 25 patients, it does provide good evidence that spinal surgeons cannot confidently rely on radiographic studies for determining fusion status. After careful and thoughtful evaluation of the other causes for persistent postoperative back pain, the surgeon may conclude that a patient will require a definitive determination of fusion status by reoperation and direct inspection.

M.-A. Perez-Espejo, M.D., Ph.D.

Intraoperative Angiography in Cerebral Aneurysm Surgery: A Prospective Study of 100 Craniotomies
Alexander TD, Macdonald RL, Weir B, et al (Univ of Chicago)
Neurosurgery 39:10–18, 1996   26–9

Introduction.—With the use of mobile C-arm image intensifiers, making intraoperative angiograms is a simple and practical matter. The effects of these studies on the surgical procedure are uncertain, however. The rate of unexpected findings was evaluated in a series of 100 consecutive intraoperative angiograms performed in patients undergoing surgery for cerebral aneurysm. Predisposing factors and complications were assessed as well.

Methods.—All patients underwent intraoperative, digital subtraction angiography after aneurysm clipping. Variables recorded included patient age and sex, intra-arterial aneurysm location and size, mode of presentation, interval between hemorrhage and surgery, and clinical grade. Immediately after clipping, the surgeons recorded whether they believed the aneurysm was occluded and whether they believed the clip occluded a major artery. All angiograms were performed with the patient's head secured in a radiolucent cranial pin head-holder. Patient positioning on a wooden spine board allowed easy access for the C-arm under the patient's head. Angiograms were performed in at least 2 planes after injection of iohexol. An additional thirty patients did not undergo angiography, most often because the aneurysm was wrapped rather than clipped.

Results.—Twelve patients had unexpected angiographic findings requiring clip adjustment. The adjustments led to restored patency of 6 major arteries and complete obliteration of 10 persistently filling, residual, or second aneurysms. Eight percent of aneurysms measuring less than 2.5 cm in diameter required clip adjustment, as did 36% of giant aneurysms. It took a mean of 30 additional minutes to perform intraoperative angiography. There was 1 cerebral infraction attributed to an embolic source, which was regarded as a complication of intraoperative angiography. Another asymptomatic infarction may also have been a complication of angiography. On logistic regression analysis, factors significantly associated with major arterial occlusion were giant aneurysm, needle aspiration or opening of the aneurysm, and aneurysm at the basilar apex. Patients with giant aneurysms and aneurysms of the posterior communicating artery were more likely to be incompletely clipped.

Conclusions.—In patients undergoing clipping of intracranial aneurysms, intraoperative angiography reveals unexpected findings requiring clip adjustment in approximately 12% of cases. The complication rate is approximately 2%, and the false negative rate is approximately 5%. Risk factors for unexpected findings include giant aneurysms and aneurysms located at the basilar apex or posterior communicating artery. Knowledge of these risk factors might make intraoperative angiography a cost-effective procedure.

▶ The article by Alexander et al. is sobering when read in the context of the ongoing, sometimes acrimonious debate with our friends and colleagues who promote the endovascular approach to the treatment of cerebral aneurysms. Some surgeons take heart in the relatively high rate of incomplete occlusion reported by our endovascular colleagues. However, this paper reiterates that incomplete surgical obliteration and, worse, inadvertent arterial occlusion, are not negligible accompaniments to the surgery of cerebral aneurysms. One advantage that the surgeon has over his or her endovascular colleague is that, usually, he or she can reposition the clip or clips to achieve complete occlusion. If this can be done during the initial surgery, then so much the better. Most surgeons would, I think, nonetheless, not favor the routine use of intraoperative angiography—the unexpected findings with regard to the posterior communicating artery notwithstanding— but would rather favor its selective use in those cases where technical difficulties are anticipated. The authors identify these difficult cases as those with giant aneurysms, with basal apex aneurysms, and with aneurysms in proximity of the posterior communicating artery. The question of cost-effectiveness is, I suppose, unavoidable. Thus, intraoperative angiography may be cost-effective only in those cases where it negates the need for postoperative angiography, but it is precisely in these selected, difficult cases that one would be concerned with the not-negligible false-negative rate of intraoperative angiography and would wish to see a high-resolution, detailed, multiple-view postoperative angiogram. Cost-effectiveness notwithstanding, the recognition of an inadvertently occluded artery and its correction before an infarct ensues is of unquestioned benefit to the individual patient.

R. Leblanc, M.D., M.S.C., F.R.C.S.C.

Fasting Improves Discrimination of Grade 1 and Atypical or Malignant Meningioma in FDG-PET
Cremerius U, Bares R, Weis J, et al (Aachen Univ, Germany)
J Nucl Med 38:26–30, 1997   26–10

Background.—Meningiomas may be affected by glucose and by drugs that influence gluconeogenesis, such as corticosteroids. Therefore, the uptake of glucose by meningiomas might differ when patients are fasting, compared with when they are not fasting. The use of positron emission tomography (PET) with labeled glucose (2[^{18}F]fluoro-2-deoxy-D-glucose [FDG]) determined whether meningioma FDG uptake does differ in the fasting and nonfasting states and whether the use of corticosteroids influences FDG-PET findings.

Methods.—Seventy-five patients (51 women and 24 men; mean age, 58 years) with meningiomas underwent FDG-PET studies. These studies were performed after an overnight fast ($n = 51$) or 3–5 hours after breakfast ($n = 24$). High-dose corticosteroids were used by 27 patients (20 in the fasting group, 7 in the nonfasting group). Standardized uptake values (threshold of 5.5) and the tumor-to-gray-matter ratio (1.05 for the 57 primary tumors and 0.85 for the 18 recurrent meningiomas) were used as indicators of FDG uptake. According to the World Health Organization (WHO) classification system, histologic examination identified 66 grade I, 6 grade II, and 3 grade III lesions.

Findings.—In all but 2 patients, the uptake of FDG was homogeneous within a patient. Based on the standardized uptake values, FDG-PET correctly identified 51 of 66 grade I tumors and 8 of 9 grade II/III tumors, which yielded a specificity of 0.77. Overall, the tumor-to-gray-matter ratio was a more sensitive indicator of tumor grade than was the standardized uptake value. Based on the tumor-to-gray-matter ratios, FDG-PET tended to be more sensitive in identifying lesions in the patients who had fasted and in patients who did not use corticosteroids. Specifically, FDG-PET was significantly more sensitive in identifying the tumor grade in the research subjects who had fasted (42 of 44, or 96%) than in the research subjects who had not fasted (16 of 22, or 73%). Furthermore, plasma glucose and insulin levels were significantly lower in the patients who had fasted than in the group that had not fasted. Insulin levels were significantly higher in the patients taking corticosteroids than in those not taking corticosteroids.

Plasma glucose levels were similar in the patients undergoing primary surgery vs. reoperation, but patients with tumor recurrences had a significantly higher standard uptake value in the reference gray matter. The standard uptake value in reference gray matter was also lower in patients taking corticosteroids.

Conclusions.—Fasting significantly improved the specificity of the tumor-to-gray-matter ratios for the grading of meningiomas. In cases in which FDG-PET overestimated the histologic grade, hyperglycemia in the patients who had not fasted probably played a role. Thus, patients who undergo FDG-PET for the estimation of meningioma grade should fast overnight before the procedure.

▶ The diagnosis and grading of meningiomas using FDG-PET requires attention to the complex physiologic factors that influence the uptake and metabolism of FDG and glucose by both normal and pathologic tissue. The authors provide a valuable insight into the importance of 1 of these factors, overnight fasting, in maximizing the specificity of FDG-PET in differentiating between atypical or malignant and grade I meningiomas. To obtain the maximum benefit from PET and other nuclear medicine imaging procedures, one must recognize that these modalities are largely predicated on physiologic rather than anatomical differentiation, and, as a consequence, meticulous attention to the details of physiology and metabolism, and ongoing medical therapy, among other factors, is necessary for deriving the maximum benefit from these procedures.

G. Pjura, M.D.

27 Neurosurgical Infections

Ventriculostomy Infections: The Effect of Monitoring Duration and Catheter Exchange in 584 Patients
Holloway KL, Barnes T, Choi S, et al (Med College of Virginia, Richmond; Univ of California, San Diego; Univ of Texas, Galveston; et al)
J Neurosurg 85:419–424, 1996   27–1

Introduction.—There is no consensus regarding the effect of the duration of intracranial pressure (ICP) monitoring on the risk of an infection in patients with ventriculostomy catheters. Another debate concerns whether replacing the old catheter with a new one at certain time intervals is beneficial. The relationship between ventriculostomy infections and ICP monitoring duration and prophylactic catheter exchange was retrospectively evaluated in 584 patients with closed-head injuries.

Methods.—Data were obtained from the Traumatic Coma Data Bank and the Medical College of Virginia Neurocore Data Bank regarding the incidence of ventriculostomy infection, the effect of catheter duration on ventriculitis and meningitis, and daily infection rates. Patients were monitored for a mean of 7.5 days.

Results.—The mean catheter duration was 5.06 days. Of 584 patients, 61 had ventriculitis (10.4% incidence rate). Of 76 patients who died during monitoring, 3 had infections. The daily infection rate (calculated for all catheters and first catheters only) peaked at days 10–12, then diminished rapidly thereafter. There was no difference in infection rate in patients whose catheters were replaced before 5 days and those whose catheters were exchanged at more than 5-day intervals. The incidence of infection in 97 patients with multiple catheter exchange was comparable for first, second, and third catheters.

Conclusion.—The risk of infection in patients with ventriculostomy catheters increased over the first 10 days, then diminished rapidly. Infection rates were lowest in the first 4 days. There were no significant differences in patients who did and patients who did not have catheter exchanges every 5 days. It is recommended that ventriculostomy catheters for ICP monitoring be removed as quickly as possible. There seems to be no benefit in catheter exchange in patients who require extended ICP monitoring.

▶ A prospective report published in the *New England Journal of Medicine* in 1984 advocated the prophylactic removal of all ventriculostomies by day 5 to decrease infection rates.[1] After this report appeared, it became standard practice to remove external ventricular drains by day 5. The authors report on their experience with a large number of external ventricular drains and infection rates. Their prospective study of 584 patients with severe head injuries indicated that there appeared to be no benefit for catheter exchange to prevent ventriculostomy infections. I am in complete agreement with this concept. Our own experience with close to 300 patients does not indicate that there was a linear correlation between the length of indwelling catheter and infection rates. Perhaps most important are the placement technique and the catheter maintenance. The authors' careful analysis of risk factors, which included craniotomy, intraventricular hemorrhage, sex, age, intracranial air, steroids, and duration of catheter in place, did not reveal any correlations to infection rate. Overall, this is an excellent report that supports the notion that automatic ventriculostomy replacement is not necessary or cost-effective.

D.F. Jimenez, M.D.

Reference

1. Mayhall CG, Archer NH, Lamb VA, et al: Ventriculostomy-related infections. A prospective epidemiologic study. *N Engl J Med* 310:553–559, 1984.

Management of Postoperative Infections After Spinal Instrumentation
Levi ADO, Dickman CA, Sonntag VKH (Mercy Healthcare Arizona, Phoenix)
J Neurosurg 86:975–980, 1997   27–2

Background.—Infections caused by spinal instrumentation occur in up to 8.5% of vertebral surgical procedures. An understanding of which factors affect the development of infection might help to control these factors and reduce this serious complication. The clinical characteristics, operative management, and outcomes in patients with spinal instrumentation who developed infections were evaluated.

Methods.—A chart review identified 452 patients who underwent spinal instrumentation, of whom 17 (3.8%; 10 men and 7 women; mean age, 57.3 years) had infections. Patients with infections before the procedure, or who had infections only at the bone-graft donor site, were excluded from the analysis. A control group of 17 patients who did not have infections was matched for the type of instrumentation used. The infection risk factors of previous surgery, steroids, diabetes, malnutrition, intercurrent infection, skin disruption, paralysis, smoking, and rheumatoid arthritis were each assigned a score of 1, and the summed risk factor score was compared between patients and controls.

Findings.—All patients underwent débridement of the infected wound, and a closed irrigation–suction system was used in 13 patients (76.5%) and left in place for a mean of 5 days. All 17 infections occurred after posterior or posterolateral spinal instrumentation procedures, but the hardware had to be removed in only 1 patient. Most infections (9, or 53%) were caused by *Staphylococcus aureus*, and 5 patients (29%) had mixed organisms; 1 patient each had infection with *Streptococcus* sp, *Proteus mirabilis*, or an unidentified organism. Also, most infections (14, or 82%) were deep infections (extending below the fascia). Patients who had infections spent an average of 16.6 extra days in the hospital (either for readmission or based on when they would have been discharged had an infection not developed). These patients also had a significantly higher mean risk factor score (2.18) than did patients in the control group (0.71). At a minimum of 8 months of follow-up, all patients are infection free.

Conclusions.—Infections are significantly more likely after procedures involving a posterior or a posterolateral approach. Most of these infections are deep, and the closed irrigation–suction system provided adequate drainage. Although some infection risk factors cannot be influenced, some can, such as nutritional supplementation for malnourishment, cessation of smoking, and so forth. In addition to improving risk factors when possible, these authors advocate operative débridement of the infected wound, IV and oral antibiotics, the use of a closed irrigation–suction system for 5 days after surgery, and maintenance of the instrumentation rather than removal.

▶ Instrumental implants have been broadly developed to treat spinal disorders in which stabilization is the main goal. These operative procedures are frequently laborious, and deep paraspinal muscle retraction is usually required. This superb article, in my opinion, precisely deals with important and practical subjects related to 1 of the most threatening problems: postoperative wound infections, which can produce catastrophic consequences in terms of the final outcome. Preoperative conditions inherent to patients and intraoperative characteristics, such as surgical time and muscle ischemia caused by excessive retraction, are categorized as risk factors for postoperative infection. The study also analyzes the standard points of the treatment to be done systematically, with a special emphasis on local irrigation–suction devices, general IV antibiotic systems, and surgical débridment; the study points out that, in the vast majority of cases, the infection can be controlled without removal of the hardware, thus maintaining good stabilization as solid bone graft fusion is achieved. The "Hamletian dilemma" (which is usually crucial in any operative procedure in which implants are used and from which an infection can occur), "to remove or not to remove," is solved in this article definitively and intelligibly.

M.-A. Perez-Espejo, M.D., Ph.D.

Primary Reconstruction for Spinal Infections

Dietze DD Jr, Fessler RG, Jacob RP (Univ of Florida, Gainesville)
J Neurosurg 86:981–989, 1997   27–3

Background.—Bone fusion is often necessary for vertebral stabilization in spinal osteomyelitis. However, when present, an infection can affect the results of fusion. The effects of infection during bone grafting and instrumentation in spinal reconstructions were examined.

Methods.—This retrospective review identified 27 spinal infections that developed in 25 patients, 35- to 76-years-old, undergoing primary vertebral reconstruction. Patients with iatrogenically acquired spinal infections were excluded from analysis. Surgical decompression was used in 26 cases, and, in 1 case, bed rest and antibiotics resolved the back pain and infection. Of the 26 surgical decompressions, 20 involved reconstruction for spinal instability by vertebral arthrodesis; 15 of these 20 also required surgical débridement and spinal instrumentation. All patients were also treated by either parenteral or oral antibiotics for 4.5 months; the 2 patients with tuberculous infections were treated with isoniazid, rifampin, and pyrazinamide for 1 year.

Findings.—Risk factors for spinal infection included immunocompromise in 8 patients, urinary tract infections in 7, diabetes mellitus in 5, obesity in 5, and smoking in 5. *Staphylococcus aureus* was identified in 60% of cases, and *Salmonella* sp, *Proteus* sp, and *Staphylococcus epidermidis* were also identified. After an average of 16 months of postoperative follow-up, radiographs showed fusion in 18 of 20 patients with vertebral arthrodesis, and 17 had an improved clinical status with improvement or resolution of axial pain. The major complications included 2 urinary tract infections, 1 deep wound infection that required débridement, 1 case of congestive heart failure, 1 case of pneumonia, and 1 case of atrial fibrillation. No recurrent spinal infections were noted during an average postoperative follow-up of 37 months.

Conclusions.—With aggressive treatment of infections, vertebral reconstruction can be performed during the primary surgical procedure. Management included surgical débridement of the infected wound, spinal reconstruction with arthrodesis and instrumentation, and prolonged antibiotic therapy. Spinal instrumentation is not contraindicated; however, its use should be reserved for clear cases of spinal instability.

► The use of autologous bone grafts has been advocated for many years as effective treatment for spinal infectious disorders. Aggressive débridement also seems to be a rational procedure for cleaning the infective focus before performing any bone grafts. This point, in my opinion, is important, no matter what type of instrumentation is going to be used to enhance stabilization on any spinal segment. I would like to emphasize this matter, because an effective débridement can produce both a safe substratum for healthy bone restoration and a good bed to receive metallic implants. Of course, the possibility of a very delayed, symptomatic, cryptic, infection caused by the instrumentation may still exist, even after the use of long-lasting, high-dosage courses of appropriate antibiotics; however, the combination of these strategies—deep focal débridement, autologous bone grafting, and aggressive medical treatment—seems to be crucial for avoiding the unnecessary removal of implants. Although more extensive series are needed to definitively prove such a hypothesis, this article gives a glimpse of that possibility as a fact in the future.

M.-A. Perez-Espejo, M.D., Ph.D.

28 Neurosurgical Work Force Issues

Work Force Requirements for Neurosurgery
Popp AJ, Toselli R (Albany Med College, NY; Univ of North Carolina, Chapel Hill)
Surg Neurol 46:181–185, 1996   28–1

Introduction.—Neurosurgeons represent less than 1% of all practicing physicians. Nonetheless, work force studies report that neurosurgery is a specialty with an oversupply of practitioners. Work force requirements for neurosurgery are discussed.

The Issues.—The present ratio of full-time equivalent (FTE) neurosurgeons to the population are 1:62,000 for unmanaged care in the United States, 1:150,000 for managed care in the United States, 1:500,000 in Great Britain, 1:132,000 in Austria, and 1:2,000,000 in India. The actual number of neurosurgeons required to offer optimal coverage for a population is controversial and depends partly on the type and intensity of patient care offered by neurosurgeons. An undersupply of neurosurgeons means suboptimal delivery of needed services. An oversupply means that there are less surgeries for each physician to perform. It has been shown that better surgical results are observed with higher volumes.

The Right Size.—In 1986, the Council on Graduate Medical Education recommended that the government should not influence the size of graduate medical training because of uncertainties in health planning. The number of physicians pursuing graduate medical education rose by more than 20% from 1988 to 1994. Despite this, neurosurgeons do not have difficulty finding employment, and areas remain for which the availability of FTE neurosurgeons to population is short, even for managed care standards. Surgical procedures yield 75% of a neurosurgeon's income but only 25% of the neurosurgeon's time. It is not possible to predict the development of new operative techniques or changes in medicine. Work force analysis is difficult and inexact in the rapidly changing medical field. Without changes in antitrust laws, the ability to limit or reduce the number of practicing neurosurgeons is not possible.

Possible Strategies.—The quality of neurosurgical practice must be maintained at its highest level. The neurosurgical community must galvanize its efforts to maintain its portion of the practice of medicine. It must speak with 1 voice. A work force study group should be created that represents all components of neurosurgery. There is a need for "right-sizing," but neurosurgeons must take an active part in the ongoing dialogue about human resources—or be dependent on the information and perception of others.

The Overproduction of Neurosurgeons Jeopardizes Future Neurosurgical Care

Stranjalis G (Hygeia Hosp, Athens, Greece)
Surg Neurol 45:314–319, 1996   28–2

Introduction.—There are too many neurosurgeons in some parts of the world (Table 2). At the present rate, there will be twice as many neurosurgeons in Greece by the beginning of the next century for the same population base. Possible ways to decrease this number in Greece include immediately reducing the number of neurosurgical units and centralizing facilities, dramatically decreasing the number of residents, having an information campaign for general practitioners and neurologists about new techniques and methods, and considering subspecialization as an immediate measure to counteract underemployment and unemployment. This analysis focuses on Greece, but is not restricted to Greece.

Commentary.—The reactions in this commentary originate from the following places:

São Paulo, Brazil.—There are too many neurosurgeons in Brazil, and many are undereducated.

London, England.—Some measure of control is the responsibility of the government.

TABLE 2.—Numbers of Neurosurgeons in Other Countries

COUNTRY	NUMBER OF NEUROSURGEONS	NEUROSURGEON/ POPULATION
USA	4,156	1:61,000*
Canada	193	1:142,000
Japan	3,561	1:35,000
Brazil	1,609	1:96,000
Mexico	280	1:377,000
Europe	6,594	1:121,000
European Union	2,200	1:160,000
Greece (1994)	160	1:62,500
Greece year 2000	280	1:36,000
Asia	9,618	1:336,000
Africa	361	1:1,900.000
World wide	23,940	1:210,000

*Clinical and nonclinical neurosurgeons included.
(Reprinted by permission of the publisher from Stranjalis G: The overproduction of neurosurgeons jeopardizes future neurosurgical care. *Surg Neurol* 45:314–319. Copyright 1996 by Elsevier Science Inc.)

New Delhi, India.—India has a paucity of neurosurgeons. This causes both an excessive clinical burden on already limited staff and long waiting lists. There is little time for academic activities and research. What is needed is a way to attract neurosurgeons from overpopulated areas to underpopulated areas. The World Federation of Neurosurgical Societies may be able to organize mutually beneficial programs.

Tokyo, Japan.—The average number of neurosurgeries per neurosurgeon is 28 per year in Japan. Patients usually treated by neurologists in Japan are being seen by neurosurgeons, as the number of neurologists is small. Young neurosurgeons are finding work in various related fields.

Multan, Pakistan.—Pakistan needs more neurosurgeons, as there is 1 per 2.4 million individuals.

Wynberg, South Africa.—Millions of individuals in Africa do not have access to neurosurgical care. The need for neurosurgery cannot be approached in isolation. It must be approached as part of a total health care system.

Conclusion.—The problem of neurosurgical care is 1 of overproduction in some areas of the world and underproduction in others. With the cooperation of the world-wide neurosurgical community, it may be possible to solve these inequalities.

Neurosurgery Workforce in Canada, 1996 to 2011
Hugenholtz H, for the Canadian Neurosurgical Society (Ottawa Gen Hosp, Ont, Canada)
Can Med Assoc J 155:39–48, 1996   28–3

Introduction.—There were 197 neurosurgeons in Canada in 1990, compared with 170 in 1995. There is concern among neurosurgeons that the demand for their time will become so high that they will need to abandon their academic and administrative responsibilities. Reported is an analysis by the Canadian Neurosurgical Society on Canadian neurosurgery human resources.

Methods.—The projected attrition, supply, and shortfall of neurosurgeons for the years of 2001 and 2011 were estimated for Canada using a resource-based analysis of need, population:physician ratios, predictions of vacant neurosurgery positions, and physician surveys.

Results.—All 174 clinically active neurosurgeons in Canada responded to the survey. An average of 76% of neurosurgeons' time was allocated to clinical practice. About 25% of neurosurgeons committed 40% of their time to administration, teaching, or research. Nearly 90% of neurosurgeons considered themselves to be working at or above their preferred capacity. Only 19 respondents reported they were available to see more patients. Neurosurgeons perform surgery an average of 15 hours per week—about one third during evenings, nights, or weekends. Almost half of neurosurgery graduates left Canada after they became certified. It is estimated that Canada will lose 62 neurosurgeons by the year 2001, and

181 neurosurgeons by the year 2011 to retirement and relocation. The top reasons for retirement and emigration were inadequate pay, institutional inflexibility, and obstacles to accessing appropriate resources. Only 5% of neurosurgeons were satisfied with the environment for neurosurgery.

Conclusion.—To make up for the current shortage of neurosurgeons, Canada must increase its neurosurgery work force by 50% in the next 5 years. Strategies must be developed for addressing the factors influencing the exodus, for providing incentives to stay, for increasing the number of physicians willing to specialize in neurosurgery, and for recruiting neurosurgeons from outside of Canada.

▶ How many neurosurgeons does the world need? Only King Solomon would be able to answer that question. Almost every country in the world is experiencing neurosurgical work force problems and issues. In many countries, there are simply too many neurosurgeons (e.g., the United States, Brazil, Greece, Spain, and probably Japan); in other countries, there are too few (e.g., Canada and countries in Asia and Africa). On 1 hand, a surplus of neurosurgeons in any country is a waste of human resources, time, and money. On the other hand, a shortage produces pain and suffering.

If King Solomon were presiding, he would no doubt advise that neurosurgeons in each country realistically study their citizens' needs and develop strategies that meet their nation's neurosurgical requirements. Once tested, successful approaches could be shared by all nations, regardless of how developed they were.

In developing countries, where neurosurgeons are usually in short supply, governments could take the lead in meeting neurosurgical needs by increasing neurosurgical training programs or by contracting with other countries to train and supply neurosurgeons. These governments would also adequately support staff neurosurgeons by providing reasonable remuneration, adequate equipment, and clinical autonomy. In countries with neurosurgical surpluses, market pressures would ultimately cut the oversupply by forcing neurosurgeons into relatively new areas of clinical practice, such as pain management, intervascular specialties, rehabilitation medicine, and further subspecialties. In addition, these neurosurgeons would reclaim clinical arenas, such as carotid artery surgery and peripheral nerve surgery, lost to other surgical subspecialists. In an effort to reduce residency slots, some governments would even pay hospitals large sums of money not to train physicians (41 New York hospitals have already volunteered to participate in such a program, sponsored by the U.S. federal government).

Clearly, this is all very complicated; inevitably, however, each nation must help itself. Furthermore, because King Solomon is not presently among us, neurosurgeons themselves must be a part of the discussion and the solution.

S. Pelofsky, M.D.

29 Pediatric Neurosurgery

Technique of Stereotactic Biopsy in a 5-month-old Child
Kondziolka D, Adelson PD (Univ of Pittsburgh, Pa)
Childs Nerv Syst 12:615–618, 1996   29–1

Objective.—Because of concerns over the risks of injury from pin fixation, stereotactic surgical techniques are rarely used in patients less than 2 years old. However, the advantages of stereotactic biopsy and radiosurgery are sometimes needed in this age group. A new method of stereotactic frame fixation for younger children that avoids the need for skull pin fixation is described.

Case Report.—The technique was developed for use in a 5-month-old girl with a growing lesion in her right thalamus. Stereotactic biopsy was indicated because of the need to obtain a histologic diagnosis. The stereotactic frame was first attached to the CT table, then the child was placed into the frame. Semirigid foam was used to support the body and the head extending out from the CT table. Fixation pins were aimed at locations associated with strong fixation. Each pin was advanced into the hollowed end of a rubber top from a Vacutainer blood sampling tube. The rubber tops were then compressed onto a 15-mm diameter area of the skin, which provided firm head fixation. There was no skull deformation, and postoperative imaging confirmed target accuracy. Biopsy specimens showed evidence of an anaplastic astrocytoma.

Discussion.—This technique provides firm head fixation without skull pin fixation, permitting stereotactic biopsy in infants and small children. Firm head control is achieved by 4-point pressure fixation, and the child's body weight is transferred directly to the CT scanner table. This procedure extends the benefits of stereotactic surgery to young infants with deep-seated brain lesions.

▶ All commercially available stereotactic neurosurgery frames have been designed for adults. Even the latest titanium-made models are too bulky and

315

heavy for the thin, malleable skull of a small child. Because of these structural features and the necessity for cranial pin fixation of the frames, young children would incur a considerable risk of head injury. Smaller and lighter "pediatric" frames can be developed, but they would be prohibitively expensive. A practical and inexpensive method for ensuring safe cranial pin fixation in children while using adult frames has been long overdue. The contribution of this article is twofold. First, small children with intracranial deep-seated lesions can now benefit from the precision of stereotactic neurosurgical management. Second, this report is an example of how solutions to practical problems in the application of medical treatment can take advantage of the potential clinical uses of an immense reservoir of instruments, tools, and materials that are available in the modern world.

D.E. Sakas, M.D.

The Relevance of Hemodynamic Factors to Perioperative Ischemic Complications in Childhood Moyamoya Disease

Iwama T, Hashimoto N, Yonekawa Y (Natl Cardiovascular Ctr, Osaka, Japan; Univ of Zürich, Switzerland)
Neurosurgery 38:1120–1126, 1996   29–2

Background.—The most common manifestation of childhood moyamoya disease (spontaneous occlusion of the circle of Willis) is cerebral ischemia. Cerebrovascular reconstructive surgery may prevent a further ischemic insult, but perioperative ischemic complications may occur. The significance of hemodynamic factors to perioperative complications in childhood moyamoya disease was investigated.

Methods and Findings.—One hundred twenty-four children younger than 15 years undergoing surgery for moyamoya disease were reviewed. Twenty-one (16.9%) had perioperative ischemic complications that could not be attributed unequivocally to surgery. Eleven of these children had infarctions, and 10 had reversible ischemic neurologic deficits without new lesions. Children with and without ischemic complications had similar mean values of intraoperative and postoperative minimum arterial carbon dioxide pressure, maximum arterial carbon dioxide pressure, and mean arterial pressure. However, the incidence of preoperative transient ischemic attacks (TIAs) and intraoperative and postoperative hypercapnia was significantly greater in patients with perioperative complications. Also, 7 of the 11 perioperative infarctions occurred in children with frequent preoperative TIAs and intra- and postoperative hypercapnia. On cerebral blood flow studies with preoperative acetazolamide loading, the new infarctions were found in regions with compromised cerebral blood flow.

Conclusions.—The occurrence of frequent preoperative TIAs is an important indicator of the instability of cerebral hemodynamics and the risk of perioperative ischemic complications. Preoperative management designed to stabilize hemodynamic status is very important for preventing these complications. Children with moyamoya disease who have frequent preoperative TIAs are at risk for ischemic brain damage caused by hypercapnia, as well as hypocapnia and hypotension. Establishing and maintaining normocapnia with normotension are important in the perioperative management of moyamoya disease in children.

▶ It is crucial for a surgeon to know the predictive factors of a good postoperative outcome. The results presented by Iwama et al. provide such information on the effects of cerebrovascular reconstructive surgery in moyamoya disease. Despite the fact that the patient population is limited to children, the authors' findings are more universal and may apply to all patients whose insufficient cerebral blood flow is surgically treated. The finding of the additive effect of preoperative TIAs and intraoperative hypotension and hypocapnia on perioperative ischemic complications is not surprising. The state-of-the-art treatment of these patients includes an avoidance of hypotension and hypocapnia; however, it is surprising and a very important finding that the number of perioperative ischemic complications dramatically increases in patients with TIAs and perioperative hypercapnia. "Steal phenomenon" is most likely responsible for the complications. This observation emphasizes the value of careful perioperative monitoring of the respiratory condition of the patients and maintenance of normocapnia. Furthermore, the excellent surgical result in the group without TIAs and hypercapnia suggests that aggressive, preventive surgery may be of value for children with moyamoya disease.

R.M. Pluta, M.D., Ph.D.

Quinolinic Acid in Tumors, Hemorrhage and Bacterial Infections of the Central Nervous System in Children
Heyes MP, Saito K, Milstien S, et al (Natl Inst of Mental Health, Bethesda, Md; Children's Natl Med Ctr, Washington, DC)
J Neurol Sci 133:112–118, 1995   29–3

Background.—Quinolinic acid (QUIN), a neurotoxic metabolite of the kynurenine pathway, accumulates in the CNS after immune activation. Whether QUIN levels are increased in the CSF in children with CNS infections, hydrocephalus, tumors, or hemorrhages was investigated.

Methods and Findings.—Fifty-one CSF samples were obtained from 43 patients' shunt implants. Patients with bacterial infections of the CNS had very high QUIN concentrations, despite treatment with antimicrobial drugs. In patients with hydrocephalus or tumors, CSF QUIN levels were increased to a lesser degree. Increases in CSF L-kynurenine levels paralleled accumulations in QUIN, which is consistent with an increase in activity of the first enzyme of the kynurenine pathway, indoleamine-2,3-dioxygenase. Patients with infections also had increases in the CSF levels of neopterin, a marker of immune and macrophage activation. The cytokines, tumor necrosis factor-α and interleukin-6, were also found in some samples, and the levels were highest in patients with infections.

Conclusions.—Quinolinic acid appears to be a sensitive marker of immune activation in the CNS. Further research is needed on QUIN as a potential contributor to neurologic dysfunction and neurodegeneration in children with CNS inflammation.

▶ This study convincingly demonstrated that QUIN, a neurotoxic metabolite of the kynurenine pathway, is elevated in the CSF of children with CNS infections. Quinolinic acid was also elevated, but to a lesser degree, in children with hemorrhages or tumors. Further studies aimed, in particular, at correlating the clinical outcome of these patients with the levels of QUIN are needed to enforce the ambitious hypothesis of the authors that this metabolite could be a contributor to neurologic dysfunction and neurodegeneration in children.

O. Vernet, M.D.

N. de Tribolet, M.D.

30 Pituitary Disorders and Surgery

SIPAP—A New MR Classification for Pituitary Adenomas
Edal AL, Skjödt K, Nepper-Rasmussen HJ (Odense Univ, Denmark)
Acta Radiol 38:30–36, 1997

30–1

Purpose.—Magnetic resonance imaging is the imaging technique of choice for diagnosis of pituitary adenomas. The need for some simple and useful MRI classification for these lesions has become increasingly apparent. An MRI classification to describe tumor delineation, the tumor's relationship to juxtasellar structures, and the tumor size is reported.

Methods.—The classification system was developed from a retrospective study of 56 patients with biochemically or surgically confirmed pituitary adenomas. The analysis included a total of 87 midfield MRI scans, including sagittal T1-weighted spin-echo and coronal T1-weighted 3-dimensional fast-field echo sequences before and after IV contrast administration. The system was designated SIPAP, an acronym for the 5 juxtasellar directions of tumor extension to or penetration into adjacent structures of the sellar-region. A 6-figure number was used to describe each adenoma, and the directions of interest were suprasellar; infrasellar; parasellar, right and left sides; anterior; and posterior. The first 4 directions were graded on coronal MRI scans, and the last 2 were graded on sagittal images.

Results.—The classification system was well adapted to the study patients. Using the SIPAP system, the authors classified all tumors except 1 postoperative remnant. The system proved useful before and after treatment, for long-term follow-up, and for comparing adenomas with different hormonal activity in terms of patient age and sex.

Conclusions.—The SIPAP system is described as a useful means of classifying pituitary adenomas from MRI scans. When used with tumor size, it provides an optimal method for registration of pituitary adenomas. It provides a broad overview of tumor extension for the neurosurgeon and can correlate the problems to be expected during surgery. The SIPAP classification is useful in classifying tumors before treatment and in following them over time.

▶ Tumors of the sellar and para-sellar regions are difficult to grade or classify, especially if they are irregular or invasive. The first attempt was made by Hardy using anatomical bony landmarks and PEG, followed by Wilson, who used grading of sellar destruction and stage of extra sellar extension, combining tumor size with its extension, based on radiographic and operative findings. This study uses the more precise MRI advantages, combining the above mentioned classifications with the 1993 Knosp-Steiner classification thus predicting the involvement of the cavenous sinus through the use of a very important landmark: the intercarotid line. However, it does not take into account the size and volume of the tumor, as proposed by Lundin and Pedersen in 1992, and these data will have to be added to the final grading. This classification will be an important addition when reporting larger series of cases pre- or postoperatively or pharmacologically treated tumors. However, for planning individual cases, the old aphorism still prevails, "A good image is worth a thousand words."

R. Marino, Jr., M.D.

Endoscopic Pituitary Surgery: An Early Experience

Jho H-D, Carrau RL, Ko Y, et al (Univ of Pittsburgh, Pa)
Surg Neurol 47:213–223, 1997

30–2

Introduction.—Based on experience with endoscopic sinonasal surgery, an endonasal endoscopic transsphenoidal approach to surgery of pituitary tumors was developed. Working under the operating microscope, the authors used a rigid fiberoptic endoscope and a sublabial, transseptal approach for operating on pituitary tumors in 4 patients. This experience prompted incisionless endoscopic transsphenoidal pituitary surgery, performed via a nostril, in 11 additional patients.

Technique.—The procedure is performed with 4-mm sinonasal rigid endoscopes, most often with 0- and 30-degree-angled lenses. The procedure is usually performed through 1 nostril, with no retractor or speculum. After outfracture of the middle turbinate, the sphenoid ostium is identified. Surgeons should hold the endoscope in their nondominant hand while performing an anterior sphenoidotomy. Once this is accomplished, the endoscope is transferred to a custom-made holder to provide a steady image and to allow the surgeon to work with both hands. The sphenoid sinus is inspected with the 30-degree-angled endoscope, but the 0-degree endoscope is mainly used to perform the operation. Pieces of removed bone are saved for reconstruction of the anterior wall. A microdrill or curettes are used to open the anterior wall. Microadenomas are removed with micropituitary rongeurs, microsuction, and pituitary curettes, and normal pituitary tissue is preserved. For macroadenomas, the 30-degree endoscope is inserted into the sella and its diaphragm, after the extrasellar extension of the tumor. The arachnoid membrane is identified, and the arachnoid plane is preserved, if possible. The tumor mass is removed carefully under direct visualization, and microsuction is applied at the tumor and pituitary interface. A free fat graft from the abdomen is used to plug the dural defect, and a watertight seal is confirmed by Valsalva maneuvers. The anterior wall of the sella is reconstructed using the previously saved pieces of bone. The sphenoid sinus is packed with absorbable gelatin film, which is also laid over the sphenoidotomy and splinted in place.

Experience.—The experience included 9 women and 6 men (median age, 43 years). Four patients had microadenomas, 4 had intrasellar macroadenomas, 3 had macroadenomas with suprasellar extension, 3 had invasive macroadenomas involving the cavernous sinus with suprasellar extension, and 1 had a metastatic adenocarcinoma. In the 13 patients with pituitary adenomas, symptoms resolved after surgery. A partial response to surgery was achieved in a patient with recurrent prolactinoma; this patient went on to have gamma knife radiosurgery. Postoperative fractionated radiotherapy was used in 2 patients, 1 because of a residual pituitary adenoma in the cavernous sinus and the other because of a metastatic adenocarcinoma. The latter patient—who was the first treated by an endonasal endoscopic approach—had a postoperative CSF leak that required endoscopic packing of a fat graft.

Conclusions.—An incisionless, endonasal endoscopic transsphenoidal approach to pituitary surgery is reported. By avoiding an open incision and postoperative nasal packing, this approach enhances postoperative recovery. It provides an excellent view of the sphenoid sinus and the sellar and suprasellar structures. Improved visualization permits more complete tumor removal, while preserving pituitary function and avoiding neuro-vascular injury.

► Although this is not the first report of endoscopic transsphenoidal pituitary surgery, the refinement and reintroduction of this technique by Jho et al. are propitious. The trend toward less invasive, short-stay surgical procedures, combined with the technological advances of stereo–video endoscopy, may place this approach among some of the most significant in the long historical development of surgical approaches to the pituitary. Sir Victor Horsley (1889) was reportedly the first to attempt removal of a pituitary adenoma through a transcranial approach in 1907, and Schloffer reported the first successful transsphenoidal pituitary resection through a lateral nasal approach. Kocher (1909) was the first to report using a submucosal approach, and Hirsch (1909–1910) used a transseptal approach with a nasal speculum. In 1910, Harvey Cushing combined the advantages of the various techniques to-date to develop the oronasal midline rhinoseptal transsphenoidal approach. Frasier (1912) introduced an intracranial transfrontal approach to the pituitary that Cushing later adopted because of the higher incidence of recurrence through the transsphenoidal approach. In 1962, Hardy refined the transsphenoidal approach using the operating microscope and intraoperative fluoroscopic guidance, and Guiot (1963) reported the first endoscopy-guided transsphenoidal adenoma resection.[1]

Although this paper describes an early experience with a relatively small number of patients, Dr. Hae-Dong Jho will likely take his place in this lineage of surgeons.

As with any procedure, patient selection for endoscopic pituitary surgery is of paramount importance. Clearly, these authors have not surmounted every obstacle that may be seen with this technique, but they have reported what appears to be a safe endonasal endoscopic transsphenoidal approach to the pituitary when performed by those skilled in the use of the endoscope.

S.R. Gibbs, M.A., M.D.

Reference

1. Palmer JD: *Neurosurgery 96: Manual of Neurosurgery.* New York, Churchill Livingstone, 1996.

Endoscopic Transseptal Transsphenoidal Surgery for Pituitary Tumors
Yaniv E, Rappaport ZH (Rabin Med Ctr, Israel; Tel Aviv Univ, Israel)
Neurosurgery 40:944–946, 1997   30–3

Background.—Operations for pituitary tumors are often performed using a transseptal, transsphenoidal approach. For wide exposure and a correct approach to the sphenoid sinus, the sublabial approach is most often used. This and the open rhinoplasty approach require removal of both nasal cartilage and the vomer; this can lead to septal perforations and dental anesthesia. The use of endoscopic nasal and sinus surgery to overcome these complications is reported.

Technique.—The procedure is performed using a 0-degree, 4-mm, rigid nasal endoscope. The endoscope is used to open the anterior wall of the sphenoid sinus. The initial incision is made in the posterior third of the septum and removes only the vomer. The vomer is saved for use in reconstructing the sellar floor. With the sphenoid sinus opened, a Hardy speculum is inserted, and the operation is performed with the operating microscope.

Experience.—The authors have used this approach in 14 patients with pituitary adenomas. None of the patients had any complications associated with the endoscopic approach, such as rhinal symptoms, nasal discharge or bleeding, or septal perforation. All had normal nasomaxillary sensation.

Discussion.—An endoscopic transseptal approach to the sphenoid sinus for pituitary surgery is reported. This simple, time-saving technique minimizes nasal operative morbidity. The operating microscope can be used with binocular vision and bimanual operation. Intrasellar inspection outside the line of sight can be carried out with angled endoscopes.

Endoscopy Assisted Transsphenoidal Surgery for Pituitary Adenoma
Jho H-D, Carrau RL (Univ of Pittsburgh, Pa)
Acta Neurochir (Wien) 138:1416–1425, 1996   30–4

Introduction.—The standard approach to surgery for pituitary adenomas is a microsurgical transsphenoidal one. On the basis of experience with endoscopic sinonasal surgery, the authors decided to apply endoscopic techniques to pituitary surgery. They described their technique of endoscopic transsphenoidal surgery for a pituitary adenoma via a nostril.

Technique.—The procedure is performed using 4-mm, 0- and 30-degree rigid endoscopes under fluoroscopic guidance. The endoscope is handheld until the anterior wall of the sella is exposed and its vertical dimension is identified by fluoroscopy. The endoscope is then mounted on a holding device. A microdrill or curettes are used to open the anterior wall of the sella, and the opening is enlarged using micro-Kerrison rongeurs. Microadenomas are removed through an opening of the anterior wall of the sella adjacent to the tumor. After being coagulated, the dura mater is opened in cruciate fashion using curved single-bladed microscissors or a scalpel. A micropituitary rongeur is used to removed enough of a specimen for pathologic analysis; the rest of the tumor is then removed while preserving normal pituitary gland tissue. After checking for CSF leakage, the surgeon closes the anterior sellar wall using a piece of bone from the septum of the sphenoid sinus.

Macroadenomas extending to the suprasellar region are removed with a 30-degree endoscope positioned at the caudal portion of the nasal cavity. Depending on the rotation of the endoscope, this provides a superior view toward the suprasellar tumor, a lateral view toward the lateral wall of the sella, and an inferior view toward the floor of the sella. Suprasellar tumors are removed circumferentially along the edge of the diaphragma sellae using a curved suction cannula. The arachnoid membrane is left intact, and normal pituitary gland tumors are preserved, if possible. The eye of the tumor, with its attached pituitary stalk, is the last to be removed. Any remaining part of the tumor is removed after careful inspection, but the intracavernous portion of the tumor is left in place. An abdominal-free fat graft is used to create a water-tight seal in the sella. Leakage of CSF or extreme extrusion of the fat graft are checked for by repeated Valsalva maneuvers and are managed appropriately.

Experience.—The authors have used their endoscopic technique in 45 patients with pituitary adenomas. Complete tumor resection was achieved in 34 patients, and subtotal resection was achieved in the rest; most of the residual tumors were located in the cavernous sinuses. The residual tumors were managed by stereotactic radiosurgery, bromocriptine, or observation.

One patient had CSF leakage, and another had postoperative sphenoidal sinusitis.

Discussion.—An endoscopic approach to transsphenoidal surgery for pituitary adenomas is reported, including 2 illustrative case reports. With experience and technical refinement, the use of approach has yielded good short-term surgical results, minimal morbidity, and a quick recovery for the patient. Endoscopy promises to play an increasingly important role in pituitary surgery and other areas of neurosurgical practice.

31 Spinal Disorders

Operative Techniques

Comparison of Lumbar Sagittal Alignment Produced by Different Operative Positions

Stephens GC, Yoo JU, Wilbur G (Univ of Kentucky, Lexington; Case Western Reserve Univ, Cleveland, Ohio)
Spine 21:1802–1807, 1996   31–1

Objective.—For patients undergoing lumbar fusion, intraoperative positioning is critical to postoperative sagittal alignment. Positions involving a lesser degree of lordosis permit better access to the spinal canal and intervertebral disks while reducing blood loss. The intraoperative position should create physiologic lordosis while maintaining the balance of the sagittal plane. Common operating positions were compared to determine which reproduce normal lumbar lordosis.

Methods and Results.—Studies were performed in normal subjects positioned on tables commonly used for lumbar fusion. With the subjects positioned on the Jackson table, radiographs indicated a mean total lumbar lordosis of 52 degrees, which was not significantly different from the standing position. With subjects on the Andrews table with the hips flexed 90 degrees, mean lumbar lordosis was 17 degrees, a 67% reduction from the standing position.

Conclusions.—For patients undergoing lumbar fusion, positioning in the prone position on a Jackson table produces a physiologic lordosis not significantly different from the standing position. Positions that reduce physiologic lordosis will lead to a positive sagittal plane balance postoperatively, which may lead to low back pain. It is important to use a position that reproduces physiologic lordosis when performing spinal fusion with instrumentation.

▶ Postoperative painful stiffness has been, particularly in earlier times, not an exceptional condition after transpedicular instrumentation and bone grafting for lumbar spinal fusion. In addition, in several cases of "overfixation," the instruments can interfere with the spine dynamics, and this could be one of the causes of persistent back pain or even of the fracture of the instrumentation itself, particularly when the standing position is resumed. In the present article, the authors seem to demonstrate the capital importance of a good and physiologic lumbar positional "recipient" of the implants, as the main goal of any lumbar fixation is to restore as much as possible the normal lordotic configuration of this spinal segment. Therefore, preoperative patient preparation and position, using a Jackson or similar surgical table, is a very important starting point for a better outcome.

M.-A. Perez-Espejo, M.D., Ph.D.

Microsurgical Anatomy of the Lateral Approach to Extraforaminal Lumbar Disc Herniations

Reulen H-J, Müller A, Ebeling U (Ludwig Maximilians Univ, Munich; Berne Univ, Switzerland)
Neurosurgery 39:345–351, 1996   31–2

Purpose.—Many groups have recommended a microsurgical "lateral" approach to extraforaminal lumbar disk herniations (ELDHs). Experience with this procedure has shown that the anatomy of the intertransverse process region may vary significantly, complicating the surgical approach. Anatomical variations of the bony structures of the lateral approach were studied.

Methods.—The cadaver study included 31 lumbar spine specimens—most consisting of 5 single lumbar vertebrae and the sacrum—from subjects who died at 30–93 years of age. Caliper and compass measurements were done to determine the relative distances and the proportions of the operative window. The findings were analyzed for relevance to the lateral approach to ELDHs.

Results.—From the L1–L2 to the L5–S1 level, the operative window became progressively smaller. Across this span, the isthmus laminae—which serves as the medial boundary of the medial intertransverse space—extended farther laterally, eventually covering the waist of the vertebral body. As the lower boundary, the facet joint was found to overlap the disk space as it moved upward and laterally. Downward movement of the transverse process—the upper boundary—was noted as well. The L5–S1 level was the most likely to show anatomical variations.

Conclusions.—The bony anatomy of the lateral approach to ELDHs is studied. From L1–L2 to L3–L4, the lateral neural foramen can be exposed by lateral retraction of the paraspinal muscles, avoiding trauma to the facet joint. A paramedian transmuscular approach can be valuable at L4–L5 and L5–S1. A plain radiograph should be obtained before surgery to analyze the potential anatomical variations and individualize the operative approach.

▶ Extraforaminal lumbar disk herniations, particularly at the lower spinal levels, are not exceptional conditions and usually require a difficult approach to avoid a neglected part of the herniated material compromising the roots. The resection of facets through a wide bone is commonly required. The authors of the present article have studied very carefully the measurements of the "lateral" intervertebral windows that can be created, with minimal muscle or bone distraction or resection to avoid damage to facet joints and periradicular tissue, with consequent postoperative pain. Using a great rationale, the authors proposed a far lateral approach, particularly in L4 to S1 extraforaminal herniated disks. I wish, finally, to emphasize the importance of the segmental innervation and vascular network of the paraspinal muscle apparatus, which can usually be preserved using the tangential route to approach those "extra"-lateral lumbosacral herniated disks, as overdistraction and sometimes authentic spinal "demolitions" would be required if the conventional midline route were used.

M.-A. Perez-Espejo, M.D., Ph.D.

A New Microsurgical Technique for Minimally Invasive Anterior Lumbar Interbody Fusion

Mayer HM (Freie Universität Berlin)
Spine 22:691–700, 1997

31–3

Background.—Anterior lumbar interbody fusion has been used for more than 60 years, yet it may be associated with unacceptable surgical trauma. Two new microsurgical techniques, 1 via a retroperitoneal approach between L2 and L5 and 1 via a transperitoneal approach to L5-S1, are suggested to achieve anterior lumbar interbody fusion.

Methods.—All 25 patients (16 females and 9 males, 16–82 years old) had disabling segmental instability and low back pain; 22 had sciatica, 12 had sensory deficits, and 10 had motor deficits. The first 20 patients underwent retroperitoneal microsurgery, in which they were placed in the right lateral decubitus position on a surgical table. The table was tilted back according to the lumbar level to be approached, and the incision was made over the craniocaudad and anteroposterior projection of the center of the disk space. All incisions were made parallel to the muscle fibers until the retroperitoneal space was exposed. After preparation of the retroperitoneal space, a spreader frame was placed on adjacent vertebral bodies to allow placement of the screws. Screws were inserted into the vertebral bodies and served as an anchor for cranial and caudal spreader valves to deflect the psoas muscle and retroperitoneal vessels. Autologous iliac bone was then grafted to complete the fusion.

The last 5 patients in the series underwent a transperitoneal microsurgical approach, in which they were placed in the Trendelenburg position with hyperextension of the lumbar spine. The surgeon stood between the patient's legs and made a 4-cm incision in the abdomen, centered over L5-S1. A surgical microscope was used for the procedure. The intraperitoneal cavity was carefully exposed, and the retroperitoneal space was retracted to expose the anterior circumference of L5-S1. Autologous iliac bone was then grafted to complete the fusion.

Findings.—For the first group, the mean operative time was 111 minutes, and the mean intraoperative blood losses were 67.8 mL at the fusion site and 78.8 mL at the donor site. For the second group, the mean operative time was 134 minutes, and the mean intraoperative blood loss was 168 mL at the fusion site and 172 mL at the donor site. None of the 25 patients required drainage at the fusion site or blood transfusions. No complications occurred, and only 6 patients required analgesics for more than 48 hours after surgery. Postoperative CT scans revealed packing of the graft at the appropriate sites in an oblique, transverse direction (for the first 20 patients) or in a sagittal direction (for the last 5 patients). All CT scans at follow-up (range, 7.8–15.3 months) showed complete fusion. Furthermore, only 6 patients reported low back pain, only 3 patients had sensory deficits (which were nonetheless improved over preoperative levels), and no patient had sciatica or a motor deficit.

Conclusions.—Both of these procedures achieved anterior lumbar interbody fusion with negligible surgical trauma, little intraoperative blood loss, and no complications. Given that all segments from L2 and S1 could be approached, these procedures may be an alternative to laparoscopic techniques. However, further research is needed to compare these results with those of traditional fusion surgery.

▶ Anterior lumbar interbody fusion was first described for the treatment of spondylolisthesis and has been used ever since for a variety of spinal lesions and deformities, generally when the pathologic condition is of the anterior spine. Some of the most common indications for this procedure include severe degenerative intravertebral disk disease and painful pseudarthrosis. Spinal infections and neoplasms, as well as corrections of spinal deformities, may warrant this approach. Traditionally, this has been through a transperitoneal or retroperitoneal approach. Dr. Mayer has presented a "minilaparotomy" approach to the L2-3 through the L5-S1 disk spaces using microsurgical modifications of the traditional approaches to the anterior lumbar spine. Although the skin incision is only 4 cm, the exposure of the anterolateral circumference of the disk space is the same as in a conventional retroperitoneal approach. He reports a mean operating time of less than 2 hours for the retroperitoneal approach and 2.25 hours for the transperitoneal operation. In addition, he reports low intraoperative blood loss and decreased incisional discomfort. This may be a technique to consider adding to the minimally invasive surgical armamentarium.

S.R. Gibbs, M.A., M.D.

Threaded Fusion Cages for Lumbar Interbody Fusions: An Economic Comparison With 360° Fusions
Ray CD (Spinal Research and Education Found, Norfolk, Va)
Spine 22:681–685, 1997   31–4

Introduction.—Solid spinal fusion can be obtained using interbody bone grafts. Various mechanical measures can be used to stabilize the graft material during fusion, and they play an important role in enhancing the rate and quality of fusion. The threaded fusion cage (TFC) is a recently developed concept of spinal fusion that is gaining acceptance. The economic aspects of the TFC technique were compared with those of the well-established pedicle screw and rod stabilization (360-degree fusion) technique.

Methods.—The study included 50 patients undergoing spinal fusion for severe, disabling back pain with diskal degeneration during a 4-year period. Ray TFCs were used for fusion in 25 patients, whereas the rest underwent anteroposterior interbody fusion using pedicle screws by the 360-degree technique. The procedures were performed by the same surgeon in the same hospital. The 2 techniques were similar in clinical efficacy and complication rates; all fusions were deemed solid by established radiologic criteria. The 2 groups were compared for surgical and hospitalization costs, operating times, and blood loss attributed to fusion at 1 and 2 lumbar levels. The costs associated with the 2 techniques were assessed in inflation-corrected 1995 U.S. dollars.

Results.—The average combined surgical, hospital, and anesthesiologist costs for 1-level TFC procedures were about $25,000 compared with nearly $42,000 for equivalent 360-degree fusion procedures. The difference was approximately 40%. For 2-level cases, the average approximate cost was $33,000 for TFC procedures and $47,000 for 360-degree fusion procedures; this was a difference of 30%. Preferential use of the TFC saved an average of nearly $15,000 per case, or $400,000 for the 25-patient subgroup. An additional cost of nearly $9,000 per case was added by the need for instrumentation removal in 10 patients in the 360-degree fusion group. None of these patients required surgery to an adjacent level for transition syndrome, however. Thus, the final difference between the 2 groups was nearly $23,000. The percentage of billed costs actually collected was 81% for the TFC cases vs. 73% for the 360-degree fusion cases. At an average follow-up of 24 months, none of the patients in the TFC group had a fusion transition syndrome requiring a second fusion procedure, and none had to have a cage removed because of instrumentation-related pain.

Conclusions.—In patients undergoing lumbar interbody fusion, the TFC technique can significantly reduce overall surgical and hospitalization costs. These cost reductions, in addition to reduced surgical time and blood loss, are a major factor in selection of the TFC method, assuming similar fusion successes, clinical outcomes, and complication rates. The authors call for further use and comparative study of the TFC technique.

Threaded Steinmann Pin Fusion of the Craniovertebral Junction
Apostolides PJ, Dickman CA, Golfinos JG, et al (St Joseph's Hosp, Phoenix, Ariz; Univ of Michigan, Ann Arbor)
Spine 21:1630–1637, 1996

31–5

Background.—Although many techniques are used to treat patients with occipitocervical instability, none have achieved universal popularity.

An experience with immediate rigid fixation via wiring a threaded Steinmann pin to the occipitocervical region is reported.

Methods.—Occipitocervical stabilization was required for 39 patients (22 females and 17 males; 8–79 years old). Causes of the instability included rheumatoid arthritis in 12 patients, congenital anomalies in 12 patients, trauma in 10 patients, tumor in 4 patients, and osteogenesis imperfecta in 1 patient. After surgical exposure, the posterior rim of the foramen magnum was enlarged, and the laminae of the cervical vertebrae were notched to improve passage of the sublaminar wires. Then, 2 or 3 burr holes were drilled into the foramen magnum to hold the Steinmann pin. The wide-diameter threaded stainless steel threaded pin was bent into a U shape and molded to fit the lordotic contour of the area. The pin was secured to the occiput and the cervical spine. Fusion was accomplished with the use of autologous iliac crest bone. In 14 patients, fusion alone was all that was required. In the other 25 patients, anterior ($n = 11$), posterior ($n = 7$), or combined ($n = 7$) decompression procedures were also needed. Basilar invagination was present in 15 patients.

Findings.—One patient died 1 month after surgery as a result of pulmonary complications. Of the 38 survivors, the occipitocervical construct was stable after an average follow-up of 38.9 months. One nonunion and 2 fibrous unions occurred, but the rest of the 35 unions were osseous. Although the 2 patients with fibrous unions had not achieved an osseous union after 34 and 40 months, respectively, neither had they had instability or subluxation. Pain improved in 37 of 38 patients (97%), and, of 31 patients with myelopathy, 30 (97%) showed substantial improvement. No patient had new, recurrent, or progressive basilar invagination, wound or graft site infections, CSF leakage, vascular injuries, or neurologic complications. Although the Steinmann pin broke in 2 patients and a wire broke in 1 patient, all these breaks occurred after osseous fusion was complete.

Conclusions.—The use of a threaded Steinmann pin was safe and effective in promoting osseous fusion in these patients with occipitocervical instability. In particular, the threads in the pin may help avoid basilar invagination of the odontoid into the foramen magnum because even the 15 patients with basilar invagination before surgery had none after surgery. This technique could be used in many patients, including those with rheumatoid arthritis, congenital anomalies, trauma, tumors, and osteogenesis imperfecta.

▶ This article is part technical note and part review of the outcome after 1 form of occipitocervical fixation very carefully carried out by a highly respected group of spinal surgeons. Their results and their honesty is to be congratulated.

After the good technical note there is a less focused results section. What I think requires emphasis is that the technique is confined to a relatively small subset of pathologic conditions in the area that cannot be treated by atlantoaxial fixation. It is the end-stage rheumatoid arthritis, the complex spinal problems, the tumors, and the very rare complicated trauma patterns that dictate that the joint "above" must be used. This use is also indicated for the patients who have had transoral odontoidectomies. I would guess, as with our own practice, that the technique can be used in less than half of the forms of fixation required in this area.

Furthermore, there are good reasons to avoid it: one of the points that the authors do not make but that is brought out in the article by Malcolm et al.[1] is that, because of the significant disability limited lateral rotation that the fixation imposes, many patients may no longer be able to drive a car.

In addition, the biomechanics have not been covered: as we understand the craniovertebral junction more, it is obvious why some form of segment saving (allowing the occiput to move on C1) may actually protect the construct and increase the chances of fusion. It is interesting that, in a surgical milieu that claims universal bone fusion in spinal surgery, 2 of their 12 patients with rheumatoid arthritis had fibrous unions despite internal and external yet did not come to grief; maybe fixation is enough.[2]

H.A. Crockard, F.R.C.S.

References

1. Malcolm GP, Ransford AO, Crockard HA: Treatment of non-rheumatoid occipitocervical instability. Internal fixation with the Hartshill-Ransford loop. *J Bone Joint Surg (Br)* 76–B:357–366, 1994.
2. Casey ATH, Crockard HA, Bland JM, et al: Surgery on the rheumatoid cervical spine for the non-ambulant myelopathic patient—too much, too late? *Lancet* 347:1004–1007, 1996.

Back Pain

Persistent Back Pain and Sciatica in the United States: Patient Characteristics

Long DM, BenDebba M, Torgerson WS, et al (Johns Hopkins School of Medicine, Baltimore, Md; Massachusetts Gen Hosp, Boston; Univ of California, Los Angeles; et al)
J Spinal Disord 9:40–58, 1996

31–6

Background.—Low back pain is common and can be seriously disabling. The characteristics of patients with persistent back pain and sciatica in the United States were reviewed.

Patient Characteristics.—Persistent low back pain occurs most commonly in persons in their mid- to late 30s and early- to mid-40s. Such patients are typically white, well educated, and generally wealthy. Most are employed, although some stop working because of their pain. Those who do quit tend to be less well educated and more likely to be involved in litigation. Typically, low back pain occurs intermittently for 10 years and is well localized. It varies considerably in severity. In addition to pain, most patients with persistent low back pain have a variety of motor and sensory deficits. Significant functional impairment at work, home, and play is associated with persistent low back pain. However, the typical patient does not experience significant psychological distress.

Most patients consult many health care providers, receive a variety of treatments, and take a range of medications to relieve their pain. A few undergo more aggressive treatment, such as surgery, intradiskal therapy, and narcotic and psychoactive drugs. None of these treatments has proved effective. Physical examination is not helpful for making a definitive diagnosis. Nonspecific manifestations, such as muscle spasm, tenderness, and trigger points, are common. Less common manifestations include motor weakness and sensory deficits in the lower extremities and reflex changes in the knees and ankles. The classic combination of reflex changes, motor weakness, and sensory deficits associated with specific protruded discs is very rare, though 1 in 3 patients has a diagnosis of disc herniation. Imaging studies show that most patients with persistent low back pain have spondylotic abnormalities involving root compression or lumbar instability. Root compression is the main cause of the complaint. The next most common diagnoses were myofascial syndrome and lumbar instability. Patients with persistent low back pain appear to be a distinct group of patient with low back pain.

▶ This work characterizes the "new" entity of persistent back pain and sciatica. It appears that the only differences between this group of patients and those carrying the label of chronic back pain relate to behavioral and psychological co-morbidities. Personally, I suspect that the basic spinal pathologic characteristics are similar for both of these groups and that it is only the coping mechanisms that differ. The demographics of the population with persistent back pain are very interesting. I am fascinated by the fact that most of these patients are in their 30s and 40s. What happens to the syndrome? As the patients get older do they improve or are they just less likely to seek medical attention? It is hoped that future reports from the National Low Back Pain Study will improve our understanding of this clinical entity.

V.C. Traynelis, M.D.

Combined Neuromuscular Electrical Stimulation and Transcutaneous Electrical Nerve Stimulation for Treatment of Chronic Back Pain: A Double-Blind, Repeated Measures Comparison
Moore SR, Shurman J (Ctr for Neurologic Study, San Diego, Calif; Scripps Mem Hosp, La Jolla, Calif)
Arch Phys Med Rehabil 78:55–60, 1997   31–7

Background.—Chronic back pain is difficult to treat, but transcutaneous electric nerve stimulation (TENS) has been found to be useful in most trials. No trials to date, however, have evaluated the use of neuromuscular electric stimulation (NMES) in these patients. These 2 methods, alone and in combination, were examined for the treatment of chronic back pain.

Methods.—Twenty-four patients (16 women and 8 men; mean age, 51 years) had chronic back pain (6 months' duration or longer; mean duration, 3.83 years) that was recalcitrant to other treatments. Treatment consisted of either conventional TENS, NMES, combined NMES–TENS, or placebo (via a modified TENS unit), self-administered over 5 consecutive hr/day for 2 days. During these 5 hours, various periods of stimulation were used: TENS and placebo were administered continuously for 5 hours, NMES was administered for three 10-minute periods with two 130-minute periods of no stimulation, and combined NMES–TENS involved one 10-minute and one 20-minute period of NMES with 3 periods of TENS stimulation. Treatments were discontinued for 2 days between treatments to minimize carry-over effects. Both before and after treatments, patients completed the Present Pain Intensity (PPI) subscale of the McGill Pain Questionnaire, a visual analog scale to measure pain intensity (VAS-I), and a visual analog scale to measure pain relief (VAS-R).

Findings.—The PPI and VAS-I measures of pain intensity decreased significantly after combined NMES–TENS treatment (by 30% for PPI and by 25% for VAS-I) compared with placebo (by 13% for PPI and by 11% for VAS-I), TENS alone (by 12% for both PPI and VAS-I), and NMES alone (by 17% for PPI and by 19%for VAS-I). Based on VAS-R scores, all 3 active treatments were significantly more effective for pain relief than placebo (combined NMES–TENS score, 59.3; TENS alone score, 47.2; NMES alone score, 48.5; and placebo score, 32.2). For both pain intensity and pain relief, combined NMES–TENS was significantly more effective than either TENS or NMES alone. Transcutaneous electric nerve stimulation alone and NMES alone provided relatively equal pain reduction and relief.

Conclusions.—A combination of NMES and TENS provided the greatest pain relief and reduction in pain intensity in these patients with chronic back pain. Transcutaneous electric nerve stimulation alone and NMES alone were equally effective for pain relief and reduction. These data should be considered preliminary, in that only conventional (not acupuncture-like) TENS was used and only three 10-minute periods of NMES were used. Nonetheless, the results with combined NMES–TENS are promising, and their combination may prove to be a valuable method for treating chronic back pain.

▶ This admittedly preliminary study may indicate some usefulness of NMES alone or in combination with TENS in the reduction of chronic back pain. This may become 1 of the nontraditional uses of NMES to be developed in the future. Neuromuscular electrostimulation has been shown to improve muscle tone and blood flow while decreasing spasticity in human patients with paraplegia.[1] At this time, however, the mechanism of reduction of pain by NMES remains unknown.

E.A. Karol, M.D.

Reference

1. Graupe D, Kohn KH: *Functional Electrical Stimulation for Ambulation by Paraplegics.* Malabar, Fl, Krieger Publishing, 1994, pp 131–151.

Work Incapacity From Low Back Pain: The Inrternational Quest for Redress

Hadler NM (Univ of North Carolina, Chapel Hill)
Clin Orthop 336:79–93, 1997   31–8

Objective.—Industrialized nations must deal with both a rapidly growing number of workers with disabling low back pain and an unsustainable increase in indemnity claims. It has even been suggested that permanent disability for nonspecific low back pain should be eliminated; however, this would reverse a century of history in providing recourse for workers who are disabled because of back pain. International trends in redress for work incapacity are reviewed, focusing on the varying adaptations of the "Prussian precedent."

The Prussian Precedent Around the World.—The Prussian precedent takes its name from the workmen's accident insurance and sickness benefits that became German law in the late 19th century. The rest of the industrialized world shortly followed suit. Although specifics vary, these plans generally refer to the Prussian paradigm, in which workers injured at work are more deserving of recompense than those who can no longer work because of non–work-related diseases. Those who have never worked are at the lowest level of entitlement. This paradigm has taken vastly different forms in different cultures around the world. In the United States, an inefficient, highly bureaucratic system has developed, with a heavy emphasis on proving causation of the injury but with no health insurance for working-age members of the population. In this situation, disability is the only medical recourse for anyone who cannot or will not work. Japan has a similar program, although it is national and is not an exclusive remedy. However, the process is much less contentious than in Western countries, perhaps because workers' compensation remains a last resort in a more flexible work environment. Other countries have taken other approaches. For example, in Switzerland and New Zealand, the issue of causation is assigned even greater importance. However, accident insurance is not exclusive to the work force. In The Netherlands, in contrast, all working adults receive benefits for work incapacity, without regard to the injury. However, the cost and percentage of the population involved are becoming less tolerable.

This situation leads the authors to question the Prussian paradigm on clinical as well as economic grounds. Experience suggests that there is no rational reason to remedy injury alone, let alone injury occurring in the workplace. The system tends to see disability as an outcome rather than a process. The outcome of consolidation is often a euphemism for the exhaustion of funds for medical intervention. Impairment ratings should also be done away with; the author believes that individuals who have to prove their illnesses cannot possibly get better.

Discussion.—The history and implications of work incapacity for injury are reviewed and focusing on redress for low back pain. Experience suggests the need to do away with the so-called Prussian paradigm, which places the highest value on workers disabled by work-related injuries. Experience has shown that this paradigm, in all its forms, is clinically unsound and ethically flawed. The author calls for sensible health care, including provisions for sick leave, and national initiatives for full employment in an environment that nurtures function and self-respect.

▶ In this essay, the author traces the present-day provision of disability insurance by industrialized countries, including the United States back to Germany in the late 19th century when Bismarck introduced public-based health care support to avoid granting wider political rights to the labor movement. The author particularly stresses the development of the workers' compensation insurance program in the United States, noting that low back pain accounts for approximately 25% of indemnity claims. He believes that, because of the widespread acceptance of general health insurance in the workplace today, the time has come to no longer view workplace injuries as something special, to dismantle the bureaucratic system that handles the claims for these injuries, and to use these administrative monies to improve the general health insurance program for workers in the United States.

C. Watts, M.D., J.D.

Outcomes

A Prospective Randomized Study Comparing Short- and Intermediate-term Perioperative Outcome Variables After Spinal or General Anesthesia for Lumbar Disk and Laminectomy Surgery

Jellish WS, Thalji Z, Stevenson K, et al (Loyola Univ, Maywood, Ill)
Anesth Analg 83:559–564, 1996   31–9

Introduction.—General anesthesia (GA) and spinal anesthesia (SA) both have benefits and disadvantages when used for patients undergoing lumbar laminectomy. The intraoperative and postoperative outcomes of GA

TABLE 2.—Intraoperative Data for Spinal Vs. General Anesthesia Groups

	Spinal	General
Total anesthesia time (min)	106.6 ± 3.2	131.0 ± 4.3*
Surgical time (min)	67.1 ± 2.8	81.5 ± 3.6*
Blood loss (mL)	133 ± 13	221 ± 32*
Intravenous fluids (mL)	1329 ± 60	1478 ± 79
Bradycardia	14.0%	22.9%
Hypertension	3.3%	26.2%*
Tachycardia	14.8%	21.3%
Hypotension	54.1%	57.4%
Ephedrine required	36.1%	22.9%

Note: Numeric data expressed as mean plus or minus standard error of the mean; bradycardia and hypotension equal decreases in heart rate and mean arterial pressure to less than 80% of baseline values; tachycardia and hypertension equal heart rate and mean arterial pressure greater than 120% of baseline values.

*P < 0.05 vs. spinal anesthesia group.

(Courtesy of Jellish WS, Thalji Z, Stevenson K, et al: A prospective randomized study comparing short- and intermediate-term perioperative outcome variables after spinal or general anesthesia for lumbar disk and laminectomy surgery. *Anesth Analg* 83:559–564, 1996.)

TABLE 3.—Short-term Recovery Outcomes in the Postanesthesia Care Unit (PACU)

	Spinal	General
Peak pain score	22 ± 3	58 ± 4*
Analgesic given	26.2%	80.3%*
Peak nausea score	12 ± 3	28 ± 5*
Vomiting	3.3%	8.2%
Antiemetic given	11.5%	22.9%
PACU time (min)	85.4 ± 4.2	80.3 ± 2.8

*$P < 0.05$ vs. spinal anesthesia group.

(Courtesy of Jellish WS, Thalji Z, Stevenson K, et al: A prospective randomized study comparing short- and intermediate-term perioperative outcome variables after spinal or general anesthesia for lumbar disk and laminectomy surgery. *Anesth Analg* 83:559–564, 1996.)

and SA were assessed in patients undergoing lumbar spine surgery to determine which technique is superior.

Methods.—A total of 122 patients were randomized to receive either GA or SA supplemented with a propofol infusion. Data from the intraoperative period through hospital discharge were recorded and compared.

Results.—The surgical time and anesthesia times were longer in the GA group than in the SA group (Table 2). Blood loss and intraoperative hypertension were greater in the GA group than in the SA group. In the postanesthesia care unit (PACU), heart rates and the mean arterial pressures were significantly higher in the GA group than in the SA group. Patients in the GA group had significantly higher peak pain scores, analgesic requirements, nausea, and antiemetic use than patients in the SA group (Table 3). On the first day after surgery, patients in the GA group had a higher incidence of nausea but did not have a similar increased incidence of vomiting (Table 4). There were no between-group differences in analgesic requirements in the 24 hours after discharge from PACU, urinary retention requiring catheterization, and time to discharge (Table 4).

Conclusion.—Findings indicate SA to be superior to GA in reducing surgical and anesthesia time and in decreasing blood loss, pain perception, the need for postoperative analgesics, nausea, and the need for antiemetics. There were no between-group differences in time to discharge. Despite these SA advantages, the tolerance for prone positioning on the frame was

TABLE 4.—Twenty-four-Hour (Intermediate) Postsurgical Outcomes

	Spinal	General
Nausea, 24 H	4.9%	24.6%*
Vomiting, 24 H	3.3	6.5%
Analgesics required	90.2%	83.6%
Urinary retention	14.8%	22.9%
Days to discharge	1.4 ± 0.2	1.7 ± 0.1

*$P < 0.05$ vs. spinal anesthesia group.

(Courtesy of Jellish WS, Thalji Z, Stevenson K, et al: A prospective randomized study comparing short- and intermediate-term perioperative outcome variables after spinal or general anesthesia for lumbar disk and laminectomy surgery. *Anesth Analg* 83:559–564, 1996.)

reduced after 2 hours, so it is imperative to perform the surgery within that time period.

▶ This prospective, randomized study with reportedly strict adherence to protocol and quite objective outcome variables admirably clarifies some potential advantages of SA over GA in this select situation. Reduced blood loss decreases patient stress and recovery time. Reduced pain and nausea improves overall patient comfort and, therefore, satisfaction. Reduced operative and anesthesia times decrease wound exposure and, of course, are more cost-effective. The surgeon needs to select patients carefully, however. Restlessness and agitation, especially in an infirm patient or with inadvertent extension of operative time, can quickly lead to disastrous complications and outcomes. Moreover, with the addition of propofol and with less thiopental sodium and nitrous oxide, the GA regimen may be better tolerated and, therefore, may further reduce the pool of willing candidates for SA.

C.P. Bondurant, M.D.

Anatomic Position of a Herniated Nucleus Pulposus Predicts the Outcome of Lumbar Discectomy

Knop-Jergas BM, Zucherman JF, Hsu KY, et al (St Mary's Hosp, San Francisco)

J Spinal Disord 9:246–250, 1996   31–10

Introduction.—Little information exists regarding the shape and position of a herniation in the spinal canal in reference to clinical outcome. The anatomical position of disk herniation with regard to postoperative success rate was retrospectively evaluated in 80 consecutively treated patients with simple disk herniations.

Methods.—Patients with central canal stenosis, foraminal stenosis, subarticular stenosis, spondylolisthesis, or reherniation were excluded. The mean patient age of the 24 women and 56 men included was 37.7 and 40.9 years, respectively. The major complaint in all patients was leg pain. Leg pain was associated with low back pain in 5% of patients. Records were reviewed for preoperative findings of CT scans after diskography and MRI of the lumbar spine. Classifications of disk herniations were: central, paracentral, intraforaminal, extraforaminal, and multiregional broad-based protrusions. The Smiley-Webster evaluation scale was used to rate clinical outcome and evaluate long-term need for pain medication. Clinical outcome was correlated with varying positions of herniations. The follow-up period ranged from 6–48 months.

Results.—Excellent, good, fair, and poor postoperative results were determined in 39 (53.4%), 9 (12.2%), 7 (9.8%), and 18 (24.6%) of patients, respectively. Excellent results were most often determined in patients with paracentral or intraforaminal herniations (Fig 3). Fair or poor (unsatisfactory) outcome was determined in 52.6% of patients with a central disk herniation, compared to 20% in patients with paracentral or intraforaminal herniation.

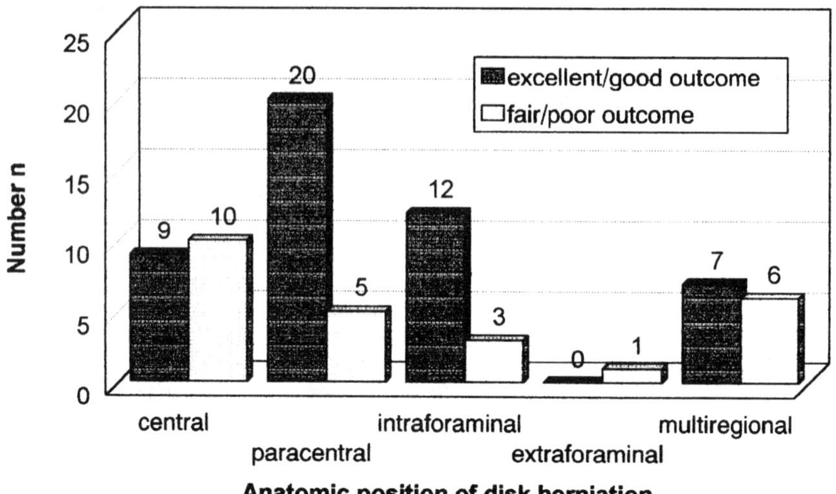

FIGURE 3.—Correlation between clinical outcome after lumbar diskectomy and anatomical position of disk herniations. (Courtesy of Knop-Jergas BM, Zucherman JF, Hsu KY, et al: Anatomic position of a herniated nucleus pulposus predicts the outcome of lumbar discectomy. *J Spinal Disord* 9:246–250, 1996.)

Conclusion.—Most patients with central disk herniations undergoing diskectomy had an unsatisfactory outcome. No patients underwent central decompression, so unsatisfactory outcome was more likely to be the result of an unstable segment than the surgical approach. The anatomical position of lumbar disk herniation was predictive of clinical outcome in patients undergoing lumbar diskectomy.

▶ Because the primary complaint in 95% of these patients was leg pain, one may assume that the authors were treating radicular symptoms. Given this setting, it is not surprising that the best results were obtained in those patient groups with intraforaminal and paracentral disk herniations. Patients with central or multiregional disk herniations frequently have collapse of the disk space, which often is associated with foraminal narrowing. I wonder whether this population would have fared better with a procedure that included not only decompression of the disk, but also a foraminotomy, reconstitution of the normal disk space height, and fusion.

V.C. Traynelis, M.D.

The Maine Lumbar Spine Study: I. Background and Concepts
Keller RB, Atlas SJ, Singer DE, et al (Maine Med Assessment Found, Augusta ; Maine Health Information Ctr, Augusta; Massachusetts Gen Hosp, Boston; et al)
Spine 21:1769–1776, 1996   31–11

Purpose.—The commonly used surgical procedures for treatment of herniated lumbar disk and spinal stenosis have not been studied in the outcomes relevant to patients. There is significant variation in the rates of surgery for these conditions, related partly to physicians' uncertainty about the best approach to these problems. This situation suggested the need for a community-based study of the outcomes of herniated lumbar intervertebral disk and spinal stenosis. The Maine Lumbar Spine study has been designed to address these issues. The design and implementation of this community-based effectiveness study were discussed.

Methods.—The prospective cohort sudy was designed to evaluate the surgical and nonsurgical treatment options for patients with herniated lumbar disk with sciatica and symptomatic spinal stenosis. It included all Maine orthopedic surgeons and neurosurgeons performing lumbar spine operations and was intended to enroll 600 patients stratified by the diagnosis of sciatica or spinal stenosis, treatment or nonsurgical treatment, and disability compensation. Initial data were collected by interview, and follow-up data, by questionnaire; imaging studies were assessed as well. A random sample of nonenrolled patients was evaluated to ensure the representativeness of the study population.

Discussion.—The study group method used in Maine Lumbar Spine study has assembled community-based practitioners to examine the appropriateness and quality of a key aspect of their practice. Community-based networks of this type can be invaluable in analyzing variations in practice patterns and in stimulating effectiveness research. Community-based effectiveness studies require mechanisms to support and implement these initiatives.

The Maine Lumbar Spine Study: II. 1-Year Outcomes of Surgical and Nonsurgical Management of Sciatica

Atlas SJ, Deyo RA, Keller RB, et al (Harvard Med School, Boston; Maine Med Assessment Found, Augusta; Eastern Maine Med Ctr, Bangor; et al)
Spine 21:1777–1786, 1996   31–12

Objective.—Patients with sciatica that does not respond to other treatments may be considered for surgery. Previous reports have noted large geographic variations in the use of lumbar spine surgery, beyond expected variations in the frequency of sciatica. These regional differences may reflect doubts about the most appropriate use of lumbar diskectomy. The Maine Lumbar Spine Study was designed to compare the results of surgical and nonsurgical treatment for patients with sciatica across the state of Maine.

Methods.—The prospective cohort study included 507 patients with sciatica recruited from the practices of orthopedic surgeons, neurosurgeons, and occupational medicine physicians. Two hundred seventy-five patients had surgery and 232 did not. All patients were interviewed at baseline; they were mailed follow-up questionnaires at 3, 6, and 12 months. The physicians provided clinical data. The 1-year outcomes evaluated were symptoms of leg and back pain, functional status, disability, quality of life, and patient satisfaction.

Results.—Baseline comparison of the 2 groups showed that the surgically treated patients had more severe sciatica through symptoms, physical signs, and imaging findings. About half of the patients in each group had symptoms rated as moderate—there were few mild cases in the surgically treated group and few severe cases in the nonsurgically treated group. Both groups were significantly improved at 1 year, but the surgically treated patients had the greater improvement. Definite improvement in back or leg pain was reported by 71% of patients in the surgically treated group and 43% of those in the nonsurgically treated group. The relative odds of definite improvement for the surgical group were 4.3, after adjustment for differences in baseline condition. Surgery gave better results for patients with moderate symptoms and normal physical examination findings. The follow-up data showed little difference in the employment vs. workers' compensation status of the 2 groups. Of patients who were receiving workers' compensation at baseline, 46% of those in the surgical group and 55% of those in the nonsurgical group were still receiving it at 1 year. One-year outcomes were similar for patients with mild symptoms in the 2 groups.

Conclusions.—Patients undergoing surgery for sciatica tend to have more severe symptoms than those treated nonsurgically. However, there is considerable overlap in symptoms between the 2 groups. One-year outcomes appear to be better for patients treated surgically, although surgery provides no apparent advantage for patients with mild symptoms at baseline. Although the study was not randomized, it provides useful information on the outcomes of surgical vs. nonsurgical treatment for sciatica. Longer follow-up is needed to see whether the differences between the 2 groups persist.

The Maine Lumbar Spine Study: III. 1-Year Outcomes of Surgical and Nonsurgical Management of Lumbar Spinal Stenosis
Atlas SJ, Deyo RA, Keller RB, et al (Harvard Med School, Boston; Maine Med Assessment Found, Augusta; Eastern Maine Med Ctr, Bangor; et al)
Spine 21:1787–1795, 1996   31–13

Purpose.—Lumbar stenosis is an increasingly diagnosed disorder—it is the most common reason for lumbar spine surgery among patients receiving Medicare. There are few data on the results of surgical vs. nonsurgical treatment for patients with lumbar spine stenosis—no randomized trials and few nonexperimental studies have addressed this issue. To compare the 1-year outcomes of surgical and nonsurgical treatment for patients with lumbar stenosis, data from the Maine Lumbar Spine Study were used.

Methods.—The prospective cohort study included 148 patients with lumbar spinal stenosis recruited from the practices of orthopedic surgeons, neurosurgeons, and occupational medicine physicians in the state of Maine. Eighty-one patients had surgery and 67 had nonsurgical treatment. All patients were interviewed at baseline; they were mailed follow-up questionnaires at 3, 6, and 12 months. The physicians provided clinical data. The 1-year outcomes evaluated were symptoms of leg and back pain, functional status, disability, quality of life, and patient satisfaction.

Results.—Baseline comparison of the 2 groups showed that the surgically treated patients had more severe lumbar spinal stenosis through imaging findings, symptoms, and functional status. A similar proportion of patients in each group had symptoms rated as moderate—there were few mild cases in the surgically treated group and few severe cases in the nonsurgically treated group. Definite improvement in the predominant symptom was reported by 55% of patients in the surgically treated group and 28% of those in the nonsurgically treated group. Among patients with moderate symptoms, those who had surgery had significantly better outcomes.

The 1-year follow-up data showed that surgical treatment was still a significant predictor of outcome, even after adjustment for baseline differences. By the 3-month follow-up evaluation, the maximal benefit of surgery already was apparent. Few patients in the nonsurgical group had their condition become worse with treatment. However, neither did they have much symptomatic or functional improvement from baseline.

Conclusions.—For patients with severe lumbar spinal stenosis, 1-year outcomes appear to be better with surgical treatment. However, it is difficult to compare the results of surgical vs. nonsurgical treatment, because patients in the different treatment groups were significantly different in their baseline characteristics. Longer follow-up is needed to see whether the differences between the 2 groups persist.

▶ This study (Abstracts 31–11, 31–12, and 31–13) confirms what conservative and thoughtful lumbar spine surgeons know: patients with lumbar radiculopathies secondary to herniated lumbar intervertebral disk disease or spinal stenosis who do not improve with judicious conservative treatment in a few weeks have a good likelihood of improvement with surgical decompression. On the other hand, patients who do not have signs and symptoms secondary to nerve root compression will not be improved by lumbar spine decompression. The authors further concluded that follow-up longer than 1 year is necessary to determine the true value of surgery. Degenerative lumbar disk disease that is seen either as a herniated lumbar intervertebral disk or lumbar spine stenosis is a progressive disease. Decompressive surgery done at 1 point in the life of the patient will not halt the progressive nature of the disease.

C. Watts, M.D., J.D.

Postoperative Management

Are Postoperative Activity Restrictions Necessary After Posterior Lumbar Discectomy? A Prospective Study of Outcomes in 50 Consecutive Cases
Carragee EJ, Helms E, O'Sullivan GS (Stanford Univ, Calif)
Spine 21:1893–1897, 1996   31–14

Introduction.—The optimal duration and necessity for postoperative restriction of activity after limited open lumbar diskectomy for a herniated lumbar disk are not known. The effect of no activity restrictions on 50

TABLE 2.—Sick Leave in 45 Employment-eligible Patients, Before and After Discectomy

	Mean (wk)	Range
Preop work loss (n = 45)	3.2	0–28
Non-Worker's comp.	2.1	0–18
Worker's comp.	5.6 ($P = 0.01$)	0–28
Postop work loss (n = 44)	1.7	0–4
Non-Worker's comp.	1.5	0–4
Worker's comp.	1.9	0–3 NS
Light work	1.4	0–4
Medium work	1.7	0–3 NS
Heavy work	2.5	0–4 ($P = 0.04$)
Postop return to full duty (44)	3.4	0–12
Non-Worker's comp.	2.6	0–8
Worker's comp.	5.3	1–12 ($P = 0.005$)
Light work	2.5	0–6
Medium work	4.7	0–8 ($P = 0.1$)
Heavy work	5.8	0–12 ($P = 0.001$)
Annual work loss since RTW	1.4	0–6
Disabled at follow-up evaluation	(1/45)	

Abbreviations: NS, not significant; *RTW*, return to work; *Preop*, preoperative; *Postop*, postoperative.
(Courtesy of Carregee EJ, Helms E, O'Sullivan GS: Are postoperative activity restrictions necessary after posterior lumbar discectomy? A prospective study of outcomes in 50 consecutive cases. *Spine* 21:1893–1897, 1996.)

consecutive patients undergoing limited open diskectomy for herniated intervertebral disks was evaluated.

Methods.—The mean patient age was 37 years. Before onset of sciatica, 45 patients were employed, 4 were students, and 1 was retired. Ten of 45 patients who were employed filed workers' compensation claims. Twenty-four patients underwent diskectomy through the interlaminar space alone, and no laminectomy was performed. Other than wound precautions, patients were given no restrictions after surgery. They were told to return to full work and domestic and recreational activities as soon as they thought they were able. They were told to expect some back and leg discomfort after surgery but were not to let it curtail activity. Patients were evaluated at a 2-year follow-up.

Results.—Of 45 patients who were employed, 44 returned to their previous work (Table 2). The 1 patient who did not return to work had been disabled for more than 6 months before surgery and received workers' compensation benefits. There was no evidence of her sciatica complaints on MRI. The mean time from surgery to return to work was 1.7 weeks. Eleven patients (25%) returned to work the next workday. The mean time to full work duties was 3.4 weeks. By 8 weeks, 43 of 44 patients (97%) returned to full duty. Patients not receiving workers' compensation returned to work significantly earlier than workers' compensation recipients. Patients with physically demanding jobs returned to work and full duties later than those with less physically demanding occupations. There were 5 complications: 1 dural tear, 1 transient foot drop that resolved in 3 weeks, 1 prolonged wound drainage that resolved without antibiotics in 3 weeks, 1 partial suprascapular nerve palsy, and 1 allergic reaction to intraoperative antibiotics. There were 3 herniations at the operative level at 14, 22, and 24 months after surgery.

Conclusion.—Early and complete return to work was possible in 98% of patients who were given no activity restrictions after lumbar diskectomy. Preoperative "demedicalization" of the process may have prevented much of the iatrogenic morbidity typically observed postoperatively.

▶ Activity restrictions after lumbar diskectomy have been firmly entrenched since early monographs. In 1953, Dr. Spurling[1] described 5–14 days of bed rest, 3 weeks of inpatient care, and 4–12 weeks away from work. He suggested, however, that prolonged bed rest and time away from work may be without benefit. Indeed, recent trends have encouraged earlier return to activity and work in both nonoperative and operative efforts, which ideally would mean less loss of conditioning. More recent cost-cutting measures have driven further attenuation of inpatient time as well as outpatient time away from work. The authors suggest that stringent postoperative restrictions may be unnecessary, thus supporting the surgeon's efforts at early mobilization of patients. For those patients mired in debates with insurance carriers, litigation, or workers' compensation, these results could force an early, therapy-free return to work that some perhaps do not wish. Those patients not so encumbered and more driven to return will likely be the big winners, as they are allowed to return more briskly, smoothly, and efficiently to everyday life.

C.P. Bondurant, M.D.

Reference

1. Spurling R: *Lesions of the Lumbar Intervertebral Disc.* Springfield, IL, Charles C. Thomas, 1953, p. 103.

Evaluation of the Contribution to Postoperative Analgesia by Local Cooling of the Wound

Brandner B, Munro B, Bromley LM, et al (UCL Hosps, London; Chase Farm NHS Trust Hosp, Middlesex, England; Royal Natl Orthopaedic Hosp, Middlesex, England)
Anaesthesia 51:1021–1025, 1996   31–15

Background.—Cryoanalgesia refers to the application of cold to block local nerve conduction of painful stimuli. There is growing interest in the use of cryotherapy in trauma care, particularly during the acute phase. The recently developed Temptek T 1000 device has proven useful for postoperative cryotherapy, applying controlled cold therapy at a constant temperature and with a pulsing rhythm using fluid-filled cooling pads. This approach to cryotherapy was tested in patients undergoing lumbar spine surgery.

Methods.—The randomized trial included 32 patients undergoing elective posterior lumbar spine surgery. Both groups received patient-controlled morphine analgesia; 1 group also received local cooling of the surgical wound using the Temptek T 1000. The cooling pad was applied immediately in the recovery unit and set to a temperature of 7.2°C to 10.0°C. Pain during the first 24 hours postoperatively was rated by a verbal analog scale. Nausea, sedation, and morphine consumption were assessed as well.

Results.—Cumulative morphine consumption was significantly reduced in the patients assigned to local cooling: 19 vs. 30 mg at 12 hours and 29 vs. 50 mg at 24 hours. Pain scores were also significantly reduced in the cryoanalgesia group; scores for nausea and sedation were lower at some times as well. Questionnaire responses indicated that the patients receiving cooling therapy were significantly more satisfied with their overall postoperative pain management.

Conclusions.—Local wound cooling appears to be a useful adjunct for postoperative pain relief in patients undergoing lumbar spine surgery. A significant improvement in pain relief and a reduction in morphine consumption are achieved when the Temptek T 1000 cooling device is used along with patient-controlled analgesia. Patient acceptability and satisfaction are high.

▶ Cold therapy may be 1 of the oldest nostrums for pain. Perhaps instinctively, we have always known the value of cooling injured tissue, as we have all at 1 time or another personally used or recommended cold therapy to reduce swelling and pain in a joint or muscle. In the acute stages after tissue trauma, cold therapy is the thermal agent of choice.

This prospective, randomized study, although not double-blind because the patient can perceive the cooling, is a simple but well-done study demonstrating the value of local cooling as an adjunctive therapy for postoperative analgesia in healthy patients undergoing lumbar spine surgery. This simple and safe noninvasive treatment resulted in significantly improved patient comfort and reduced consumption of narcotics during the first 24-hour postoperative period.

The only caution that I would offer is that this is a very short-term study, and it did not follow up the condition of the surgical wound after local cooling was applied. It is well known that the physiologic response to cold therapy is a decrease in blood flow and tissue metabolism, which may have the beneficial effect of reducing bleeding and inflammation; however, it may also reduce the chemotactic gradient for macrophage delivery. Consequently, future studies should address surgical wound surveillance, and the infection rates should be reported for comparison.

S.R. Gibbs, M.A., M.D.

Miscellaneous

Smoking and the Human Vertebral Column: A Review of the Impact of Cigarette Use on Vertebral Bone Metabolism and Spinal Fusion
Hadley MN, Reddy SV (Univ of Alabama, Birmingham; Valley Med Ctr, Fresno, Calif)
Neurosurgery 41:116–124, 1997   31–16

Background.—Despite its serious and varied ill effects on health, smoking continues to be an important public health problem. Relatively little is known about the effects of smoking on the appendicular and axial skeleton; few studies have examined the mechanisms by which smoking influences bone metabolism and healing. The available evidence on smoking's effects on bone and bone metabolism is reviewed, with special reference to its negative impact on spinal fusion.

Smoking and Back Pain.—Epidemiologic data find that smokers are at increased risk of back pain, sciatica, and spinal degeneration. Back complaints become more frequent with the increasing number of pack-years smoked. Other studies have linked smoking to an increased risk of disk and spinal degeneration and an increased rate of bone mineral loss. Surgeons have linked smoking to delayed bone healing and formation of pseudarthrosis after spinal fusion. These effects may be particularly dramatic in smokers undergoing lumbar spinal fusion, in whom the rate of symptomatic fusion failure may be elevated 3–5 times. Many studies have found that smoking has an adverse effect on bone mineral density and bone mineral content, especially for women who continue to smoke after menopause. Clinical observations suggest that postmenopausal women who smoke are at increased risk for vertebral compression fractures. There are 3 main mechanisms by which smoking could negatively affect bone metabolism: an adverse effect on bone mineral density through accelerated osteoporosis, impairment of bone blood flow, and inhibition of osteoblast cellular metabolism.

Smoking and Spinal Fusion.—Smoking adversely affects spinal fusion in patients undergoing vertebral arthrodesis. These effects are most apparent in the early and middle phases of spinal fusion. The processes of fusion—from initial capillary ingrowth through revascularization, cartilage and bone formation, remodeling, and further bone formation—are delayed and limited in smokers. Fusion does occur, but smokers have a high failure rate, are at risk for delayed nonunion, and form less strong bone than nonsmokers. The authors propose a multifactorial mechanism for these effects, based on the suboptimal environment for potential fusion in smokers. Fusion rates may be especially poor when allograft bone is used as the fusion substrate; autograft bone should be the preferred substrate in smokers.

Discussion.—Smoking has adverse effects on bone and bone metabolism, and these are reflected in the suboptimal results of spinal fusion in smokers. Through multiple mechanisms, smokers have weaker, mineral-deficient vertebrae with a reduced blood supply and less functional bone-forming cells. Smoking raises the risk of advanced bony degradation, degenerative disease of the spinal column, and susceptibility to traumatic vertebral injury. For various biological, physiologic, and mechanical reasons, spinal fusion procedures are less likely to be successful in smokers than in nonsmokers.

▶ This is an important article for spinal surgeons. The authors have provided an excellent review of the deleterious effects of smoking on bone metabolism and bone healing as it relates to spinal fusion procedures.

The spinal surgery literature is peppered with a variety of reports relating smoking to failed spinal fusion, but the precise mechanisms have not been well elucidated.

Spinal fusion requires a host response to osteoinductive signals from the bone graft substrate for promotion of angiogenesis and the ingrowth of osteoblasts; however, the toxic breakdown products from tobacco incineration impair these factors.

Because these patients have accelerated osteoporosis, impaired bone blood flow, and impaired osteoblast metabolism, they are clearly at higher risk for pseudoarthrosis, and the consent process for the operation should address this. The authors point out that allograft bone is less osteoinductive and has no osteogenic capability compared with autograft bone. In smokers, autograft bone appears to be a superior fusion substrate because the trophic factors, bone morphogenic proteins, and osteoinductive cytokines remain intact.

S.R. Gibbs, M.A., M.D.

A System for Reporting the Size and Location of Lesions in the Spine
Wiltse LL, Berger PE, McCulloch JA (Long Beach Mem Med Ctr, Calif; Northeast Ohio Univ, Rootstown)
Spine 22:1534–1537, 1997   31–17

Introduction.—There is no standardized nomenclature for use in communicating the findings of CT and MRI scans among professionals involved in the care of patients with spinal disorders. As a result, radiologists' reports are often much longer and less precise than they should be. A new standardized system for reporting the size and location of lesions in the lumbar or thoracic spine is reported.

Methods.—The new system was developed by 12 leading physicians— including radiologists, orthopedic surgeons, neurosurgeons, and physiatrists—from 11 different centers. The goal of the new nomenclature was to make reports of CT or MRI scan findings simpler and more accurate. The nomenclature used aspects of various other systems reported over the previous decade.

Results.—Areas in the axial plane were designated "zones," whereas those in the craniocaudal direction were called "levels." From medial to lateral, the zones were called the central canal zone, the subarticular zone, the foraminal zone, and the extraforaminal zone. The craniocaudal levels, from above downward, were the suprapedicle level, the pedicle level, the infrapedicle level, and the disk level. The lesion size could be described as normal, mild, moderate, moderately severe, or severe. Alternatively, the lesion size could be rated using the numbers 1–5, with 1 indicating normal and 5 indicating severe.

Discussion.—A standardized nomenclature for reporting the size and location of spinal lesions is proposed. The system is illustrated by some typical cases and the reports of the reading radiologist. It provides a means of describing the absolute size of the abnormality, its relative size in relation to the size of the spinal canal, and the location of the lesion. The authors hope their system will facilitate communications among all health care professionals who care for patients with spinal disorders.

▶ *Herniation, rupture, extrusion, bulge, protrusion,*—do each of these words have a specific meaning or are they used synonymously? The issue is that there is no standardized nomenclature used in communicating spinal findings. The prevailing language may vary depending on the venue and the specialist. The neurosurgeon, the orthopedic surgeon, the neurologist, the neuroradiologist, and the rehabilitation physician each use their own spinal vernacular. Fardon *et al.*[1] noted there were 52 terms used by English-speaking surgeons to describe "degenerative" diseases of the intravertebral disks. The North American Spine Society has presented a spinal nomenclature, but, unfortunately, no system to date has been broadly adopted.

The authors present a system of zones and levels to describe lesions in relation to normal vertebral anatomical landmarks. In addition, they have presented a numerical grading system for words used as graded descriptors of size and/or severity. Their system is logical, simple, and easy to recall. Perhaps, because of this, this system will be more readily and widely adopted, thereby reducing the litany of ill-defined descriptors currently in use.

S.R. Gibbs, M.A., M.D.

Reference

1. Fardon D, Pinkerton S, Balderston R, et al: Terms used for diagnosis by English-speaking spine surgeons. *Spine* 18:274–277, 1993.

Lumbar Motion Segment Pathology Adjacent to Thoracolumbar, Lumbar, and Lumbosacral Fusions
Schlegel JD, Smith JA, Schleusener RL (Univ of Utah, Salt Lake City)
Spine 21:970–981, 1996   31–18

Background.—Alhough surgeons may believe that the segment next to a fused spinal motion segment can break down, such occurrences have not been well documented in the literature. Patients with segmental abnormalities adjacent to previously fused spinal segments were reviewed in the current study.

Methods.—Fifty-eight patients free of symptoms at an average of 13.1 years after thoracolumbar, lumbar, or lumbosacral fusion were assessed. All had consulted 1 of 2 spinal surgeons because of abnormalities adjacent to a previously fused thoracic or lumbosacral segment.

Findings.—Spinal stenosis, disk herniation, or instability at the adjacent segment were noted. Segments next to the adjacent segment were almost as likely to break down. Seventy percent of 37 patients followed up for more than 2 years had good or excellent outcomes. Seven of these 37 patients needed additional surgery. Sagittal and coronal imbalances appeared to contribute to the breakdown.

Conclusions.—This is the largest reported series of patients with adjacent segment breakdowns. The segment next to the adjacent segment was almost as likely to break down. Sagittal and coronal alignment seemed to play a role in abnormalities of adjacent segments. Seventy percent of the patients in this series had good outcomes.

▶ The effects of arthrodesis on the threshold for injury of adjacent motion segments of the spine has long been an area of concern for spinal surgeons, although there has been no definitive documentation of a causal relationship.

The literature is replete with case reports, and one cannot attend a spine meeting without anecdotes to this effect. In patients with recurrent lower extremity symptoms who have previously had fusion of the spine, the breakdown of the segment adjacent to a fused segment is commonly among the differential diagnoses.

The authors have reported the largest series of patients evaluated with segmental abnormalities adjacent to previously fused spinal segment(s).

Spondylosis is a degenerative process, and, as the authors have noted, this study documenting adjacent segment disease may only be documenting the natural history of a disease process that may have developed otherwise irrespective of the fusion. The authors made other observations that lacked statistical power but that seemed to suggest that sagittal and coronal imbalances were factors in symptomatic spondylosis of adjacent segments. Interestingly, spinal stenosis was the most common finding among patients seen after a long symptom-free period after their spinal fusion.

Although this study does not show a causal relationship between lumbar fusion and delayed, symptomatic degeneration at an adjacent segment, it does provide some useful information for forecasting the probable outcome for these patients.

If a causal relationship does exist, perhaps, in the future, we will see less of this with the advent of more minimally invasive fusion techniques that avoid disruption of midline structures and fascial attachments to the spine. Spinal mechanics is exceedingly complex; however, through our improved understanding of this, a functional restoration (artificial disk) of a diseased or damaged motion segment may make this long-debated issue moot.

S.R. Gibbs, M.A., M.D.

Administration of Methylprednisolone for 24 or 48 Hours or Tirilazad Mesylate for 48 Hours in the Treatment of Acute Spinal Cord Injury: Results of the Third National Acute Spinal Cord Injury Randomized Controlled Trial
Bracken MB, for the National Acute Spinal Cord Injury Study (Yale Univ, New Haven, Conn; Natl Inst of Neurological Disorders and Stroke, Washington, DC; Johns Hopkins Univ, Baltimore, Md)
JAMA 277:1597–1604, 1997   31–19

Purpose.—The National Acute Spinal Cord Injury Study (NASCIS) 2 found that high-dose methylprednisolone for 24 hours improved neurologic outcomes after acute spinal cord injury. This treatment is likely to work by suppressing lipid peroxidation and hydrolysis, which destroy neuronal and microvascular membranes. These processes extend beyond the 24-hour period after an injury. Another trial evaluated the use of a 48-hour maintenance dose of methylprednisolone. It also examined the use of the lipid peroxidation inhibitor tirilazad mesylate in the hope of reducing complications compared with high-dose methylprednisolone.

Methods.—The randomized, double-blind, clinical trial included 499 patients with acute spinal cord injuries treated at 16 North American NASCIS centers. All patients were treated within 8 hours after injury. Treatment began with an IV bolus of 30 mg/kg methylprednisolone. The patients were then randomized into 3 groups. Those in the 24-hour group received a methylprednisolone infusion of 5.4 mg/kg/hr for 24 hours. Those in the 48-hour group received methylprednisolone at the same dose rate for 48 hours. Those in the tirilazad group received tirilazad mesylate in one 2.5 mg/kg bolus infusion every 6 hours for 48 hours. The 3 groups were compared for motor function changes from baseline at 6 weeks and at 6 months after injury. They were also evaluated for changes in Functional Independence Measure (FIM) at 6 weeks and at 6 months.

Results.—Motor recovery at 6 weeks and at 6 months was significantly better in the 48-hour methylprednisolone group than the 24-hour methylprednisolone group. At both times, these differences were significant for patients who started treatment at 3–8 hours after injury. For patients starting treatment within this time, the 48-hour methylprednisolone infusion significantly increased the chances of improving by 1 full neurologic grade at 6 months and increased the chances of improvement in FIM at 6 months. These patients also had more severe sepsis and pneumonia than the other 2 groups. However, other complications and mortality rates were similar among groups. Outcomes for patients in the tirilazad group were comparable with those in the 24-hour methylprednisolone group.

Conclusions.—The results of the NASCIS 3 trial show that patients with spinal cord injuries in whom treatment is started within 3 hours of the injury should receive high-dose methylprednisolone for 24 hours. For those starting treatment within 3–8 hours, methylprednisolone treatment should be extended to 48 hours. The study finds no rationale for the use of tirilazad, although further study with different dosing regimens may be indicated.

▶ As I have written previously, the lipid peroxidation process plays a crucial role in the evolution of the secondary changes in the injured spinal cord. This fact has been linked to the microvascular damage and hypoperfusion that occurs after an injury. Therefore, the importance of prompt treatment (less than 8 hours and preferably 3 hours after trauma) has been recognized (NASCIS 2 study). The methylprednisolone analogues and, particularly, the aminosteroids and lazaroids (tirilazad mesylate was used in this cooperative study) have also shown a powerful action as lipid peroxidation inhibitors. This article addresses the importance of the duration of treatment after trauma, which can even influence the dosing schedule of the aforementioned compounds. This fact is of no small importance, as, in the case of methylprednisolone treatment, larger doses (treatment for 48 hours after the injury)—associated with a significant increase in secondary complications such as pneumonia—are required to achieve the same therapeutic effects as 24 hours of treatment, even if this treatment is started only 3 hours after the spinal cord injury. The study also suggests the possibility of using new dosing regimens of tirilazad. This possibility should be considered cautiously but, nonetheless, is exciting, as this compound could inhibit, as the authors say, posttraumatic lipid peroxidative pathophysiologic conditions more effectively and with less secondary effects.

M.-A. Perez-Espejo, M.D., Ph.D.

Patterns of Anterior Spinal Canal Involvement by Neoplasms and Infections

Schellinger D (Georgetown Univ, Washington, DC)
AJNR 17:953–959, 1996

31–20

Background.—The anatomy of the anterior epidural space is the leading factor in how tumoral and infectious processes spread into the anterior spinal canal. Whether the invasion pattern of neoplasms and infections can be predicted based on the epidural space and spinal anatomy present was determined.

Methods.—A total of 58 patients with subtotal spinal canal compromise caused by neoplasms ($n = 44$) or infections ($n = 14$) were imaged at 140 levels (15 cervical, 87 thoracic, 38 lumbar) to determine retrovertebral growth patterns. Imaging consisted of MRI, CT, and/or CT myelography in 6 patients.

Findings.—Retrovertebral disease extension patterns were similar at all 3 spinal levels studied. Of the 140 levels imaged, 136 images showed that the diseased mass was smooth, marginated, and bilobulated and that it grew against the posterior surface of the vertebra. In 108 cases, the mass was symmetric, and in 28, it was asymmetric. A bilobulated mass was more likely with more advanced invasion, particularly when the mass extended rostrally or distally directly behind the vertebra. Detachment of the midline septum from the vertebral body (observed in 20 levels) was characteristic of more progressive canal compromise. In the other 4 levels imaged, the diseased mass was unilobulated and did not extend beyond the midline. This pattern occurred in cases of advanced osseous involvement.

Conclusions.—The anterior epidural space is defined by the posterior longitudinal ligament, which is anchored to the vertebral body by a midline septum, and by the ligament's associated lateral membranes. Diseases in this area conform to this anatomical compartment, and bilobular diseases cross over the septum. Furthermore, the anterior epidural space freely communicates with the perivertebral space at the exit foramina, which offers a route of spread for neoplastic and infectious processes. Ultimately, understanding the anatomy of the anterior epidural space will add to our understanding of disease processes in this region.

▶ The authors continue their microanatomical studies of the spinal canal using CT and MRI scans to define compartments that have not been emphasised previously in standard anatomical textbooks. Their thesis is that migrating disk fragments and advancing neoplasms and infective processes go down the "paths of least resistant," which are determined by various potential spaces—the attachment of ligaments in the spinal canal; therefore, the type of compression is predictable. They draw attention particularly to the anterior epidural space, which has a midline septum and leaf-like extensions of the membrane to each side. The growth of an infective cranioplastic process is down the path of least resistance; therefore, because of the thick midline structure, there may not be a central bulge of tumor or pus.

Although this is an important additional piece in the jigsaw of the anatomical pathologic process, at this stage, it does not add significantly to the management of the lesions. We await the next article from this group.

H.A. Crockard, F.R.C.S.

32 Trigeminal Neuralgia

Trigeminal Evoked Potential: Monitored Thermorhizotomy: A Novel Approach for Relief of Trigeminal Pain
Leandri M, Gottlieb A (Univ of Genoa, Italy; Istituto Tumori, Genoa, Italy)
J Neurosurg 84:929–939, 1996   32–1

Purpose.—For patients with trigeminal neuralgia, radiofrequency coagulation is the most selective rhizotomy technique and provides the best lesional control. This technique has been underused, however, because of the need to rely on the patient's subjective feedback in terms of needle positioning and monitoring the extent of the lesion. Trigeminal evoked potentials (TEPs) have been suggested for use in monitoring this procedure, but the technique has never been fully developed. A reliable method of using TEPs to monitor thermorhizotomy for trigeminal neuralgia was reported.

Technique.—The TEPs used in this procedure are produced by stimulation of the supraorbital, infraorbital, and mental nerves and recorded by electrodes at the scalp and trigeminal nerve. The thermorhizotomy cannula is specially modified to create a concentric bipolar electrode that can both record TEPs and create lesions. In the initial step, baseline scalp TEPs are recorded from the derivation of the cervical vertex to C7. This is done to prove correct placement of the various stimulating electrodes. Next, the peripheral nerve trunks are stimulated, and TEPs are recorded from the trigeminal electrode to determine where the electrode is relative to the root bundles. Next, cutaneous trigger points or painful areas are stimulated, and root activity is recorded for fine positioning of the trigeminal electrode. The position of the trigeminal electrode in terms of the motor root is then determined by stimulating the nerve through the electrode and assessing the response of the masseter motor. Finally, thermolesions are made and the scalp TEPs are recorded immediately before and after. Repeated lesions are made to reach a 20% to 50% reduction in the amplitude or a 0.30–msec delay of the scalp-recorded W_2 wave. The authors have used this technique to very good effect in 30 patients with trigeminal neuralgia of the second branch.

Conclusion.—This thermorhiztomy technique is guided exclusively by objective electrophysiologic data, and there is no need for patient cooperation. The immediate results in clinical practice have been very good; further studies will describe the long-term pain relief and will provide a quantitative analysis of sensitivity. The best results are achieved when the monitoring data show satisfactory positioning of the trigeminal electrode and a suitable lesion with little or no masticator weakness.

▶ We congratulate Leandri and Gottlieb for refinement of the technique confirming that sensory and motor TEPs during percutaneous thermocoagulation (PTC) are valuable in localizing trigeminal electrodes, as they hypothesized and we demonstrated in previous publications.[1, 2] Speed, as a goal, has been deleterious, particularly in PTC. I would seriously hesitate to accept the medicolegal implications of PTC "quickly performed without needing cooperation from the patient," exclusively under general anesthesia.

Residual morbidity from PTC is becoming increasingly unnecessary and unacceptable, and it may be minimized by the following measures: (1) a systematic micrometric evaluation of the somatotopic organization of the trigeminal ganglion and rootlets in every patient using a multi-array electrode,[3] (2) the recording of verbal responses in the awake patient after low-voltage stimulation, which is invariably painless and, although subjective, generally very precise, (3) the constant clinical examination of the awake patient, (4) the clinical use of the blink reflex, as described by Sindou et al.,[4] (5) the use of TEPs, and (6) straight and curved thermocouples small enough to make small low-temperature lesions that cannot exceed the intended target.

E.A. Karol, M.D.

References

1. Karol EA, Sanz OP, Rey RD: Sensory and motor trigeminal evoked potentials to localize the position of trigeminal electrodes. *Acta Neurochir (Wien)* 108:110–115, 1991.
2. Leandri M, Karol EA: Letter to the Editor. *Acta Neurochir (Wien)* 109:163–165, 1992.
3. Karol EA, Sanz OP, Gonzalez La Riva FN, et al: A micrometric multiple electrode array for the exploration of gasserian and retrogasserian trigeminal fibers: Preliminary report. *Neurosurgery* 33:154–158, 1993.
4. Sindou M, Keravel Y, Abdennebi B, et al: Traitement neuro-chirurgical de la nevralgie trigeminale. Abord direct ou methode percutanee? *Neurochirurgie* 33:89–111, 1987.

The Long-term Outcome of Microvascular Decompression for Trigeminal Neuralgia
Barker FG II, Jannetta PJ, Bissonette DJ, et al (Massachusetts Gen Hosp, Boston; Univ of Pittsburgh, Pa)
N Engl J Med 334:1077–1083, 1996

32–2

Introduction.—A syndrome characterized by paroxysmal facial pain, trigeminal neuralgia, or tic douloureux, can be treated with carbamazepine. Operative treatments include neurectomy of trigeminal-nerve branches outside the skull, percutaneous ablations, injection of glycerol, or physical compression. Most reports provide only short-term follow-up information about several surgical procedures of treating trigeminal neuralgia. Patients with trigeminal neuralgia who had microvascular decompression of the trigeminal-nerve root during a 20-year-period were studied.

Methods.—Microvascular decompression of the trigeminal nerve for medically intractable trigeminal neuralgia was provided to 1,185 patients. The procedure involved a small retromastoid craniectomy, through which the trigeminal nerve is examined microsurgically for vascular compression at or near its point of entry into the brain stem. Repositioning with stents was accomplished with any compressive arteries and some veins. Patients filled out questionnaires annually on the presence and nature of any facial pain and the details of any subsequent treatment for tic.

Results.—The median follow-up for the 1,185 patients was 6.2 years. In the first 2 years after surgery, most postoperative recurrences of tic took place. Recurrences of tic occurred with 30% of patients, and 11% had second operations for the recurrences. Excellent final results were found for 70% of patients 10 years after surgery. These patients reported they were free of pain without medication for tic. Another 4% indicated they had occasional pain, but did not require long-term medication. The annual rate of recurrence of tic was less than 1% 10 years after surgery. In 82% of patients, immediate postoperative relief from tic was complete. In 16%, it was partial and in 2%, relief was absent. Significant predictors of eventual recurrence were female sex, venous compression of trigeminal-root entry zone, symptoms lasting more than 8 years, and lack of immediate postoperative cessation of tic. If a trigeminal ganglion lesion had been created with radiofrequency current before microvascular decompression, patients were more likely to have burning and aching facial pain. A patient's likelihood for having a cessation of tic after microvascular decompression was not lessened by a previous ablative procedure. Complications included 2 deaths before the operation (0.2%) and 1 brain stem infarction (0.1%). Ipsilateral hearing loss occurred in 16 patients (1%).

Conclusion.—For trigeminal neuralgia, microvascular decompression is a safe and effective treatment. The long-term success rate is high.

► Since the discovery of vascular compression as a common cause of trigeminal neuralgia, the only etiologic treatment is the microvascular decompression. It is therefore surprising that so many methods, based on the destruction of the nervous tissue, like avulsions and chemical and thermal lesions to the ganglion, still enjoy great popularity. An outpatient procedure is certainly more attractive for the patient than the proposal for craniotomy, especially if the patient is unaware of the rate of recurrent pain after these procedures and the dangers of anesthesia dolorosa.

The long-term results in this article are excellent and would suggest that microvascular decompression is the method of choice. However, these results are evidence of skillful surgeons. An occasional operator may have less satisfactory results, and this may be the reason for still so many parallel ways of treatment.

B. Klun, M.D., Ph.D.

Three-dimensional Imaging for Presentation of the Causative Vessels in Patients With Hemifacial Spasm and Trigeminal Neuralgia
Kumon Y, Sakaki S, Kohno K, et al (Ehime Univ, Japan)
Surg Neurol 47:178–184, 1997

32–3

Objective.—The cause of hemifacial spasms and trigeminal neuralgia is vascular compression of the root exit or root entry zone (REX) of the facial or trigeminal nerve. Preoperative appreciation of these relationships is essential for maximizing the chances of good operative results. Magnetic resonance imaging has been used for this purpose but is not always successful in demonstrating the causative vascular structure. High-speed MRI using spoiled gradient recalled acquisition in the steady state (SPGR) clearly shows vessels as high-intensity areas, thus showing the causative vessels; however, it does not always show the courses of the vessels and nerves on the same plane. Three-dimensional (3-D) reconstruction of SPGR MRI data was performed for preoperative evaluation of hemifacial spasms and trigeminal neuralgia.

Methods.—The study included 20 patients with hemifacial spasms and 6 with trigeminal neuralgia. All patients underwent SPGR MRI and MR angiography. Three-dimensional images were constructed by the surface-rendering method using the data from SPGR MRI. The goal of obtaining the imaging studies was to demonstrate the 3-D relationship between the causative vessels and the REZ of the facial or trigeminal nerve as clearly as possible.

Results.—In each patient, the SPGR MRI scan showed that the causative vessel was compressing or in contact with the root exit or REZ of the facial or trigeminal nerve. The MR angiography and 3-D imaging studies permitted identification of the causative vessels. The anatomical relationship of the causative vessels and the nerve REZ was clearly depicted by the 3-D reconstructions, which were confirmed by the intraoperative findings. Surgery successfully relieved symptoms in all patients with trigeminal neuralgia and in 18 of 20 with hemifacial spasms. Postoperative SPGR MRI revealed adequate decompression of the involved nerve.

Conclusions.—In patients with hemifacial spasms or trigeminal neuralgia, SPGR MRI, MR angiography, and 3-D imaging are very useful in depicting the causative blood vessel. The 3-D images, reconstructed from the SPGR MRI data, are especially useful for simulating the planned operative procedure. Cerebral angiography appears necessary mainly when the MRI findings suggest cerebrovascular disease.

▶ Kumon et al. applied an elegant technique of MR 3-D imaging to show neurovascular contacts in 20 patients with hemifacial spasms and in 6 with trigeminal neuralgia; the resultant images after surgical decompression were interesting. For several years, I have systematically studied MRI serial crude thin sections showing vessels at the dorsal REZ of the trigeminal nerve in patients with trigeminal neuralgia, and, I have studied lately, multiplanar reconstruction in an oblique projection. I have seen a high incidence of neurovascular contacts in patients with trigeminal neuralgia. In addition, I have frequently seen an absence of vessels on the side with trigeminal pain and intimate vascular contact on the opposite side; I have also seen this latter situation in patients with unrelated pathologic conditions. Thus, given the limitations of our MRI technique, I believe that the demonstration of neurovascular contact is not enough to suspect, predict, or exclude a clinically significant neurovascular compression or conflict. It is hoped that studying a large enough number of patients and controls with sophisticated MRI as in this study, will help to establish if and when neurovascular imaging is clinically relevant.

E.A. Karol, M.D.

Stereotactic Radiosurgery for Trigeminal Neuralgia: A Multiinstitutional Study Using the Gamma Unit

Kondziolka D, Lunsford LD, Flickinger JC, et al (Univ of Pittsburgh, Pa; Northwest Hosp Gamma Knife Ctr, Seattle; Good Samaritan Hosp, Los Angeles)
J Neurosurg 84:940–945, 1996   32–4

Purpose.—Some patients with persistent or recurrent typical trigeminal neuralgia—many of whom are elderly and with co-morbid conditions—need a minimally invasive approach to treatment. The authors hypothesized that stereotactic radiosurgery, with lesion localization by stereotactic high-resolution MRI, could relieve the pain of trigeminal neuralgia while preserving facial sensation. This multicenter study assessed the technique, dose-selection parameters, and results of gamma knife stereotactic radiosurgery in patients with trigeminal neuralgia.

Methods.—The analysis included 50 patients with trigeminal neuralgia treated at 5 hospitals. Surgery had been performed previously in 32 patients; the mean number of procedures done per patient was 2.8. Radiosurgery consisted of a single 4-mm isocenter targeted at the nerve root entry zone, with a target dose of 60–90 Gy. The patients were followed up for a median of 18 months. The results were classified as excellent (freedom from pain), good (50% to 90% relief), or treatment failure.

Results.—Magnetic resonance imaging was highly successful in depicting the proximal trigeminal nerve and root entry zone. Treatment produced excellent results in 58% of patients and good results in 36%; the treatment failure rate was 6%. Pain relief was achieved in a median of 1 month. In 94% of patients, the response to treatment persisted through up to 3 years after radiosurgery. The exceptions were 3 patients with recurrent pain at 5–10 months. Fifty-four percent of patients were free of pain at 2 years. Eighty-eight percent reported 50% to 100% pain relief. Complete pain relief was achieved in 72% of patients receiving a maximum radiosurgical dose of 70 Gy or greater compared with 9% of patients receiving a lower dose. Facial paresthesia developed after radiosurgery in 6% of patients. This side effect resolved completely in 1 of the 3 patients and partially in another. There were no other nerve deficits and no cases of deafferentation pain.

Conclusions.—Although longer term follow-up is needed, gamma knife radiosurgery appears to be an effective treatment for trigeminal neuralgia that does not respond to medical or surgical treatment. It is a minimally invasive technique that avoids the risks of open surgery and reduces the chances of loss of normal nerve function. The proximal trigeminal nerve and its root entry zone appears to be an appropriate radiosurgical target. This treatment warrants further study as treatment for recurrent trigeminal neuralgia or as a primary treatment for elderly patients or those in poor medical condition.

▶ I had the privilege to discuss with Dr. Leksell a stereotactic but nonradiosurgical approach to the gasserian ganglion in an unusual patient with trigeminal neuralgia secondary to van Buchem's syndrome, an osteosclerotic disorder precluding all conventional neurosurgical treatment.

Based on a critical analysis by the authors of Lindquist et al.[1] and Rand et al.[2] experience, the revival of radiosurgery in the neurosurgical armamentarium for treatment of trigeminal neuralgia, is welcomed, particularly after the suggested shift of the target from the gasserian ganglion (where more selective techniques are being developed)[3] to the dorsal root entry zone. This excellent multi-institutional study demonstrates an unexpected early relief of pain after radiosurgery and shows promising early results.

A long-term follow-up is anxiously awaited because the technique may become a less invasive alternative to neurovascular decompression and, perhaps, to percutaneous procedures, in which morbidity is still significant.

E.A. Karol, M.D.

References

1. Lindquist C, Kihlström L, Hellstrand E: Functional neurosurgery: A future for the gamma knife? *Stereotact Funct Neurosurg* 57:72–81, 1991.
2. Rand RW, Jacques DB, Melbye RW, et al: Leksell Gamma Knife treatment of tic douloureux. *Stereotact Funct Neurosurg* 61:93–102, 1991.
3. Karol EA, Sanz OP, Gonzalez La Riva FN, et al: A micrometric multiple electrode array for the exploration of gasserian and retrogasserian fibers: Preliminary report. *Neurosurgery* 33:154–158, 1993.

Comparison of Surgical Treatments for Trigeminal Neuralgia: Reevaluation of Radiofrequency Rhizotomy

Taha JM, Tew JM Jr (Univ Cincinnati, Ohio; Mayfield Clinic, Cincinnati, Ohio)
Neurosurgery 38:865–871, 1996

32–5

Background.—Authorities disagree on the best surgical treatment for trigeminal neuralgia. The outcomes of radiofrequency rhizotomy and the efficacies of other surgical procedures for this disorder were assessed.

Methods.—Five hundred patients with trigeminal neuralgia underwent radiofrequency rhizotomy at 1 center between 1981 and 1986. Outcomes from this series were compared with those of previously reported patients undergoing radiofrequency rhizotomy (6,205 patients), glycerol rhizotomy (1,217 patients), balloon compression (759 patients), microvascular decompression (MVD) (1,417 patients), and partial trigeminal rhizotomy (250 patients).

Findings.—Microvascular decompression had the lowest rate of technical success. The highest rates of initial pain relief and the lowest rates of pain recurrence were associated with radiofrequency rhizotomy and MVD. The greatest rate of pain recurrence was associated with glycerol rhizotomy. Balloon compression had the highest rate of trigeminal motor dysfunction and the lowest rate of corneal anesthesia or keratitis, the latter also being low after MVD. The rates of facial numbness and dysesthesia were lowest with MVD. The rates of dysesthesia were similar after all percutaneous procedures. Posterior fossa exploration was associated with the highest rates of permanent cranial nerve deficits, intracranial hemorrhages or infarctions, and perioperative morbidity and mortality.

Conclusions.—Percutaneous techniques and posterior fossa exploration have advantages as well as disadvantages. For most patients undergoing initial surgery, radiofrequency rhizotomy is the procedure of choice. For healthy patients with isolated pain in the first ophthalmic trigeminal division or in all 3 trigeminal divisions and for patients who wish to avoid a sensory deficit, MVD is the recommended procedure.

▶ The number of methods for the treatment of trigeminal neuralgia is a clear proof that the ideal 1 has not yet been found. Obviously, the authors of the paper have a great deal of experience in radiofrequency lesions; therefore, they regard it as the most satisfactory method. In addition, the majority of patients are usually quite happy in accepting the proposal of a small procedure, often done on an outpatient basis, vs. a major surgical operation.

However, the main objection against this and other methods (MVD is an exception) is the destruction of the nervous tissue and not the removal of the offending factor, which is, in a high percentage, an abnormally positioned vessel. The more severe the sensory loss, the more convincing the abolishment of the pain is; however, the likeliness of a recurrence is not eliminated. In addition, there is a considerable difference in the point of view between the surgeon and the patient. Although the first one sees only the excellent result, the other one may be quite unhappy about the numb face. As soon as there is a sensory loss, the risk of anesthesia dolorosa, regardless how small, should constantly be kept in mind. Finally, recurrences would require additional lesions, and cases with bilateral pain could prove to be a real problem.

B. Klun, M.D., Ph.D.

33 Vascular Malformations

Arteriovenous Malformations

Hemorrhage Risk After Stereotactic Radiosurgery of Cerebral Arterio-venous Malformations

Pollock BE, Flickinger JC, Lunsford LD, et al (Univ of Pittsburgh, Pa)
Neurosurgery 38:652–661, 1996

33–1

Background.—Stereotactic radiosurgery can obliterate about 80% of arteriovenous malformations (AVMs) of less than 3 cm in mean diameter within a latency period of 2–3 years. The main disadvantage of this procedure is that patients remain at risk for bleeding during this latency period, until the AVM is obliterated. The effect of stereotactic radiosurgery on the hemorrhage rate of AVMs was analyzed.

Methods.—The clinical and angiographic characteristics of 315 patients with AVMs before and after radiosurgery were reviewed. A total of 263 bleeds occurred in 196 patients in 10,939 patient-years before radiosurgery, yielding an annual nonfatal hemorrhage rate of 2.4%. Two hundred ninety-five patients were followed up for 24 months or longer.

Findings.—Arteriovenous malformation bleeds occurred in 21 patients at a median of 8 months after radiosurgery. Another 2 patients had 3 aneurysmal bleeds at 5–32 months postoperatively, yielding a 7.4% total risk of hemorrhage per patient. Actuarial bleeding rate until AVM obliteration was 4.8% per year in the first 2 years after radiosurgery and 5% per year for the third to fifth years after radiosurgery. In a multivariate analysis, the presence of an unsecured proximal aneurysm was associated with an increased risk of postradiosurgical hemorrhage. None of the 7 patients with intranidal aneurysms had AVM hemorrhages. Radiation doses of 25 Gy or more to the AVM margin did not confer a protective effect compared with doses of less than 25 Gy to the AVM margin. None of the 140 patients with angiographically confirmed complete obliteration had bleeding after this confirmation, and none of the 19 patients without residual nidus had an early draining vein.

Conclusion.—In this series, stereotactic radiosurgery was not associated with a significant change in the hemorrhage rate of AVMs during the latency period before obliteration. There was no protective benefit for patients with incomplete nidus obliteration within 60 months of radiosurgery. Aneurysms in patients with unsecured proximal aneurysms should be obliterated before radiosurgery or at the time of surgical AVM resection.

▶ This study provides information of major importance in the management of AVMs of the brain. With this large series of 314 AVMs, the Pittsburgh team demonstrate very clearly that postradiosurgery hemorrhage risk (7.4%) of the AVM before the obliteration reflects the natural history of AVM. The absence of hemorrhage after angiographic complete occlusion (or early draining vein without residual nidus) confirms the justification for using radiosurgery in AVM.

The absence of a protective effect against hemorrhage for patients with incomplete nidus obliteration and an obliteration rate of only 67% confirm the evidence that radiosurgery must be strictly limited to AVMs not amenable to microsurgical resection.

Such an accurate estimation of the risk–benefit ratio is required for the other techniques so that the treatment options can be discussed and quantifiable patient information can be gathered.

J. Regis, M.D.

Prediction of Obliteration After Gamma Knife Surgery for Cerebral Arteriovenous Malformations

Karlsson B, Lindquist C, Steiner L (Karolinska Hosp, Stockholm; Univ of Virginia, Charlottesville)
Neurosurgery 40:425–431, 1997

33–2

Background.—Several reports have addressed the importance of various parameters for angiographic and clinical outcomes of stereotactic radiosurgery for arteriovenous malformations (AVMs). However, there have been no systematic studies to evaluate the capability of these parameters to predict the success rate and complications of radiosurgery. The predictive factors for radiosurgical obliteration of cerebral AVMs are analyzed.

Methods.—The study included 945 patients undergoing gamma knife radiosurgery for AVMs from 1970 to 1990. Various factors were analyzed for their effect on obliteration of the AVM nidus, including patient factors, AVM volume and location, angiographic factors, and dosimetry and treatment parameters.

Results.—As the minimum dose (i.e., lowest peripheral dose) and the average dose increased, so did the obliteration rate. As the AVM volume increased, the obliteration rate decreased. The major dose factor in the success or failure of treatment was the minimum dose to the AVM, that is, the higher the minimum dose, the better the chance of total AVM obliteration. In the logarithmic curve that describes this relationship, the incidence of obliteration increased with the minimum dose up to 87%. The higher the average dose, the shorter the latency period to obliteration.

Among obliterated AVMs, the larger the lesion, the lower the minimum dose used. The K index—the product (minimum dose) · (AVM volume)$^{1/3}$—was used to relate the obliteration rate to the product minimum dose. A linear increase in obliteration rate was noted up to a K index value of approximately 27. Beyond this point, the value of the obliteration rate remained constant at approximately 80%. For 273 patients receiving a dose of at least 25 Gy, the obliteration rate at a 2-year latency period was 80% and had a 95% confidence interval of 75% to 85%. Including obliterations occurring beyond that point, the obliteration rate was 85% (95% confidence interval, 81% to 89%).

Conclusions.—In patients undergoing gamma knife radiosurgery for AVMs, the likelihood of AVM obliteration is related to the lowest dose administered to the AVM and to the volume of the AVM. This relationship, described by the K index, can be used to calculate the probability of obliteration. Until a prospectively proven predictive method is available, it is probably better to use the K index than to perform no assessment of the probability of obliteration.

▶ This important study, a 20-year experience using stereotactic radiosurgery to treat a series of 1,319 patients, represents the results of treatment of approximately one fourth of AVMs worldwide (2,400 of the 10,000 irradiated AVMs in the world have been treated by the present authors). Because this series was started without previous reports to rely on, this is a unique contribution. The authors found that the minimum dose was most important: the higher the minimum dose, the higher the obliteration rate, up to 25 Gy. The obliteration rate in a 273-patient subset with this minimum dose was 81%. The authors also suggest that larger AVMs require less of a peripheral dose to obliterate. This very large and long-term report will certainly guide future AVM stereotactic radiosurgery for many years to come.

R. Marino, Jr., M.D.

Surgical Resection of Large Incompletely Treated Intracranial Arteriovenous Malformations Following Stereotactic Radiosurgery
Steinberg GK, Chang SD, Levy RP, et al (Stanford Univ, Calif)
J Neurosurg 84:920–928, 1996   33–3

Background.—Radiosurgery is effective in obliterating small arteriovenous malformations (AVMs). However, its success rate for obliterating larger AVMs is not as good. One experience with the microsurgical resection of AVMs was reported.

Methods.—Thirty-three patients, aged 7–64 years, undergoing microsurgery for AVMs were followed up for 1–11 years. Initial lesion volumes ranged from 0.8 to 117 cm³, and the mean was 21.6 cm³. Doses ranged from 4.6 to 45 GyE. Ten of 27 AVMs located in eloquent or critical areas were in language, sensory, or visual cortex; 11 were in the basal ganglia/thalamus; 3 were in the corpus callosum; and 1 each was in the brain stem, hypothalamus, and cerebellum. Venous drainage was deep in 13 lesions, superficial in 12, and both in 8. Spetzler-Martin grades were II in 1 patient, III in 12, IV in 16, and V in 4. Eight patients had recurrent bleeding after radiosurgery but before surgery. Radiation necrosis developed in 3 patients, and endovascular embolization was done before surgery in 25 patients.

Findings.—Compared with AVMs in patients who had not had radiosurgery, the AVMs in the current patients were found to be markedly less vascular, partially thrombosed, and more easily resected at surgery. Pathologic study demonstrated endothelial proliferation with hyaline and calcium in vessel walls. Some AVM vessels showed partial or complete thrombosis. Evidence of vessel and brain necrosis was noted in many patients. The resection was complete in 28 patients and partial in 5. Thirty-one patients had excellent or good clinical outcomes. Two patients died from recurrent bleeding from residual AVMs. The condition of 4 patients worsened after microsurgical resection. For the most part, final clinical outcomes were associated with the pretreatment grade.

Conclusions.—In this series, microsurgery or embolization plus microsurgery after incomplete obliteration of the AVM after radiosurgery was useful in treating some AVMs, especially when patients had recurrent bleeding from residual lesions. In some patients, stereotactic radiosurgery before microsurgical resection can transform large, complex AVMs into resectable lesions. Combined embolization and radiosurgery in the treatment of portions of large AVMs in the deep and eloquent areas of the brain may be a useful strategy.

▶ The role of radiosurgery in the treatment of large AVMs not considered for microsurgical resection is not clear today. We know that, for AVMs larger than 3 cm (maximum diameter), the doses must be decreased to avoid normal brain injury, which, at the same time, dramatically decreases the success rate. What can we expect when treating so large a lesion by radiosurgery? How do we treat these lesions to achieve a reasonable obliteration rate and an acceptable complication rate?

We do know that, in this population, a great percentage of AVMs will not be obliterated completely. Now we also know from this paper from Steinberg et al. that further microsurgery is not compromised by previous radiosurgery and is certainly facilitated by radiosurgery in the majority of cases. This is a very important contribution that strongly supports the argument for decision making when faced with a large AVM that has little chance of being obliterated using radiosurgery.

J. Regis, M.D.

Embolization of Cerebral Arteriovenous Malformations: Part 1. Technique, Morphology, and Complications
Wikholm G, Lundqvist C, Svendsen P (Univ Hosp, Göteborg, Sweden)
Neurosurgery 39:448–459, 1996   33–4

Background.—Improved outcomes have been reported for surgery and stereotactic irradiation in patients with cerebral arteriovenous malformations (AVMs). However, data on the frequency and severity of complications and outcomes are often difficult to interpret. An experience from 1 center, where embolization is the main treatment of AVMs, was analyzed.

Methods and Findings.—One hundred fifty of 192 patients referred to the center were eventually treated. Eighty-five percent of the AVMs were Spetzler-Martin grade III or higher. Total embolization was done in 13% of the patients. In 66%, total embolization or embolization followed by stereotactic irradiation or surgery was achieved. Combined treatment with stereotactic gamma radiation was the most important aspect of the treatment strategy. The procedure-associated mortality rate was 1.3%. Although the total incidence of complications after embolization was high— 40%—only 6.7% were considered severe. Large size and the presence of deep feeders were the only angiographic features that predicted failure to achieve full treatment. Seventy-one percent of the 14 AVMs with volumes of less than 4 cc were embolized completely. The total embolization rate for the 20 AVMs 4–8 cc in volume was 15%. The full treatment rate in combination with gamma treatment was 75% in this subgroup, and 10% of these patients underwent surgery after embolization. Fifteen percent of the patients had severe complications, although there were no complications after November, 1990.

Conclusions.—Two thirds of these AVMs, most of which were considered unsuitable for surgical excision, were decreased to a size suitable for gamma knife treatment or totally occluded by embolization alone. Although the total complication rate was high, the combined death and serious complication rate was 8%, which is comparable to that after about 3 years without treatment.

Embolization of Cerebral Arteriovenous Malformations: Part II. Aspects of Complications and Late Outcome
Lundqvist C, Wikholm G, Svendsen P (Sahlgrenska Univ, Götoborg, Sweden)
Neurosurgery 39:460–469, 1996   33–5

Background.—The main goal of arteriovenous malformation (AVM) treatment is to eliminate the risk of cerebral bleeding. However, all methods of eliminating the AVM are associated with a risk of complications. The risk of complications and late outcomes associated with embolization were analyzed.

Methods and Findings.—In 20 patients, AVMs were eliminated by embolization alone, and, in 14, they were eliminated by embolization and supplementary surgery. In another 66 patients, AVMs were embolized to a size suitable for supplementary stereotactic irradiation. These 100 patients had a stable clinical course. Outcomes were less favorable in another group of 50 patients, who had had embolization and were only partially treated. Headaches and epilepsy responded positively to treatment. A history of cerebral bleeding did not affect the prognosis of recurrent bleeding. Conversely, AVMs with feeder or nidus aneurysms were associated with a greater risk of bleeding. The prognosis was worse for patients with histories of bleeding and large, partially treated AVMs.

Conclusions.—Patients with AVMs in eloquent areas or with lesions too large for stereotactic radiosurgery can be treated by embolization alone or combined with other therapies. Such treatments offer the possibility of eliminating the AVM. A history of bleeding indicates the need for a more aggressive treatment approach in patients with large AVMs.

▶ The group assessing and treating cerebral AVMs at the Sahlgrenska University Hospital provide a paradigm of how multidisciplinary groups should function and, in the 2 papers under review (Abstracts 33–4 and 33–5), good examples of the valuable data that can be generated with this approach. There is 1 point that should be mentioned at the outset: when the authors refer to "full treatment," they do not mean complete obliteration of a cerebral AVM but only that the patient underwent the proposed treatment protocol, including embolization and surgery or stereotactically focused radiosurgery as required, in its entirety. Indeed, a majority of fully treated patients had residual, partially treated AVMs. These 2 papers do not, then, report on the obliteration rate of cerebral AVMs treated by this group but on the early complications of their treatment protocol related specifically to embolization. Their systematic approach in the assessment and treatment of patients with an AVM and the detailed analysis of their results within the limitations already mentioned are the reasons why these papers are of interest. The authors report on their evaluation and treatment of 150 patients with cerebral AVMs judged by 1 or more neurosurgeons to be inoperable and also believed to be inappropriate for stereotactically focused radiotherapy as a primary treatment, presumably because of their size. After a multidisciplinary conference, all the patients underwent embolization using a variety of endovascular devices and embolic material. Those patients whose embolization did not result in complete obliteration then underwent extirpative surgery or stereotactically focused radiosurgery. The 100 patients completing the proposed treatment plan were considered to be fully treated, whereas the 50 patients in whom partial obliteration by embolization was not amenable to other treatment modalities were considered to be partially treated. It is only with attentive reading of these 2 papers that the reader can get some approximation of the obliteration rate resulting from their treatment regimen; thus 20 patients had complete obliteration by embolization, and 14 had extirpative surgery after embolization. Of the 66 patients in whom embolization was followed by stereotactically focused radiosurgery, 44 had angiograms at 2 years after the last treatment, and, of these, 34 had complete or almost complete obliteration of their AVMs. If one considers, as

I do not, that almost complete obliteration is equivalent to complete obliteration, then their complete obliteration rate is based on 68 of 124 patients assessed at 2 years after last treatment and is 55%. Bearing in mind that these patients' AVMs were deemed inoperable, this is not a negligible result. The real gist of their papers, however, is a detailed analysis of the complications related to the embolization produced to achieve this less-than-ideal result. These are comprised of 2 deaths and 10 "severe," 23 "moderate," and 26 "slight" complications, mainly in the form of hemorrhagic or ischemic strokes. Delayed complications related to radiotherapy are not addressed. Neurosurgeons will be interested to read that the features that make up the now widely used Spetzler-Martin system for grading operative risk are not indicative of the increased risk of embolization. Thus, such features as the size of the AVM, its relationship to eloquent cortex, and the presence of deep venous drainage were not predictive of hemorrhagic or ischemic complications after embolization. However, the size of the malformation and the presence of deep feeding arteries were associated with partial completion of the protocol, within the definition of the authors. A history of a prior hemorrhage as the presenting symptom was not associated with an increased risk of hemorrhaging related to the treatment; however, a large AVM, especially 1 involving the central region, or the presence of 1 or more aneurysms within the nidus of the malformation or on 1 or more arteries supplying the AVM was related to an increased risk of treatment-related hemorrhaging. Especially sobering is the observation that patients with large AVMs that were first seen with cerebral hemorrhages and whose malformations could only be partially treated were at a higher risk of death within this protocol.

That embolization can completely obliterate small AVMs, as was the experience of the authors, and that extirpative surgery can successfully follow the incomplete obliteration of an AVM that was previously judged too risky to operate on are, these days, mundane observations. I look forward to the reporting by this group and by other groups on the effects of stereotactically focused radiotherapy on partially embolized AVMs still not believed to be amenable to direct surgery after embolization.

R. Leblanc, M.D., M.S.C., F.R.C.I.C.

Miscellaneous

A Founder Mutation as a Cause of Cerebral Cavernous Malformation in Hispanic Americans
Günel M, Awad IA, Finberg K, et al (Yale Univ, New Haven, Conn; Univ of New Mexico, Albuquerque; Stanford Univ, Palo Alto; et al)
N Engl J Med 334:946–951, 1996   33–6

Background.—Cerebral cavernous malformation is characterized by abnormal vascular spaces with a lining of a single layer of endothelium and no intervening neural parenchyma or mature vessel-wall elements. It can cause headaches, seizures, and cerebral hemorrhage. Both familial and sporadic cases have been found, particularly among Hispanic Americans of Mexican descent. Previous studies have discovered a causative gene on the long arm of chromosome 7. A linkage study was performed with segregation of genetic markers in patients with both familial and sporadic disease.

Methods.—Genomic DNA was extracted from the venous blood of 57 patients with cerebral cavernous malformation, diagnosed with either surgery or MRI and of 47 unrelated, healthy controls. Of the 57 patients, 47 were members of 14 kindreds with familial cavernous malformation and 10 were patients with sporadic cases. The genotypes on chromosome 7q were determined with polymerase chain reaction, and haplotypes were constructed.

Results.—All of the affected members, but none of the unaffected members of 1 family inherited allele 6 of locus D7S657. Markers D6S492 and D7S479 were not completely cosegregated, indicating disease gene location in a 7-cm segment between D7S492 and D7S479, found in all 47 chromosomes from the kindreds, but only 4 of the 98 chromosomes from the Hispanic controls. Identical haplotypes were found in affected patients from 10 kindreds, with the affected patients from the other 4 kindreds having haplotypes with a portion of the interval that contained the cavernous-malformation gene. In addition, the entire conserved haplotype was found in 33 asymptomatic subjects from the kindreds. Eight of the 10 patients with sporadic disease also had the entire conserved haplotype, and the other 2 had part of the conserved haplotype containing the cavernous-malformation gene.

Conclusion.—Virtually all cases of either familial or sporadic cavernous malformation in Hispanic Americans of Mexican descent were caused by inheritance of the same mutation from a common ancestor. Further study is needed to identify the mutation, which can form the basis of a genetic screening test.

▶ The identification of a gene causing cerebral cavernous malformations in individuals of Hispanic descent illustrates the power of current genetic neurobiological techniques and has propelled a routinely encountered neurosurgical pathologic lesion, cavernous angiomas, out of the 19th century realm of descriptive neurology into the 21st century era of potential molecular neurobiological manipulation. Less than a decade after the demonstration that cerebral cavernous angiomas cluster within Hispanic families, not only has the causative gene been mapped to chromosome 7 but non–Hispanic familial clusters have been identified where the same genetic loci have been implicated. The present study further narrows the site of the cavernous malformation gene to a much shorter segment of the long arm of chromosome 7 than was previously known, and indicates that this gene is operant not only in familial cases but also in patients of Hispanic descent with sporadic cavernous malformations. As pointed out by the authors, this augers well for the future development of a sensitive and specific diagnostic test that could identify individuals at risk before clinical manifestation. The subsequent demonstration by this group that the loci implicated in Hispanic cases are not involved in some non–Hispanic families attests to the heterogenic complexity of this malformation, which initially appeared deceptively simple.

R. Leblanc, M.D., M.S.C., F.R.C.I.C.

Growth, Subsequent Bleeding, and De Novo Appearance of Cerebral Cavernous Angiomas
Pozzati E, Acciarri N, Tognetti F, et al (Bellaria Hosp, Bologna, Italy)
Neurosurgery 38:662–670, 1996   33–7

Background.—As more and more cavernous angiomas are recognized in patients with less severe clinical manifestations, it is increasingly important to understand the natural history of these lesions. Their biological behavior appears relatively benign, although there is clearly potential for recurrent bleeding and growth. Certain familial, sexual, and racial factors may influence the natural history of cavernous angiomas. Eighteen patients whose cavernous angiomas exhibited aggressive biological behavior are described.

Patients.—The 18 patients were identified from a series of 145 patients with brain cavernous angiomas treated during a 16-year period. The patients were 13 women and 5 men (mean age, 29 years). The aggressive behavior consisted of recurrent overt bleeding, growth, or de novo appearance. Cavernomas were located in the cerebellum for 3 patients, in the brain stem for 1 patient, in the thalamus for 4 patients, in the caudate nucleus for 2 patients, in the diencephalon for 1 patient, and in the white matter of the cerebral hemispheres for 7 patients. Three patients had familial or multiple cavernous angiomas, 2 patients were pregnant, 3 had undergone radiotherapy for other tumors, and 1 had undergone radiosurgery.

Treatment and Outcomes.—Six patients had new cavernous malformations not previously demonstrated. Ten patients had recurrent hemorrhages developing a mean of 11 months after a previous bleeding. Treatment was surgical in 11 patients and conservative in 7. Progressive hypothalamic dysfunction caused death in 1 patient with a diencephalic cavernoma. Repeated symptoms developed in 3 nonsurgically treated patients, causing additional neurologic deficits. Surgery led to an improved outcome in 4 patients but to no change in 7.

Conclusions.—A series of cavernous angiomas with aggressive biological behavior is reported. A number of different factors may be related to this aggressive behavior, including pregnancy, familial or multiple cavernomas, previous whole brain irradiation or radiosurgery, incomplete removal, the location of the lesion within the brain, and associated venous malformations. Aggressively behaving cavernous angiomas are more prevalent in women than in men, which suggests a possible hormonal influence. More research is needed to confirm the more aggressive behavior of cavernomas in female patients and to determine the effects of irradiation on the growth and de novo genesis of these lesions.

▶ Once again, this group has contributed significantly to the growing literature on cavernous malformations, and they especially confirm Robinson et al.'s[1] findings of a predominant occurrence among females and of pregnancy as a significant risk factor for agressive behavior of these lesions. Regarding the latter, some have suggested that this may be caused by an expanded intravascular volume and/or endocrine factors that promote vascular proliferation during pregnancy.

The prognosis with this subcategory of vascular malformations is not easily forecasted because the pathophysiologic characteristics and hemorrhagic potential are so variable.

Since the advent of MRI, more lesions are being identified nearer the lesser end of the clinical spectrum; consequently, this allows for the possibility of early intervention.

Stereotactic radiosurgery has been advocated for the management of some of these lesions.[2] However, these authors have reported that previous wholebrain or stereotactic radiotherapy has correlated with a more aggressive behavior of the lesion. This issue should be further investigated in terms of dosimetry to determine the threshold in these lesions for hemorrhagic dysnagiogenesis and hemorrhage. Any rational treatment plan for cavernous angiomas should take into account the risk factors identified in this report.

S.R. Gibbs, M.A., M.D.

References

1. Robinson JR, Awad IA, Little JR: Natural history of the cavernous angioma. *J Neurosurg* 75:709–714, 1991.
2. Kondziolka DJ, Lunsford LD, Kestle JRW: The natural history of cerebral cavernous malformations. *J Neurosurg* 83:820–824, 1995.

Occult Cerebrovascular Malformations After Irradiation
Pozzati E, Giangaspero F, Marliani F, et al (Bellaria Hosp, Bologna, Italy)
Neurosurgery 39:677–684, 1996   33–8

Introduction.—Occult cerebrovascular malformations (OVMs) can take a number of forms, although most requiring clinical attention are cavernous malformations. Recent reports have described the development of hemorrhagic lesions resembling OVMs in patients who have undergone cerebral irradiation. Five patients who had de novo OVMs after radiotherapy of the brain are reported.

Patients.—The patients were 4 females and 1 male. Four patients had received "standard" or focused irradiation for brain tumors; the other had been treated for a deep cavernous angioma. Four of the patients were less than 15 years old when they underwent irradiation. All of the OVMs developed within the radiation ports; they appeared between 3 and 9 years after radiotherapy. Acute symptoms, such as headaches, vomiting, or focal signs, led to the diagnosis of OVM in 4 patients. The other patient was asymptomatic. The findings of serial MRI scans were available in 4 patients.

Findings.—The OVMs initially appeared as hypointense foci on T1- and T2-weighted images. This was followed by focal or multifocal hyperintensity on T1-weighted images and mixed signal intensity on T2-weighted images. On late follow-up, a ring of decreased signal intensity developed. Four patients were managed surgically, and the other was managed by neuroradiologic monitoring. The surgical specimens showed clusters of closely packed vascular spaces with the appearance of cavernous malformations. In some cases, these spaces were associated with a thrombosed, thick-walled vein with intense hemosiderin deposits and fibroblastic proliferation. Areas of the brain adjacent to the lesions showed changes of telangiectasia. All patients recovered and were well at follow-up.

Discussion.—Occult vascular malformations can occur as late complications of cerebral irradiation. They are most likely to occur in children undergoing radiotherapy. These lesions need close neuroradiologic surveillance; depending on the circumstances, surgery should be considered. Although more cases must be studied, postirradiation OVMs may exhibit more aggressive behavior than spontaneous lesions.

▶ High venous pressure has been reported in developmental venous anomalies (DVA) associated with cavernous malformations seen with hemorrhages.[1] De novo formation of a cavernous malformation in close association with a DVA with stenosis of its collector vein has also been observed.[2]

Thus veno-occlusive disease seems to be associated with hemorrhages, and the development and growth of OVMs.

Irradiation has been shown to preferentially affect the cerebral veins, and endothelial proliferation has eventually led to venous occlusive disease, hemorrhages, and also proliferation of telangiectasia.[3]

This mechanism can explain the de novo formation of OVMs in patients irradiated at a young age. These malformations, which seem to show a more aggressive behavior, should be looked for, recognized, and treated promptly before life-threatening hemorrhages occur.

P.P. Maeder, M.D.

N. de Tribolet, M.D.

References

1. Dillon WP, Wilson CB, Hieshima GB, et al: Hemorrhagic venous malformations: The role of venous restriction. Presented at the 30th Annual Meeting of the American Society of Neuroradiology, St. Louis, June 1992.
2. Maeder PP, Gudinchet F, Meuli RA, et al: Development of a cavernous malformation of the brain. *AJNR*, in press.
3. Gaensler EHL, Dillon WP, Edwards MSB, et al: Radiation-induced telangiectasia in the brain simulates cryptic vascular malformations at MR imaging. *Radiology* 193:629–636, 1994.

34 Miscellaneous

Projection of the Lumbar Pedicle and Its Morphometric Analysis
Ebraheim NA, Rollins JR Jr, Xu R, et al (Med College of Ohio, Toledo)
Spine 21:1296–1300, 1996   34–1

Background.—Posterior transpedicular screw fixation is most commonly used to treat an unstable lumbar spine. Although several studies of pedicular anatomy have been done, there are few quantitative data on the location of the lumbar pedicle axis for each level.

Methods and Findings.—Fifty dry lumbar specimens, including 150 lumbar vertebrae, were analyzed. No significant differences in dimension were noted between men and women. The mean distance from the projection point to the midline of the transverse process changes consistently from L1 to L5. The mean projection point in both sexes above L4 was 3.9 mm for L1, 2.8 mm for L2, and 1.4 mm for L3 superior to the midline of the transverse process. At L4, this point was near the midline of the transverse process. The projection point at L5 was a mean of 1.5 mm inferior to the midline of the transverse process.

Conclusion.—The mean distance from the projection point of the lumbar pedicle axis to the midline of the transverse process varies consistently at different levels. Knowledge of these values may be useful for screw placement in the lumbar pedicle.

▶ The unique finding of this study was that the "entry site" for lumbar pedicle fixation varies from level to level. The change is gradual and consistent, as one may expect. The transition point appears to be L4; rostral to this level, the entry point is superior to the midline of the transverse process, and it is inferior to this landmark at L5. There has been a growing interest in the use of frameless stereotactic techniques in spinal surgery. Although elegant, such guidance systems are currently expensive and cumbersome. More importantly, advanced technology is not a substitute for a sound understanding of anatomy. Those surgeons who place lumbar pedicle screws should be familiar with this work.

V.C. Traynelis, M.D.

The Cerebellum: Movement Coordinator or Much More?
Barinaga M
Science 272:482–484, 1996

34–2

Purpose.—Patients with lesions of the cerebellum have difficulty with movement tasks, which suggests that the cerebellum functions to help the brain coordinate movements. However, a growing body of evidence suggests that it participates in many other brain functions as well—even cognition. The evidence for different nonmotor functions of the cerebellum is reviewed.

Nonmotor Functions of the Cerebellum?—Neuroanatomical studies have shown extensive connections between the cerebellum and "higher" brain structures. The cerebellum appears to be involved in many nonmotor functions, including analysis of sensory information, telling time, and solving puzzles. During the 1990s, several studies have suggested cerebellar involvement in cognitive tasks, including verb-generation and puzzle-solving tests. Work by researchers at the University of California, Berkeley, suggests that the cerebellum assists not only in timing motor control of fine movements but also in sensory discrimination and other brain activities. These experiments suggest that the cerebellum is necessary for various types of mental timing for nonmotor as well as motor functions. However, other researchers suggest that the cerebellum's apparent roles in cognition and timing simply reflect its motor-related functions—it is activated when someone is planning or even thinking about movements.

One research group is trying to discover whether the cerebellum is involved in coordinating the acquisition of sensory information needed for the brain to accomplish various tasks. Studies using functional MRI scans indicate that the cerebellum is more involved in sensory acquisition than in movement, as such. Other researchers suggest that the cerebellum may be activated in anticipation of difficult tasks requiring high-quality sensory information. There is some evidence that the cerebellum may help the brain to focus attention on sensory stimuli, and that research subjects with cerebellar damage are slower to shift attention. Beyond sensory discrimination, it has even been suggested that the cerebellum may help prepare various brain systems to operate at maximal efficiency. This could explain why patients with cerebellar damage do not seem badly impaired but do show deficiencies on specialized tests.

Discussion.—There is ongoing controversy as to whether the cerebellum acts mainly to coordinate motor function or whether it has other roles as well. More research is needed to see whether the cerebellum is involved in cognitive function, timing, general preparedness, or sensory discrimination—or all of these—in addition to motor coordination.

▶ *Cerebellum* the diminutive of cerebrum, describes the organ that, by weight, constitutes only 10% of the total brain, yet the cerebellum contains more than half of all the neurons in the brain. Under the overhang of the occipital lobes and crouched below the tentorium, the motor and sensory homunculi are mapped onto the cerebellum and are protected in the deepest recess of the calvaria. Nevertheless, some have judged that, because its complete destruction produces no sensory impairment or diminution of muscle force, the cerebellum is nothing more than a mass of insubstantial electricity.

The cerebellum learns and makes adjustments in ongoing movements as well as in central motor programs based on comparisons of external and internal sensory feedback. The cerebellum depends on experience for its success.

More recently, some investigators have demonstrated that the cerebellum is activated during cognitive tasks, such as verb generation, that is, a test in which a noun is presented and a verb related to the noun must be generated. In addition, others have proposed that the cerebellum is involved in other nontraditional functions like timing and sensory discrimination.

The cerebellum, although dwarfed by the lofty presence of the cerebrum, may be more than the bower of accuracy and precision of movement.

S.R. Gibbs, M.A., M.D.

Lesions of the Calvaria: Surgical Experience With 42 Patients
Wecht DA, Sawaya R (Univ of Texas, Houston)
Ann Surg Oncol 4:28–36, 1997   34–3

Introduction.—The skull is a rare site of primary malignancies and benign tumors. The management of skull masses is a challenging problem in neurosurgical practice, and there is little guidance provided by the literature. Key issues include the best means of radiologic evaluation, the need for preoperative biopsy, the type of surgical repair, if any, and the postoperative results expected. A 13-year experience with the surgical management of lesions of the calvaria is reported.

Methods.—The experience included 42 patients (age range, 13–82 years,) who had surgery for lesions of the calvaria. Patients with lesions of the skull base and those with primary lesions of the scalp or brain secondarily involving the calvaria were excluded. Indications for surgery included uncertain diagnosis; a benign lesion with a good chance for total removal; a malignant lesion appearing as the only manifestation of a systemic malignancy in remission at the time; and a lesion that was rapidly enlarging, causing significant symptoms, or not responding to radiotherapy or chemotherapy.

Findings.—The pathologic diagnosis was malignancy in 23 patients, a benign lesion in 16, and uncertain in 5. Most patients had a palpable mass on the scalp, whether of recent occurrence or long-standing. The most common locations were the frontal and parietal bones. Computed tomography was the most effective study for characterizing the lesions and was often the only study necessary. In 22 patients, preoperative needle biopsy was performed to establish a definitive diagnosis and to clarify the treatment plan. A biopsy was of greater diagnostic value for malignant than benign lesions. Sixteen patients were managed by craniectomy alone, and 26 were managed with craniectomy plus cranioplasty. In 35 patients, gross total excision of the lesion was possible. Postoperative complications developed in 6 patients, including 2 cases of complete loss of function of the frontalis branch of the facial nerve and 2 cases of postoperative seizures. The operative mortality rate was 0. At a follow-up of at least 2 years, 23 patients were still alive.

Discussion.—A large series of patients with primary lesions of the calvaria is reviewed. The initial diagnosis can be made by clinical examination and plain radiographs; soft-tissue and bone window CT scanning provides useful preoperative information. Preoperative needle biopsy provides useful information when these studies provide no reasonable diagnosis and when there is a suspicion of malignancy. The experience suggests some indications for surgery. Resection and repair of calvarial lesions is usually relatively simple and well tolerated.

▶ As Richard Selzer said in *Mortal Lessons: Notes on the Art of Surgery,*[1] "Ah, but there is more to the skull than helmet to the brain..., like the flesh, bone is subject to defect and disease." This is an interesting paper because these authors have assimilated the largest series to date of pathologic lesions primarily involving the calvaria. The management of a patient with a skull mass presents a very real challenge to the practicing neurosurgeon, and these authors have provided a succinct diagnostic and management outline borne of their 13-year experience. The authors identify 4 main reasons to operate on an individual with a lesion of the calvaria: (1) to establish a firm diagnosis; (2) to obtain a complete exicision of a presumed benign mass; (3) to remove the only apparent residual of a known (and tracked) systemic disease; and (4) to give symptomatic relief to the patient with an enlarging lesion and poorly controlled systemic disease. I would add a fifth reason—cosmesis. Some of these lesions, especially fibrous dysplasia and osseous meningiomas, may become quite large and disfiguring.

S.R. Gibbs, M.A., M.D.

Reference

1. Selzer R: *Mortal lessons: Notes on the art of surgery.* New York, Simon and Schuster, 1976.

Subject Index

H

Author Index

A

Acciarri N, 369
Adams HP Jr, 40
Adamski E, 82
Adelson PD, 315
Adour KK, 22
Akai F, 281
Akman NM, 83
Albright RE Jr, 242
Aldape K, 245
Aldrich MS, 159
Alexander TD, 301
Allard P, 136
Allen NB, 153
Amar K, 182
Amini R, 109
Andersen O, 187
Andreasen NC, 180
Apostolides PJ, 329
Arndt S, 180
Arnold AC, 201
Asano T, 227
Aschoff A, 37
Atkinson RP, 53
Atlas SJ, 338, 339, 340
Aull S, 173
Avoni P, 107
Awad IA, 367

B

Baca V, 120
Bakay RAE, 271
Ballard DJ, 71
Barboriak DP, 153
Bares R, 303
Barinaga M , 374
Barker FG II, 355
Barkovich AJ, 116
Barnes T, 305
Baron MS, 271
Barr-Hamilton RM, 164
Bassetti C, 159, 160
Bauer J, 105
Baumgartner C, 173
Bazil CW, 158
Beech R, 72
Behrmann R, 226
BenDebba M, 331
Berg AT, 111
Berger MS, 238
Berger PE, 346
Bertolino A, 145
Besag FMC, 113

Bichard WD, 219
Bissonette DJ, 355
Blanchet PJ, 136
Blatt J-L, 135
Blond S, 135
Bogaev CA, 275
Bono F, 7
Bordessoule D, 192
Bouillot P, 244
Boyett JM, 248
Braakman R, 282
Bracken MB, 348
Brandner B, 343
Brannagan TH III, 208
Brashear A, 21
Breneman JC, 242
Brew BJ, 93
Brismar J, 291, 292
Broderick J, 65
Brodie HA, 277
Bromley LM, 343
Brott T, 65
Brott TG, 40
Butler K, 280

C

Calligaro KD, 254
Camfield CS, 119
Camfield PR, 119
Campbell G, 145
Capen DA, 300
Carolei A, 175
Carragee EJ, 341
Carrau RL, 320, 323
Castillo M, 143
Chabriat H, 60
Chadwick D, 106
Chang SD, 363
Chervin RD, 159
Chia L, 15
Chiesi A, 89
Choi S, 305
Christopher S, 246
Cipolotti L, 179
Clark AW, 23
Cleator GM, 101
Cobbs CS, 245
Cohen BH, 248
Colledge NR, 164
Couldwell WT, 285
Cremerius U, 303
Cruz J, 38
Cruz-Flores S, 166
Cunha L, 53

D

Dacey RG Jr, 223
Dagher AP, 148
Dally LG, 89
Dam M, 78
Daube JR, 25
Davies L, 13
de Boni A, 78
Defebvre L, 135
Deletis V, 249
Delgado JA, 174
De Mascarel HA, 192
De Michele G, 31
Deyo RA, 339, 340
Dickman CA, 306, 329
Diener HC, 53
Dietze DD Jr, 308
Di Maio L, 31
Diringer H, 95
Diringer MN, 223
Doherty C, 67
Doig GS, 108
Dolliff G, 24
Donnan GA, 50
Dougherty MJ, 254
Duarte J, 174
Dulac O, 113
Dyck PJ, 10, 17

E

Ebeling U, 326
Eberwine J, 32
Ebraheim NA, 373
Edal AL, 319
Ehsan T, 221
Elliott JP, 222
Engelter S, 149
Erşahin Y, 274

F

Farber MO, 21
Feeser BR, 58
Fernandez A, 15
Fessler RG, 308
Filla A, 31
Finberg K, 367
Fischer E, 82
Fisher RS, 221
Fisher WS, 259